Atlas of Cronkhite-Canada Syndrome

Ryota Hokari • Tadakazu Hisamatsu
Editors

Atlas of Cronkhite-Canada Syndrome

Springer

Editors
Ryota Hokari
Department of Internal Medicine
National Defense Medical College
Tokorozawa, Japan

Tadakazu Hisamatsu
Department of Gastroenterology and Hepatology
Kyorin University School of Medicine
Mitaka, Tokyo, Japan

ISBN 978-981-19-0654-1 ISBN 978-981-19-0652-7 (eBook)
https://doi.org/10.1007/978-981-19-0652-7

This book is a translation of an original Japanese edition. The original publication was publicly released on the website http://www.ibdjapan.org/pdf/doc014.pdf in 2021. The translation has been facilitated using machine translation (by the service DeepL.com) followed by authors revising, editing and verifying the translated manuscript.

This Springer imprint is published by the registered company Springer Nature Singapore Pte Ltd.
The registered company address is: 152 Beach Road, #21-01/04 Gateway East, Singapore 189721, Singapore

Preface

Cronkhite–Canada Syndrome (CCS) is a rare hyperplastic gastrointestinal (GI) polyposis syndrome manifested by various GI symptoms, alopecia, and onychodystrophy of unknown etiology. Since it was first reported by Cronkhite and Canada, more than 400 cases of CCS have been reported worldwide, with 75% reported from Japan. However, there have been no published systematic investigations based on endoscopic features. In Japan, this disease is designated as an intractable disease by the Ministry of Health, Labor and Welfare (MHLW). The "Research on Intractable Inflammatory Bowel Disease" group (IBD group), funded by MHLW, has been engaged in data collection, educational activities, and development of diagnostic criteria and severity criteria for this disease.

This atlas describes 88 cases, including not only endoscopic photographs but also clinical findings, laboratory findings, clinical course, and pathological images. The pathogenesis and treatment of this disease have not yet been established. As a first step, it is important to raise awareness of this disease among clinicians. We hope that the widespread use of this endoscopic atlas will increase the awareness of this disease, and that the accumulation of cases will lead to the elucidation of its pathogenesis and the development of treatment methods in future.

I would like to express my sincere gratitude to all the experts who contributed to this project and to all the doctors who provided us with cases. In addition, I would like to express my sincere gratitude to the members of Springer Nature who devoted great effort for publishing the book.

Finally, we hope this review article can give abundant benefits to a lot of readers in this field.

Tokyo, Japan | Tadakazu Hisamatsu

Project Members

Principal Investigator: Tadakazu Hisamatsu (Department of Gastroenterology, Kyorin University School of Medicine)

Research Assignor: Ryota Hokari (Department of Internal Medicine, National Defense Medical College)

Project Members

- Takayuki Matsumoto (Division of Gastroenterology, Department of Internal Medicine, Iwate Medical University)
- Kazuki Kakimoto (Second Department of Internal Medicine, Osaka Medical and Pharmaceutical University)
- Naoki Hosoe (Center for Diagnostic and Therapeutic Endoscopy, Keio University School of Medicine)
- Makoto Ooi (Division of Gastroenterology, Department of Internal Medicine, Kobe University Graduate School of Medicine)
- Hideaki Hozumi (Self-Defense Force Sendai Hospital)
- Tomonori Yano (Department of Medicine, Division of Gastroenterology, Jichi Medical University)
- Rintaro Moroi (Division of Gastroenterology, Tohoku University Hospital)
- Masanao Nakamura (Department of Gastroenterology and Hepatology, Nagoya University Graduate School of Medicine)
- Tadayuki Oshima (Department of Gastroenterology and Hepatology, Hyogo College of Medicine)
- Naoki Ohmiya (Fujita Health University)
- Masaaki Higashiyama (Department of Internal Medicine, National Defense Medical College)

Collaborators

- Mikihiro Fujiya (Gastroenterology and Endoscopy, Division of Metabolism and Biosystemic Science, Gastroenterology, and Hematology/Oncology, Department of Medicine, Asahikawa Medical University)
- Katsuyoshi Ando (Gastroenterology and Endoscopy, Division of Metabolism and Biosystemic Science, Gastroenterology, and Hematology/Oncology, Department of Medicine, Asahikawa Medical University)
- Shunichi Yanai (Division of Gastroenterology, Department of Internal Medicine, Iwate Medical University)
- Fukunori Kinjo (Center for Gastroenterology, Urasoe General Hospital)
- Kazuhide Higuchi (The Second Department of Internal Medicine, Osaka Medical College)
- Noriko Kamata (Osaka Metropolitan University Graduate School of Medicine)
- Ichiro Hirata (Osaka Central Hospital)
- Sakiko Hiraoka (Department of Gastroenterology and Hepatology, Okayama University Graduate School of Medicine, Dentistry and Pharmaceutical Sciences)

- Keita Harada (Department of Gastroenterology and Hepatology, Okayama University Graduate School of Medicine, Dentistry and Pharmaceutical Sciences)
- Kingo Hirasawa (Division of Endoscopy, Yokohama City University Medical Center)
- Shuji Kanmura (Kagoshima University Graduate School of Medical and Dental Sciences)
- Miwa Sada (Department of Gastroenterology, Kitasato University School of Medicine)
- Kiyonori Kobayashi (Research and Development Center for New Medical Frontiers, Kitasato University School of Medicine)
- Masaru Nakano (Department of Gastroenterology and Hepatology, Kitasato University Kitasato Institute Hospital)
- Jiro Watari (Memorial Tower Hospital)
- Takehiro Torisu (Department of Medicine and Clinical Science, Graduate School of Medical Sciences, Kyushu University)
- Junji Umeno (Department of Medicine and Clinical Science, Graduate School of Medical Sciences, Kyushu University)
- Yuji Naito (Department of Gastroenterology, Graduate School of Medicine, Kyoto Prefectural University of Medicine)
- Ken Inoue (Department of Gastroenterology, Graduate School of Medicine, Kyoto Prefectural University of Medicine)
- Mari Hayashida (Department of Gastroenterology and Hepatology, Kyorin University School of Medicine)
- Keiichi Mitsuyama (Inflammatory Bowel Disease Center, Division of Gastroenterology, Department of Internal Medicine, Kurume University School of Medicine)
- Shinichiro Yoshioka (Inflammatory Bowel Disease Center, Division of Gastroenterology, Department of Internal Medicine, Kurume University School of Medicine)
- Takanori Kanai (Department of Internal Medicine (Gastroenterology), Keio University School of Medicine)
- Yuzo Kodama (Department of Gastroenterology, Graduate School of Medicine, Kobe University)
- Hiroshi Nakase (Department of Gastroenterology, Sapporo Medical University School of Medicine)
- Tsukasa Yamakawa (Department of Gastroenterology, Sapporo Medical University School of Medicine)
- Akira Andoh (Department of Medicine, Shiga University of Medical Science)
- Shigeki Bamba (Division of Digestive Endoscopy, Shiga University of Medical Science)
- Kan Uchiyama (Division of Gastroenterology and Hepatology, Department of Internal Medicine, The Jikei University School of Medicine, Kashiwa Hospital)
- Hironori Yamamoto (Department of Medicine, Division of Gastroenterology, Jichi Medical University)
- Shunji Ishihara (Department of Internal Medicine II, Shimane University Faculty of Medicine)
- Katsuyuki Fukuda (Department of Gastroenterology, St. Luke’s International Hospital)
- Masakazu Nagahori (Department of Gastroenterology, Tokyo Medical and Dental University Hospital)
- Teppei Omori (Institute of Gastroenterology, Tokyo Women's Medical University)
- Yasuo Suzuki (Ginza Central Clinic)
- Katsuyoshi Matsuoka (Toho University Sakura Medical Center)
- Atsushi Masamune (Division of Gastroenterology, Tohoku University Graduate School of Medicine)
- Sohachi Nanjo (Third Department of Internal Medicine, University of Toyama)
- Mitsuhiro Fujishiro (Nagoya University, The University of Tokyo)
- Fumikazu Koyama (Department of Surgery, Division of Endoscopy, Nara Medical University)
- Ken Sugimoto (Hamamatsu University School of Medicine)

- Hiroto Miwa (Department of Gastroenterology and Hepatology, Hyogo College of Medicine)
- Fumihito Hirai (Department of Gastroenterology, Fukuoka University School of Medicine)
- Takashi Hisabe (Department of Gastroenterology, Fukuoka University Chikushi Hospital)
- Masahiro Kishi (Inflammatory Bowel Disease Center, Fukuoka University Chikushi Hospital)
- Reiko Kunisaki (Inflammatory Bowel Disease Center, Yokohama City University Medical Center)
- Tetsu Kinjo (Department of Endoscopy University of the Ryukyus Hospital)
- Naoto Shirai (JA Shizuoka Koseiren Enshu Hospital)

Contents

Cronkhite–Canada Syndrome

Ryota Hokari, Tadakazu Hisamatsu,
and Masaaki Higashiyama

1 Overview of Cronkhite–Canada Syndrome

1.1 Overview

Cronkhite–Canada Syndrome (CCS) is a non-hereditary disorder characterized by multiple non-neoplastic polyps in the gastrointestinal tract. CCS is considered to be a rare disease worldwide, but the majority of reported cases are from Japan (Fig. 1). Polyps are frequently detected particularly in the stomach and colon, and in more than half of cases, polyps are also detected in the small intestine. Cutaneous manifestations such as alopecia, onychodystrophy, and hyperpigmentation, as well as dysgeusia, are also characteristic. Corticosteroids are highly effective in the treatment of this disease. However, relapses occur in some cases and the incidence of gastrointestinal malignancies is higher than in the general population. Therefore, early induction and maintenance of remission as well as regular observation over a long period are necessary [1].

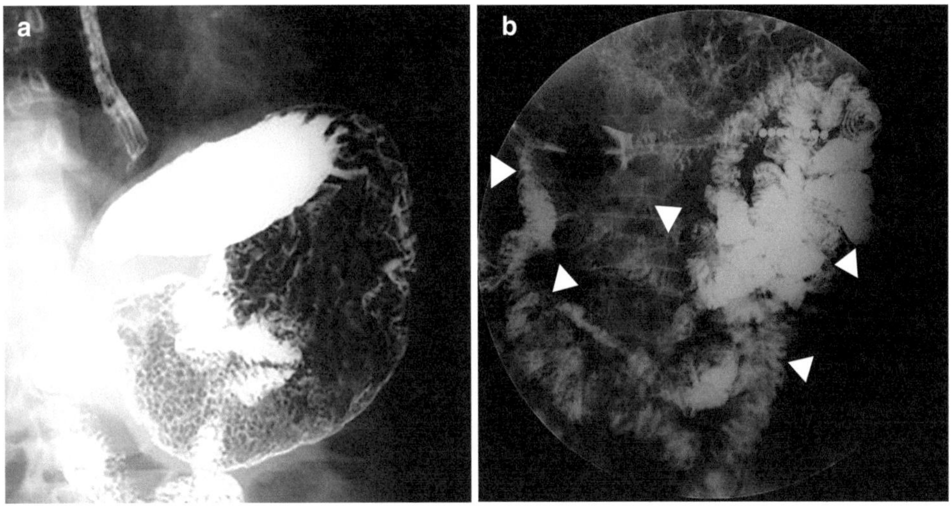

Fig. 1 Barium X-ray radiography. (**a**) Stomach: Multiple moderate-sized radiolucent circular images are observed. (**b**) Small intestine: Multiple radiolucent circular images are observed (arrow heads)

R. Hokari (✉) · M. Higashiyama
Department of Internal Medicine, National Defense Medical College, Tokorozawa, Saitama, Japan
e-mail: ryota@ndmc.ac.jp; masaakih@ndmc.ac.jp

T. Hisamatsu
Department of Gastroenterology and Hepatology, Kyorin University School of Medicine, Mitaka, Tokyo, Japan

R. Hokari, T. Hisamatsu (eds.), *Atlas of Cronkhite-Canada Syndrome*, https://doi.org/10.1007/978-981-19-0652-7_1

1.2 Epidemiology

Since the first two cases were reported by Cronkhite and Canada in 1955, only about 500 cases have been reported worldwide, of which about 75% are from Japan. The mean age at diagnosis is 63.5 years, and the male to female ratio is 1.84:1, with a predominance of males. In the 1980s, nearly half of the deaths were due to malnutrition and gastrointestinal bleeding, but recent studies suggest that the number of deaths due to malnutrition is low [2].

However, the complications of gastrointestinal tumors are higher than in the general population (Fig. 2). Gastric adenoma, gastric carcinoma, colorectal adenoma, and colorectal carcinoma are reported in 5–15%, 5–10%, 15–70%, and 15–20%, respectively, and the majority of cases are already complicated at the time of diagnosis. As for the small intestine, reports of adenoma and carcinoma complications are rarer than in other parts of the body [3].

1.3 Etiology

The etiology of this syndrome remains unclear. However, there are common features such as a high response rate to corticosteroids, inflammatory cell infiltration to polyps and intervening mucosa, and reversibility of polyps by treatment. In addition, there are reports of cases in which exposure to drugs is thought to be the trigger for the onset of the disease, suggesting the involvement of immunological abnormalities [2].

1.4 Clinical Features

1. Symptoms

   Gastrointestinal symptoms include abdominal pain, diarrhea, and decreased appetite. Particulary, diarrhea is observed from the beginning and is often nonhematogenous. In older patients, the symptoms are less severe and may be overlooked. The main findings, skin triad (alopecia, onychodystrophy, and hyperpigmentation) (Fig. *3*a–c) and dysgeusia, are not always present in the early stages of the disease (50–60%) and often appear during its course. Although hair loss is seen throughout the body, it often occurs first, especially in the hair of the head (alopecia). Hyperpigmentation is often seen on the palms and fingers. Other complications include gastrointestinal bleeding and intussusception, as well as neoplastic lesions and protein losing enteropathy (PLE) [4] (Fig. *3*d, e).

2. Clinical examination and laboratory findings

   Although blood test shows elevated CRP level, hypoalbuminemia, hypogammaglobulinemia, electrolyte abnormalities, anemia, etc, none of these findings are specific to CCS. However, because of the high rate of complications of PLE, the clinical significance of hypoalbuminemia is high. Fecal alpha1-antitrypsin clearance test and 99mTc-human serum albumin scintigraphy are helpful tests for PLE (Fig. 4), but protein leakage can be confirmed among only half of PLE cases by these tests. In addition, Helicobacter pylori infection may be involved in the disease. H. pylori IgG antibodies in the blood, H. pylori antigen in the stool, and urea breath test have been conducted to confirm the presence of infection [2].

3. Endoscopic findings

   In CCS, multiple polyps are found in the stomach and colon in almost all cases, but small polyps and erythematous and edematous mucosa may also be seen in the esophagus and small intestine (see chapter "Endoscopic Images per Organ"). Although CCS might be easily suspected based on the findings of white light observation, a combination of small bowel endoscopy, chromoendoscopy, and image-enhanced endoscopy with high magnification can provide a more detailed picture of the disease (see chapter "Endoscopic Images of Small Bowel Capsule Endoscopy, Balloon-Assisted Enteroscopy and Image-Enhanced Endoscopy").

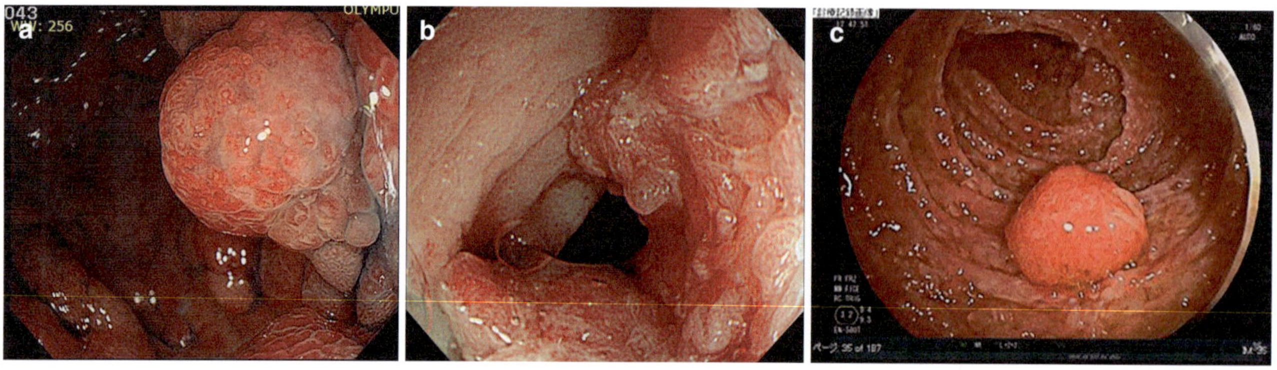

Fig. 2. Coincident cases of CCS with intestinal tumor. (**a**) Gastric cancer. (**b**) Colorectal cancer. (**c**) Small intestinal adenoma

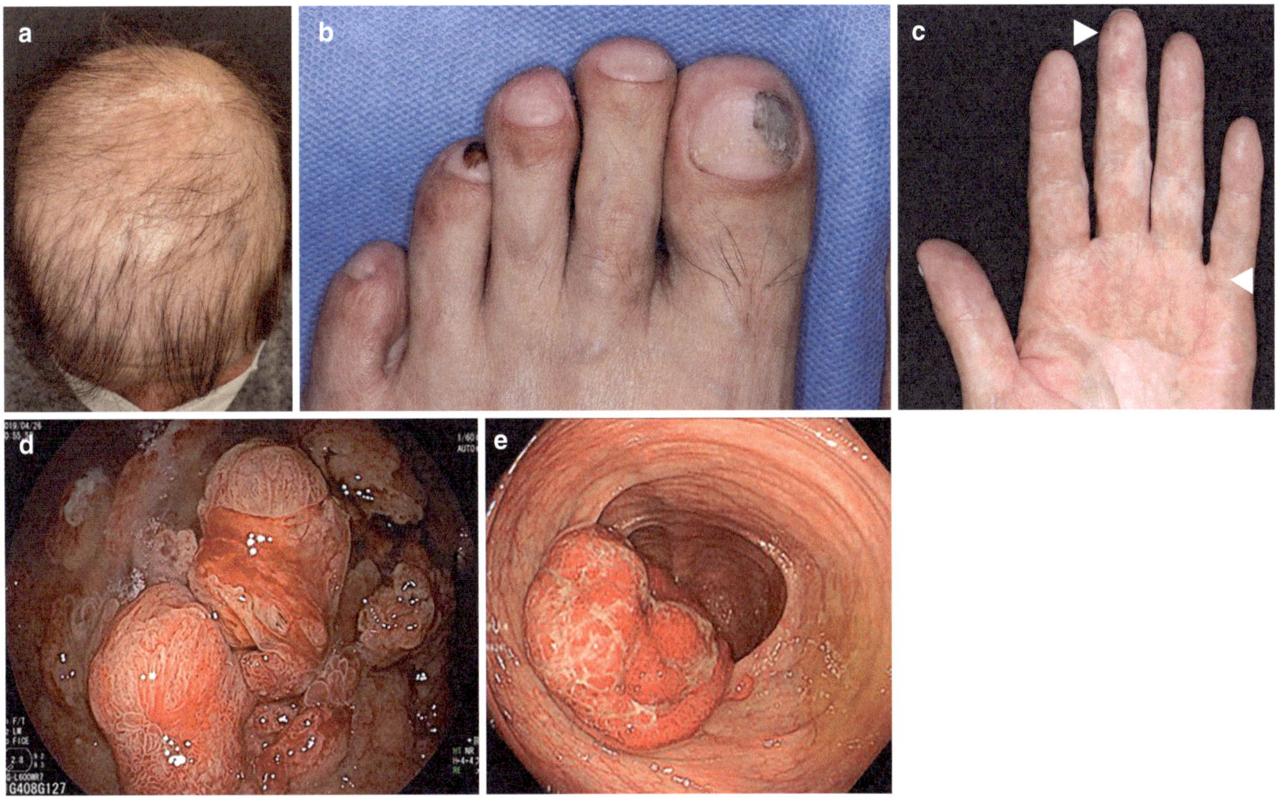

Fig. 3 (**a**)–(**c**) Skin triad. (**a**) Alopecia, (**b**) onychodystrophy, (**c**) hyperpigmentation (arrowheads). (**d**) Gastrointestinal bleeding. (**e**) Ileocecal intussusception induced by small intestinal polyp

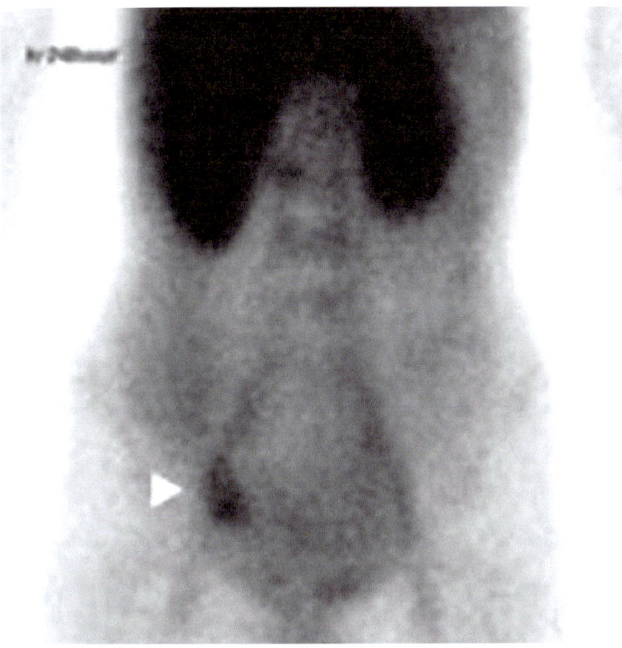

Fig. 4 99mTc-human serum albumin scintigraphy. There is an abnormal leakage of radio-labeled albumin in the ileocecal region (arrow)

Furthermore, there are not a few cases of coincident adenoma/carcinoma in this disease. It is not easy to detect neoplastic polyps before treatment. However, it has been reported that magnified endoscopic observation using image-enhanced endoscopy may be able to differentiate inflammatory hyperplastic polyps from neoplastic lesions (See chapter "Endoscopic Images of Coincident Carcinoma and Adenoma to Differentiate from Non-neoplastic Polyps").

4. Pathological findings

   The pathological findings of polyps are classified as non-neoplastic. They present as hyperplasia with cystic dilatation and tortuosity of the mucosal gland, which may show serrated protrusion into the lumen. The dilated glandular ducts are filled with protein-rich mucus. In some cases, there is a marked infiltration of inflammatory cells, and the inflammatory cells are predominantly lymphocytes, eosinophils, and plasma cells, with fewer neutrophils. Compared with other non-neoplastic polyposis diseases, this disease is characterized by the presence of marked inflammatory findings from the mucosa to the lamina propria in the intervening mucosa between polyps.

   In addition, adenomatous polyps, especially in the colon are often coincident with CCS. It may be difficult to differentiate between adenomas, juvenile polyps, and inflammatory polyps based on either endoscopic findings or histopathological findings individually. Therefore, it is desirable to diagnose based on the combination of endoscopic and histopathological findings (see chapter "Comparison of Pathological and Endoscopic Images (per Organ)").

1.5 Treatment

1. Medical treatments
   (a) Corticosteroids

   Predonisolone (PSL) of 30 mg/day or more are usually effective, and oral doses of 30–50 mg/day are appropriate for inducing remission. Although higher initial doses tend to make earlier clinical responses, use of doses greater than 60 mg/day increases the frequency of serious adverse events such as sepsis and thrombosis.

   If the patient responds to treatments, remission of diarrhea will occur in about 2 months (average of 51 days), and remission of dysgeusia will occur in about 3 months (84 days). This is followed by improvements in nutritional deficits, such as weight loss, and cutaneous manifestations in a few months to 6 months.

   The time it will take for improvement of endoscopic findings is the longest among other clinical findings (around 8 months), and some cases take several years. Since a rapid dose reduction of corticosteroid may cause relapse, sufficient improvement in clinical symptoms and endoscopic findings should be necessary before discontinuation or reduction of medication [2].

   (b) Nutritional therapy

   Nutritional therapy is important as a supportive therapy because the disease is more common in the elderly, who are at increased risk of malnutrition, and highly immunocompromised because of the high prevalence of PLE and the potential impact of corticosteroids on the immune system. Total parenteral nutrition (TPN) and semi-digestion nutrition agents have been shown to improve response to corticosteroids therapy and shorten the time to remission, but their efficacy has not been fully elucidated [2, 5].

   (c) Alternative therapies for refractory cases

   In some refractory cases, the use of cyclosporine A [6], azathioprine [6] and anti-TNFα antibodies including infliximab (IFX) [7] has been reported to achieve remission. There have been other reports of the use of antibiotics, histamine H2 receptor antagonists [8], and Helicobacter pylori eradication therapy [9], but the number of cases is small and the efficacy of all these agents has not been fully verified.
2. Endoscopic and surgical treatments

   Coincident malignant tumor can be treated endoscopically or surgically. Hemorrhage from polyps can be treated by endoscopic hemostasis and colonic polyps located at occlusion point of intussusception can be resected surgically. The diagnosis of coincident adenoma or carcinoma is difficult to make because of the large number of polyps and the erythematous and edematous intervening mucosa. The detection rate increases when the polyps have regressed and the mucosal edema has improved thanks to successful treatments. After initial treatments, it is recommended that the patient should be monitored using image-enhanced endoscopy, chromoendoscopy, and magnifying endoscopy. The incidence of carcinoma after the polyps have disappeared is not known, but regular surveillance endoscopy is recommended [4].

1.6 Differential Diagnosis

Other polyposis such as non-neoplastic polyposis (juvenile polyposis, Peutz–Jegher syndrome, Cowden syndrome) and adenomatous polyposis (Gardner syndrome, Turcot syndrome) are listed in the differential diagnosis [10, 11] (Table 1). For diagnosis, in addition to the distribution pattern and pathological findings of polyps, careful history taking and confirmation of skin and mucosal findings are important. It should also be noted that there are sporadic cases of hereditary diseases, and the absence of a family history cannot exclude the diagnosis of hereditary diseases [12].

2 Diagnostic Criteria for Cronkhite–Canada Syndrome

Major Criteria

1. Multiple non-neoplastic polyposis in the gastrointestinal tract, especially in the stomach and colon.
2. Gastrointestinal symptoms, mainly chronic diarrhea.
3. Characteristic cutaneous manifestation (Triad), including alopecia, onychodystrophy, and hyperpigmentation (at least one cutaneous manifestation).

Minor Criteria

4. Hypoproteinemia (hypoalbuminemia) with protein leakage.
5. Impaired taste (dysgeusia) or weight loss and nutritional deficiencies.
6. Endoscopic features: gastrointestinal polyposis characterized by stalkless diffuse polyposis.
   - Stomach: Edematous elevated lesions with ill-defined margin.
   - Colon: Strawberry-like polypoid lesions with well-defined margin.

Table 1 Differential diagnosis of gastrointestinal polyposis

Diseases	Histology	Inheritance pattern	Susceptible age group	Favorite site for polyps	Complications
Familial adenomatous polyposis	Adenoma	Autosomal dominant	10s	Colon > stomach > small intestine	Osteoma, dental anomaly, congenital hypertrophy of retinal pigment epithelial cell, soft tissue tumor, desmoid tumor, goiter, pancreatic cancer
Gardner's syndrome		Autosomal dominant	20s–30s	Colon > stomach > small intestine	Colorectal cancer, mandibular osteoma
Turcot syndrome		Autosomal recessive		Colon > stomach > small intestine	Central nervous system tumor
Peutz–Jeghers syndrome	Non-neoplastic	Autosomal dominant	10s–20s	Stomach, small intestine, colon	Hyperpigmentation, intussusception, melena
Cowden syndrome		Autosomal dominant (PTEN gene mutation)	20s	Whole digestive tract (Pharyngeal and esophageal polyposis is highly specific)	Oral mucosal papilloma, skin lesions (trichilemmoma, cutaneous papilloma, keratosis of distal extremities), thyroid cancer, breast cancer, uterine cancer, renal cell carcinoma, colorectal cancer
Juvenile polyposis		Autosomal dominant	Childhood	Whole digestive tract	Congenital malformation, intussusception, ileus, melena
Von Recklinghausen syndrome		Autosomal dominant	50s	Small intestine	Glioma
Cronkhite–Canada syndrome,		Non-hereditary	60s	Whole digestive tract	Skin lesions (alopecia, hyperpigmentation, onychodystrophy), gastrointestinal cancer
Inflammatory polyposis	Regenerative epithelium			Colon	Ulcerative colitis, colorectal cancer
Benign lymphoid polyposis	Lymphoid tissue			Small intestine, colon	None
Serrated polyposis syndrome	Diverse (six types such as hyperplastic, serrated adenoma, adenoma, etc.)		50s–60s	Colon	Colorectal cancer

7. Histological features (non-neoplastic polyps): Inflammation of the mucosal lamina propria with cystic dilatation of the glands, mucosal, edema, and inflammatory cell infiltration. Inflammation/edema of the intervening mucosa is also present. It is sometimes classified as hamartomatous polyps (juvenile-like polyps).

Diagnositic Criteria
Major critera 1 is essential for diagnosis.

Definite
- All major criteria: *1 + 2 + 3*.
- Two major criteria including 1 with minor criteria 4: *1 + 2 + 4*, or *1 + 3 + 4*.
- Two major criteria including 1 with minor criteria 6 and 7: *1 + 2 + 6 + 7*, or *1 + 3 + 6 + 7*.

Possible
- Major critera 1 with other criteria but insufficient to diagnose as definite.

Notes on the application of diagnostic criteria
It is acceptable to use clinical symptoms of the patients at any time during the disease course to diagnose the disease.

3 Type, Stage, and Severity of Cronkhite–Canada Syndrome

3.1 Classification of Disease Stage

- *Active stage*
- *Remission stage*

Note 1: The active stage is characterized by characteristic cutaneous manifestations, complaints of gastrointestinal symptoms, decreased serum albumin levels and increased CRP levels, and endoscopic findings of polyps in the gastrointestinal tract and inflammation of the intervening mucosa.

Note 2: The remission type is subdivided as follows.

<complete remission>

Resolution of characteristic cutaneous manifestation and gastrointestinal symptoms, normalization of serum albumin and CRP levels, and endoscopic resolution of polyps in the gastrointestinal tract and inflammatory findings in the mucosa.

<partial remission>

A condition in which there are improvements in response to treatments, but not yet complete remission.

3.2 Classification by Clinical Severity

- *Mild disease*
- *Moderate disease*
- *Severe disease*

The severity criteria are shown in Table 2.

Table 2 The severity criteria

Item	Points	Criteria
1. Stool frequency/day	0	Normal for patient
	1	1–2 times/day more than normal
	2	3–4 times/day more than normal
	3	More than 5 times/day more than normal
2. Serum albumin level	0	>3.5 g/dL
	1	3.5 g/dL≥, >3.0 g/dL
	2	3.0 g/dL≥, >2.5 g/dL
	3	2.5 g/dL≥
3. Edema	0	None
	1	Mild (obvious pitting edema)
	2	Moderate (indistinct veins and bones)
	3	Severe (obviously swollen)
4. Physician's overall assessment	0	Normal (complete remission)
	1	Mild illness
	2	Moderate illness
	3	Severe illness
5. Weight loss (5 kg/6 months or more)	0	None
	1	Applicable
6. Anemia (hemoglobin: 12 g/dL or less in male, 10 g/dL or less in female)	0	None
	1	Applicable
7. Bloody stool	0	(–): None
	1	(+): Slightly mixed blood in less than half of the defecation
	2	(++): Obvious bloody stool in every defecation
8. Other findings	1 point per item	• Cutaneous manifestations (alopecia, onychodystrophy, or hyperpigmentation, plus 1 point if any of them applies) • Dysgeusia • Intussusception

Note 3: The total score calculated from each item is used to evaluate the activity and therapeutic effects.

Disease activity

- *Severe disease:* Item 2 ≥2 points and the total score ≥10 points.
- *Moderate disease*: Intermediate between severe and mild disease.
- *Mild disease*: All Items from 2 to 7 = 0 point and a total score ≤3 points.

Therapeutic effects

- *Improvement*: Total Score decreased by 2 points or more
- *Exacerbation*: Total score increased by 2 points or more

Clinical remission/relapse

- *Clinical remission*: Total score ≤1
- *Relapse*: Total score ≥2

Note 4: It is recommended to confirm which method is used for measuring serum albumin value because measuring methods might be different from each facility.

Note 5: It is acceptable to use clinical symptoms of the patients at any time during the disease course to diagnose the disease.

Note 6: The diagnosis is made based on the severest findings among the endoscopic findings observed. The endoscopic examination should be performed in a short period of time, and it is not necessary to observe the entire gastrointestinal tract. The disease activity should not be determined based on the number and size of polyps because their changes are very slow.

3.3 Classification of Polyps by Endoscopic Findings

1. Number of polyps
   - Small numbers: <10 per gastrointestinal tract
   - Moderate number: 10–100 per gastrointestinal tract
   - Large number: >100 per gastrointestinal tract
2. The features of the polyp
   (a) Size of polyps
      - Small: <5 mm
      - Medium: 5–10 mm
      - Large: >10 mm
   (b) Mucosal change of polyps (Fig. 5)
3. Distribution type of polyps
   (A) Stomach and colon
      - A-1. Sparse type (Fig. 6).

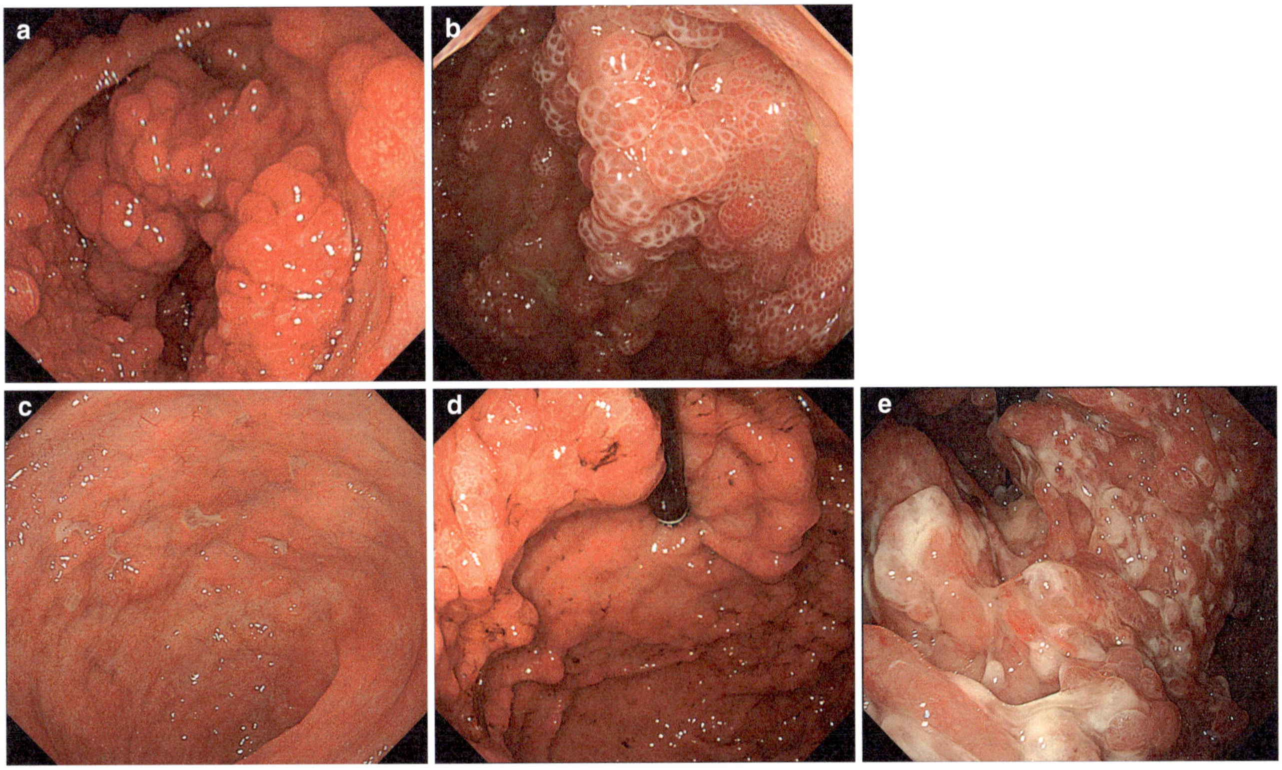

Fig. 5 Mucosal change of polyps. (**a**) Erythematous. (**b**) Edematous. (**c**) Erosive. (**d**) Hemorrhagic. (**e**) Whitish mucus adhered

Fig. 6 Sparse type: Polyps are intervened by healthy mucosa. There is no inflammation or edema in the intervening mucosa

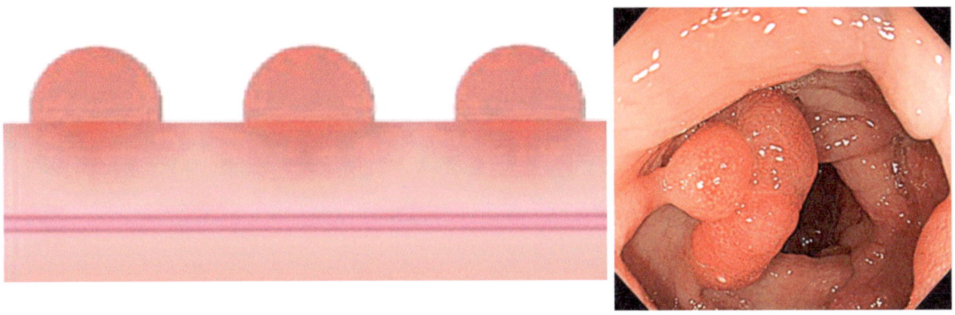

Fig. 7 Confluent type: Polyps are dense with little intervening mucosa

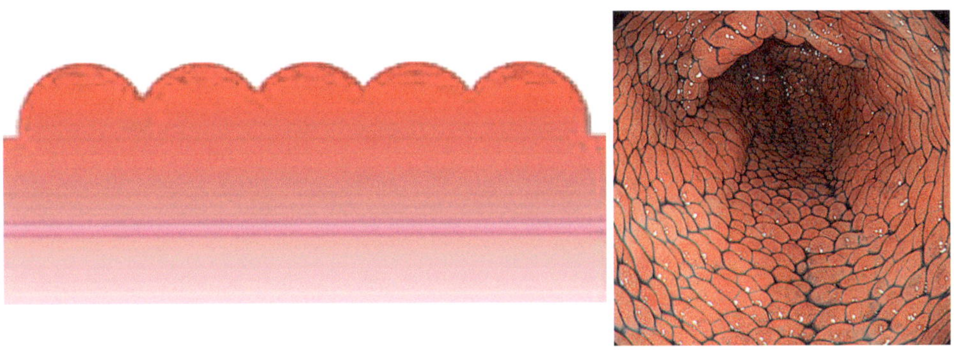

- A-2. Confluent type (Fig. 7).
  <Confluent subtype>
- A-2-1. Semi-confluent type: Intervening mucosa between polyps has inflammatory and edematous changes (Fig. 8).
- A-2-2. Thickening type (Fig. 9).

(B) Duodenum and small intestine
- B-1. Fold thickening type (Fig. 10).
- B-2. Polyp formation type (Fig. 11).
  (The distribution type of polyps such as confluent, semi-confluent, and sparse type is the same as for gastric and colorectal polyps.)

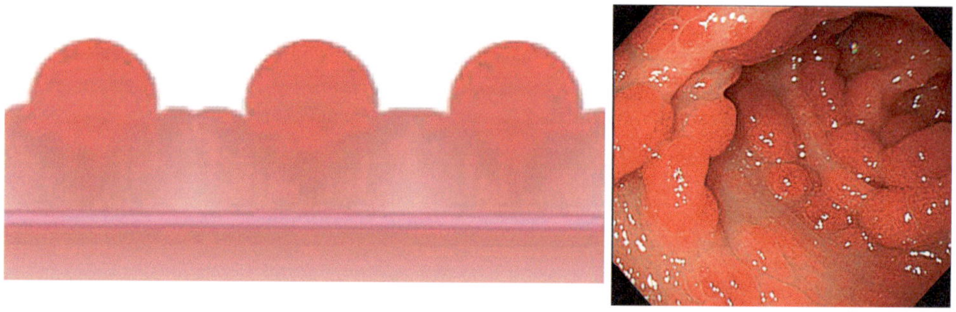

Fig. 8 Semi-confluent type: Intervening mucosa between polyps has inflammatory and edematous changes

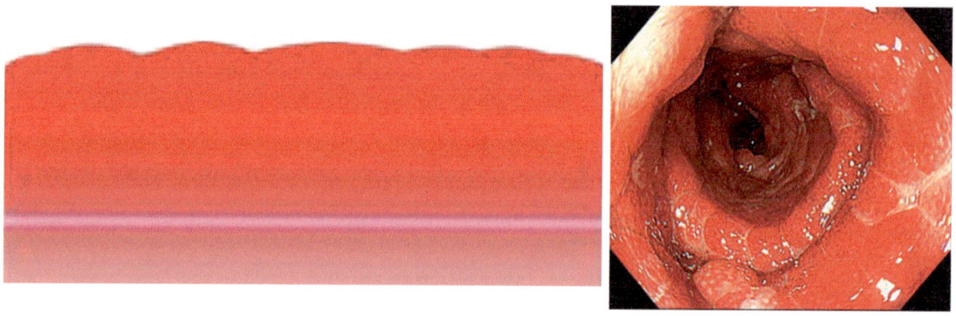

Fig. 9 Thickening type: The shape and size of the polyps cannot be determined, but lumen are narrowed due to diffuse thickened mucosa with inflammatory or edematous changes

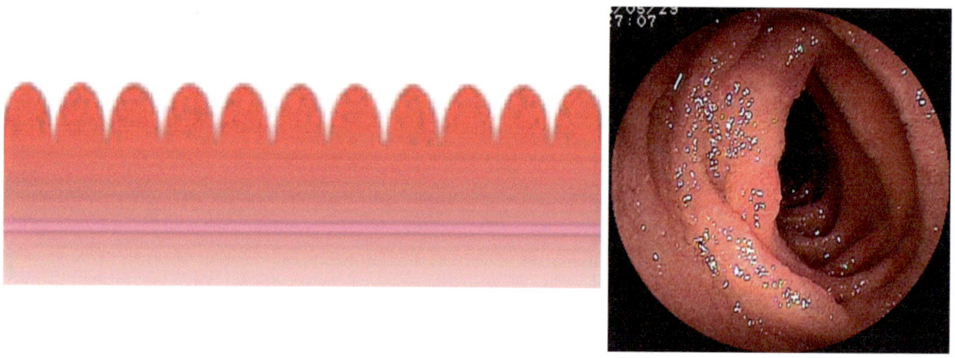

Fig. 10 Fold thickening type: The villi are enlarged and shortened and there are edematous changes in the mucosa. In more severe cases, the villi may be indistinct and the entire fold may appear thickened. In some cases, thickened villi become polypoid appearance

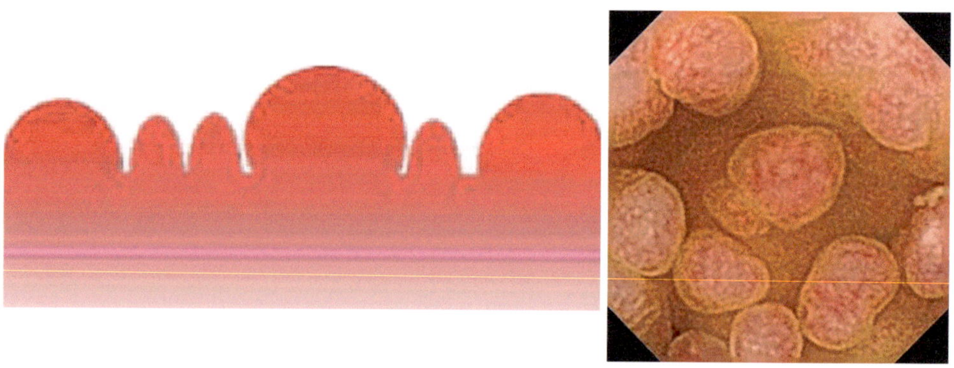

Fig. 11 Polyp formation type: Polyps with different shape from enlarged villi are observed

Table 3 Endoscopic activity criteria

Endoscopic activity	Inflammatory findings of the mucosa (intervening mucosa, polyp surface)
Mild	Erythematous
Moderate	Edematous, hemorrhagic (contact bleeding), fold thickening
Severe	Thickening, hemorrhagic (spontaneous), whitish mucus adhered

4. Features of the intervening mucosa
   - Normal
   - Erythematous
   - Edematous
   - Erosive
   - Hemorrhagic
   - Whitish mucus adhered

The size, distribution, and features of the polyps should be classified based on the predominant findings.

5. Classification by endoscopic activity
   - Mild
   - Moderate
   - Severe

The endoscopic activity criteria are shown in Table 3.

3.4 Classification by Clinical Course

- Spontaneous remission type
- Relapse-remitting type
- Chronic continuous type
- First attack type

Note: Spontaneous remission is a remission without any treatment.

Note: Chronic continuous type is an active phase for more than 12 months after the first attack.

Note: The first attack type is one attack only.

3.5 Classification by Responsiveness to Corticosteroids

Clinical response classification:

- Good early clinical response: Improvement within 2 months from initial treatments.
- Good early clinical remission: Remission within 2 months from initial treatments.

3.6 Definition of Refractory Cronkhite–Canada Syndrome Based on Treatment Responsiveness

1. Cases that are on strict corticosteroid therapy but meet one of the following criteria.
   (a) Steroid-resistant cases (no improvement even after initial treatments by PSL 30–40 mg and following treatments by PSL 15–20 mg 2 months later).[1]
   (b) Steroid-dependent cases (relapse during tapering or soon after discontinuation of steroid).
2. Frequent relapses or chronic persistent cases while under strict medical treatments other than coriticosteroids.

[1]In severe cases, the effect of corticosteroids should be assessed early after the initiation of steroids, and if there is no effect at all, another treatment should be considered within 2 months. The clinical symptom that shows the earliest change is the frequency of defecation [2].

3.7 Special Complication Cases

- Gastrointestinal adenoma complication
- Gastrointestinal cancer complication

References

1. Comprehensive study on epidemiology, pathogenesis, diagnosis, and treatment of intestinal rare intractable diseases from the viewpoint of homology and difference.
2. Watanabe C, Komoto S, Tomita K, Hokari R, Tanaka M, Hirata I, Hibi T, Kaunitz JD, Miura S. J. Endoscopic and clinical evaluation of treatment and prognosis of Cronkhite-Canada syndrome: a Japanese nationwide survey. Gastroenterol. 2016;51:327-336.
3. Kato S, Tajiri T, Tanaka S. Gastrointestinal lesions associated with Cronkhite-Canada syndrome. Journal of the Japanese Medical Association. 2005;1:46-47.
4. Watanabe Chikako, Hotaru Ryota, Miura Soichiro. Other Polyposis Diseases - With Special Reference to Cronkite Canada Syndrome -. Journal of the Japanese Medical Association. 2017;114:431-437.
5. Russell DM, Bhathal PS, St John DJ. Complete remission in Cronkhite-Canada syndrome. Gastroenterology. 1983;85:180-5.
6. Ohmiya N, Nakamura M, Yamamura T, Yamada K, Asuka N, Yoshimura T, Hirooka Y, Matsumoto T, Hirata I, Goto H. Steroid-resistant Cronkhite-Canada syndrome successfully treated by cyclosporine and azathioprine. J Clin Gastroenterol. 2014;48:463-4.

7. Watanabe D, Ooi M, Hoshi N, Kohashi M, Yoshie T, Ikehara N, Yoshida M, Yanagita E, Yamasaki T, Itoh T, Azuma T. Successful treatment of Cronkhite-Canada syndrome using anti-tumor necrosis factor antibody therapy. Endoscopy. 2014;46(Suppl 1):476-7.
8. Allbritton J, Simmons-O'brien E, Hutcheons D, Elizabeth W. Cronkhite-Canada syndrome: report of two cases, biopsy findings in associated alopecia, and a new treatment option. Cutis. 1998;61:229-32.
9. Okamoto K, Isomoto H, Shikuwa S, Nishiyama H, Ito M, Kohno S. A case of Cronkhite-Canada syndrome: remission after treatment with anti-Helicobacter pylori regimen. Digestion. 2008;78:82-7.
10. Matsumoto T, Iida M: Genetic abnormalities in hereditary colorectal cancer and clinical hereditary polyposis of the gastrointestinal tract: clinical picture and genetic abnormalities. J Digest 2000; 97: 1007-1016.
11. Tamura K, Tomita T. Classification and characteristics of gastrointestinal polyposis. J Digest 2017; 114: 403-41.
12. Blumenthal GM, Dennis PA. PTEN hamartoma tumor syndromes. Eur J Hum Genet 2008; 16: 1289-1300.

Endoscopic Images per Organ

Ryota Hokari, Tadakazu Hisamatsu, and Masaaki Higashiyama

1 Gastric Polyps

Typical gastric polyps observed by esophagogastroduodenoscopy (EGD) are described as "red cavir like," which is characterized by findings of dense distribution of small hemispheric, edematous, and erythematous polyps without intervening mucosa between adjacent polyps. Glandular duct orifices (pits) are dilated in many cases. Polyps are predominantly located from the gastric antrum to pylorus and less frequently in the gastric body.

R. Hokari (✉) · M. Higashiyama
Department of Internal Medicine, National Defense Medical College, Tokorozawa, Saitama, Japan
e-mail: ryota@ndmc.ac.jp; masaakih@ndmc.ac.jp

T. Hisamatsu
Department of Gastroenterology and Hepatology, Kyorin University School of Medicine, Mitaka, Tokyo, Japan

R. Hokari, T. Hisamatsu (eds.), *Atlas of Cronkhite-Canada Syndrome*, https://doi.org/10.1007/978-981-19-0652-7_2

1.1 Confluent type (A-2) (Fig. 1)

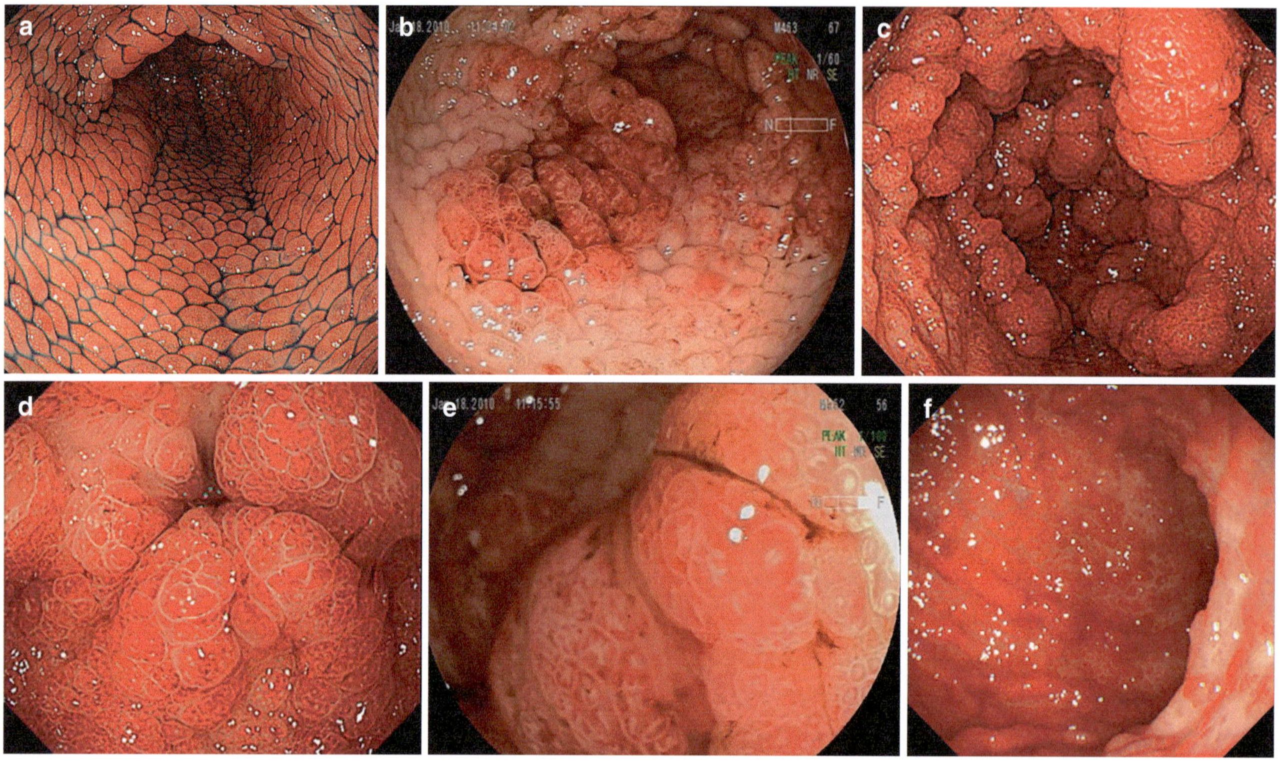

Fig. 1 (**a**) Confluent type. Small, erythematous polyps in the antrum with little or no intervening mucosa. (**b**) Confluent type. Small, partially erythematous polyps with dilated pits in the antrum. (**c**) Confluent type. Medium to large, erythematous polyps in the antrum. (**d**) Confluent type. Large erythematous polyps with partially dilated pits in the antrum. (**e**) Magnified image. Polyps with round to star-shaped pits. (**f**) Confluent type. Small polyps are densely located longitudinally along the gastric folds at the body of greater curvature

1.2 Confluent subtype: Semi-confluent type (A-2-1) (Fig. 2)

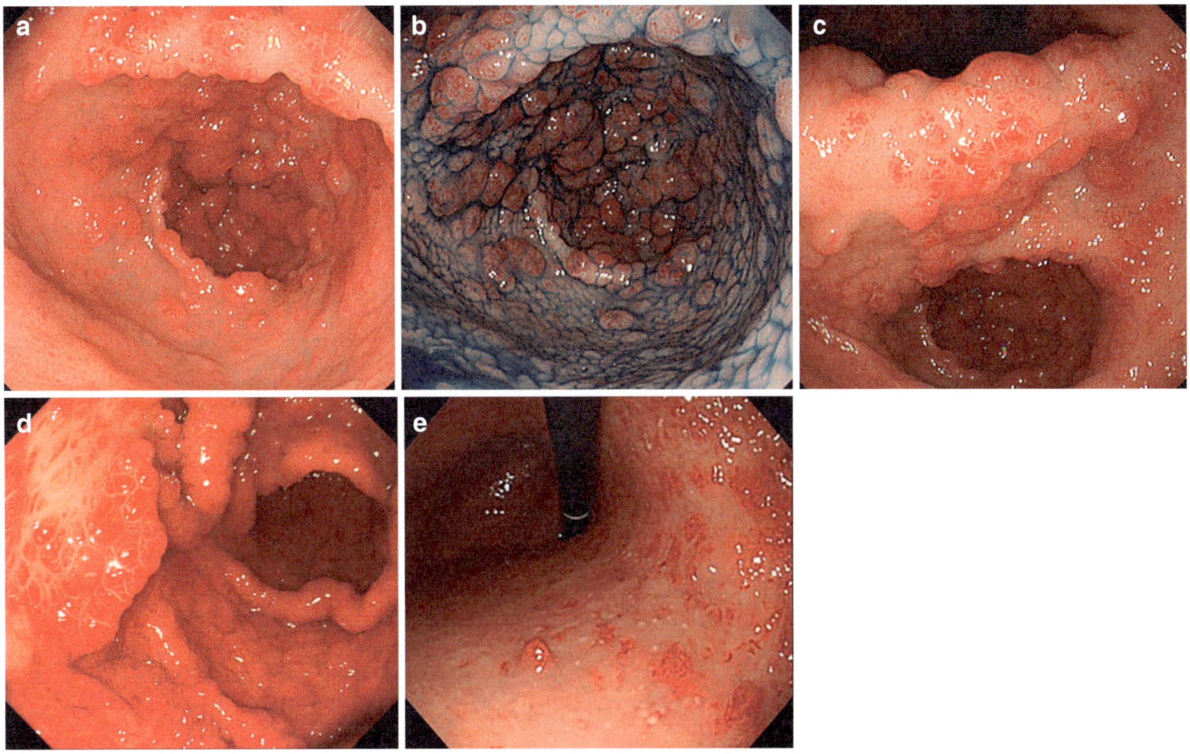

Fig. 2 (**a**) Scattered, small, erythematous polyps with mildly edematous intervening mucosa in the antrum. (**b**) Indigo carmine dyeing of (**a**). Mildly elevated lesions in the intervening mucosa are clarified. (**c**) Small polyps at gastric angle. The intervening mucosa is also edematous and partially erythematous. (**d**) Small polyps of the anterior wall of the lower part of the body. The anterior wall at the lower part of the body shows a submucosal tumor (SMT)-like elevation partly covered with white mucosa, flat erythematous elevation, and fused small polyps. A small area of intervening mucosa is also erythematous. (**e**) Scattered, low erythematous polyps located longitudinally at the lesser curvature of the body. The intervening mucosa is edematous and whitish, and the regular arrangement of collecting venules (RAC) has disappeared

1.3 Confluent subtype: thickening (A-2-2) (Fig. 3)

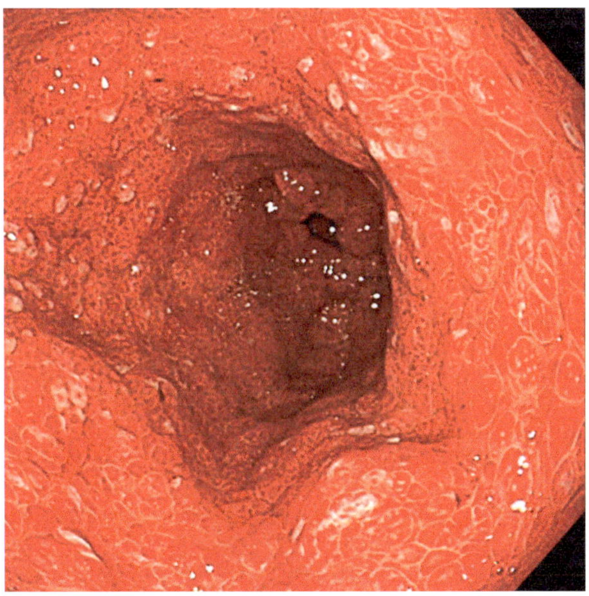

Fig. 3 Gastric antrum. The entire mucosa is thickened with redness and edema. The borders of the individual polyps are indistinct, and it is difficult to distinguish their shape and size

1.4 Sparse type (A-1) (Fig. 4)

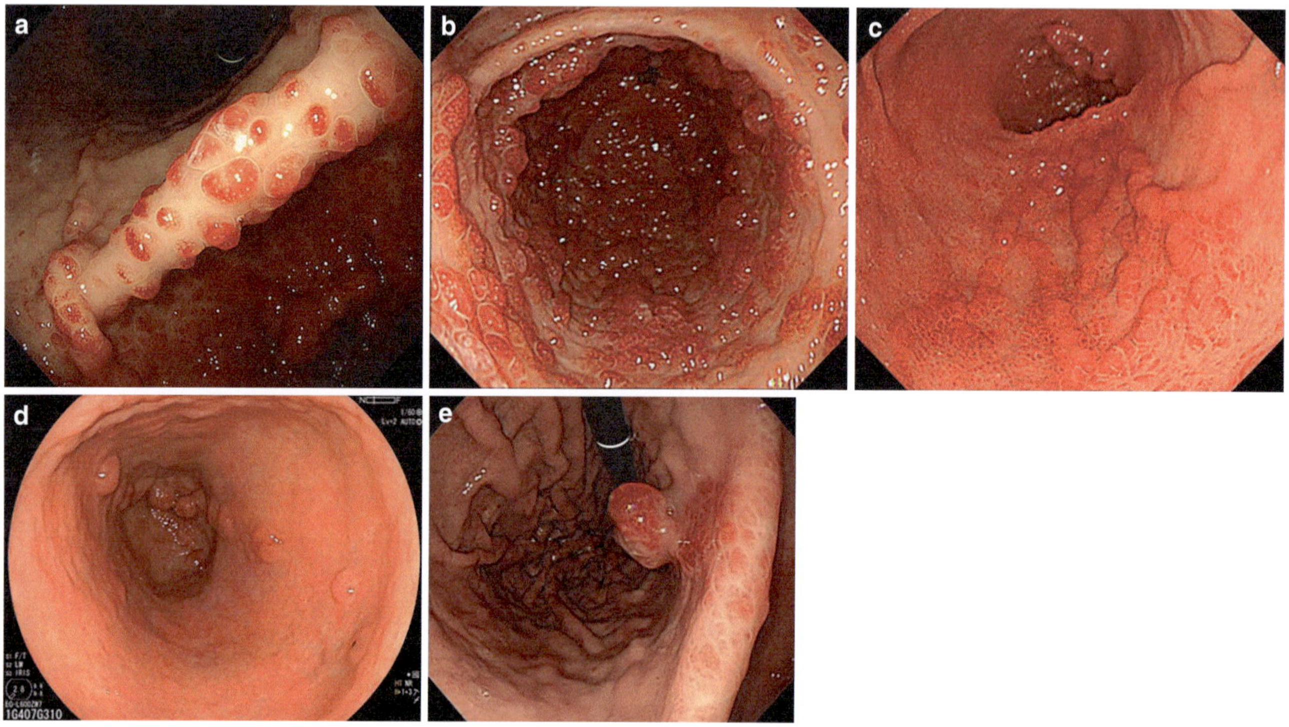

Fig. 4 (**a**) Scattered small, erythematous polyps in the gastric angle. The intervening mucosa is completely devoid of erythema. (**b**) Circumferentially scattered small, erythematous, and edematous polyps with no inflammatory findings in the intervening mucosa in the antrum. (**c**) Small erythematous polyps are distributed along the gastric fold in the lower part of the body to antrum. There are no inflammatory findings in the intervening mucosa. (**d**) Small, less erythematous and edematous polyps in the antrum. The intervening mucosa is normal. (**e**) Medium, Yamada type III (sub-pedunculated) polyps with normal intervening mucosa in the gastric angle

2 Colorectal Polyp

Multiple, medium-sized polyps with an erythematous surface and a whitish glandular orifice (pit) with an intervening flat mucosa are observed by colonoscopy (CS), the typical presentation of which is described as "strawberry like" appearance. However, they may sometimes have mild erythematous and strong edematous mucosa, whose interstitium surrounding glands are widen and whiten. These color patterns provide red and white reversal from strawberry-like pattern, which is described as "bubble tea like" appearance. In addition, the intervening mucosa may be apparently normal, but microscopic changes in the arrangement of the pit and surrounding capillaries may be visible on higher magnified observation.

2.1 Sparse type (A-1) (Fig. 5)

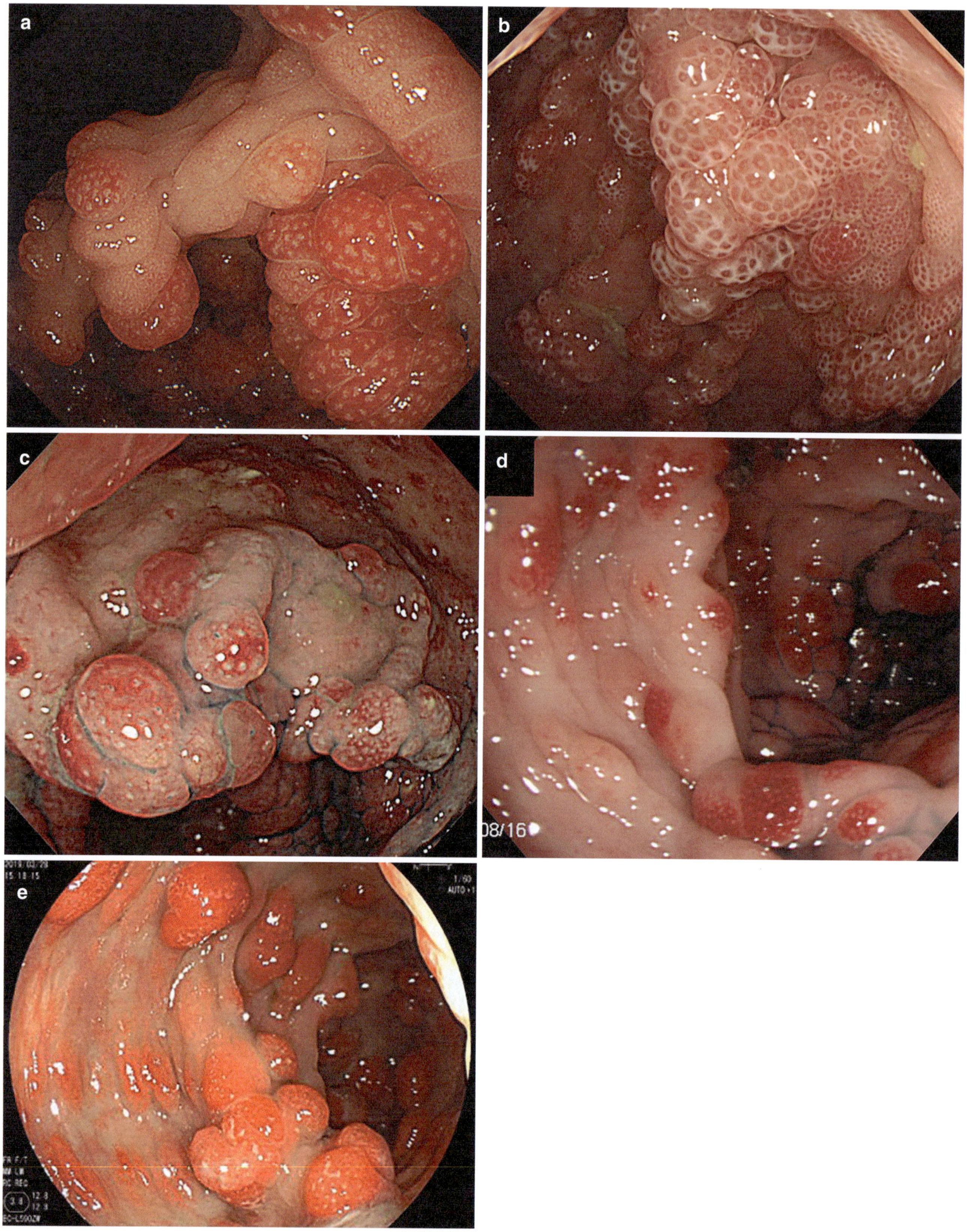

Fig. 5 (**a**) Small to medium-sized, mainly erythematous polyps with a "strawberry-like" appearance of white dots at the glandular duct orifice. (**b**) Medium-sized, slightly erythematous polyps, whose interstitium surrounding glands becomes wide and white, looking a "bubble tea like" appearance. (**c**) Scattered, small polyps on the surface of a SMT-like elevation. The small polyps are unevenly erythematous and the distance between pits are broadened. (**d**) The small, flat polyps are aligned circumferentially and have intense erythema with a well-defined border looking like a cherry red spot. There is no change in the intervening mucosa. (**e**) Medium-sized, erythematous, high polyps are longitudinally aligned. There is no change in the intervening mucosa

2.2 Confluent type (A-2) (Fig. 6)

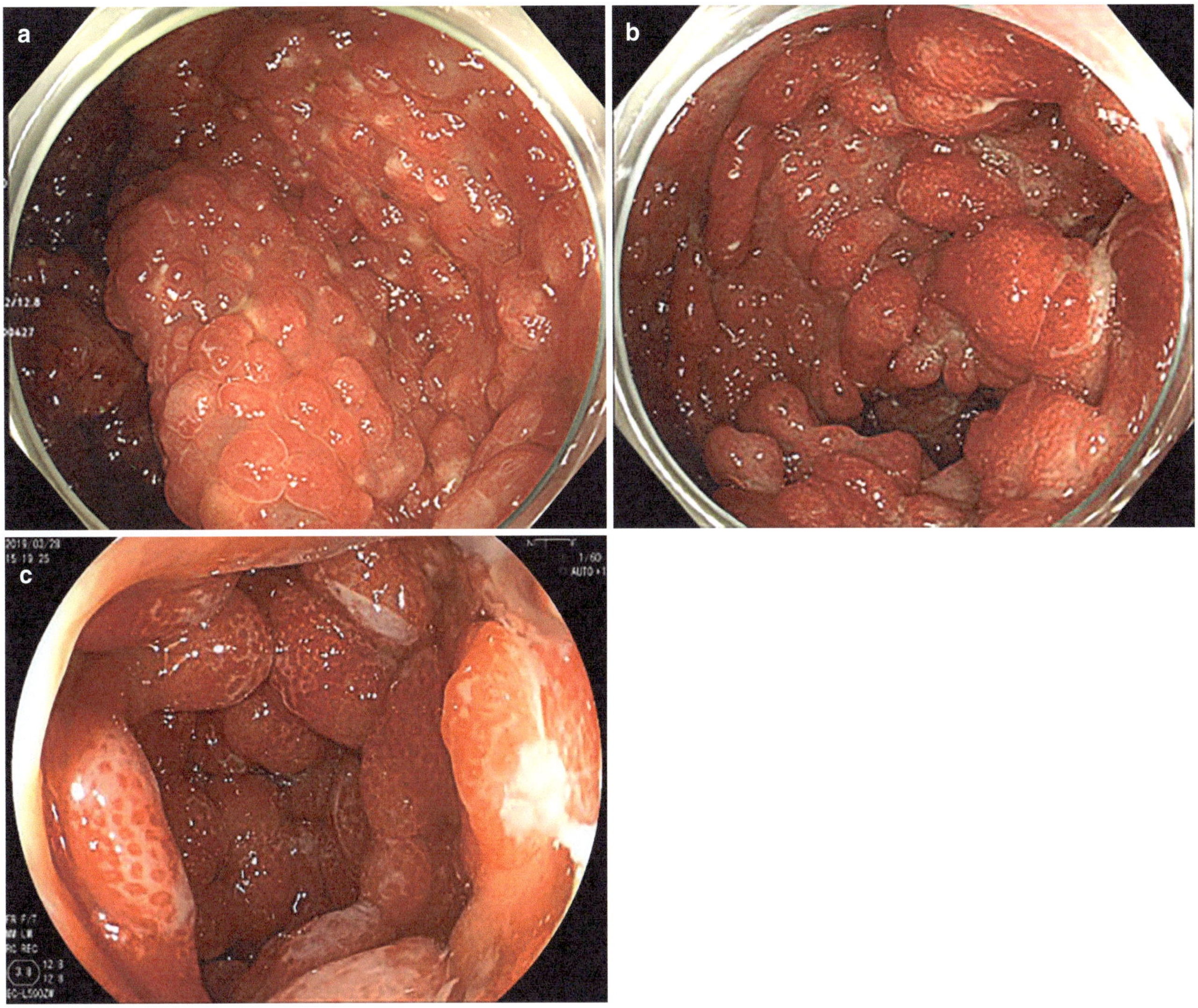

Fig. 6 (**a**) Small, mildly erythematous polyps, which have some scattered white spots with no obvious dilated pits. There is no intervening mucosa. (**b**) Medium to large, erythematous polyps. (**c**) Large polyps. Lumen was narrowed probably due to mucosal thickening

2.3 Confluent subtype: Semi-confluent type (A-2-1) (Fig. 7)

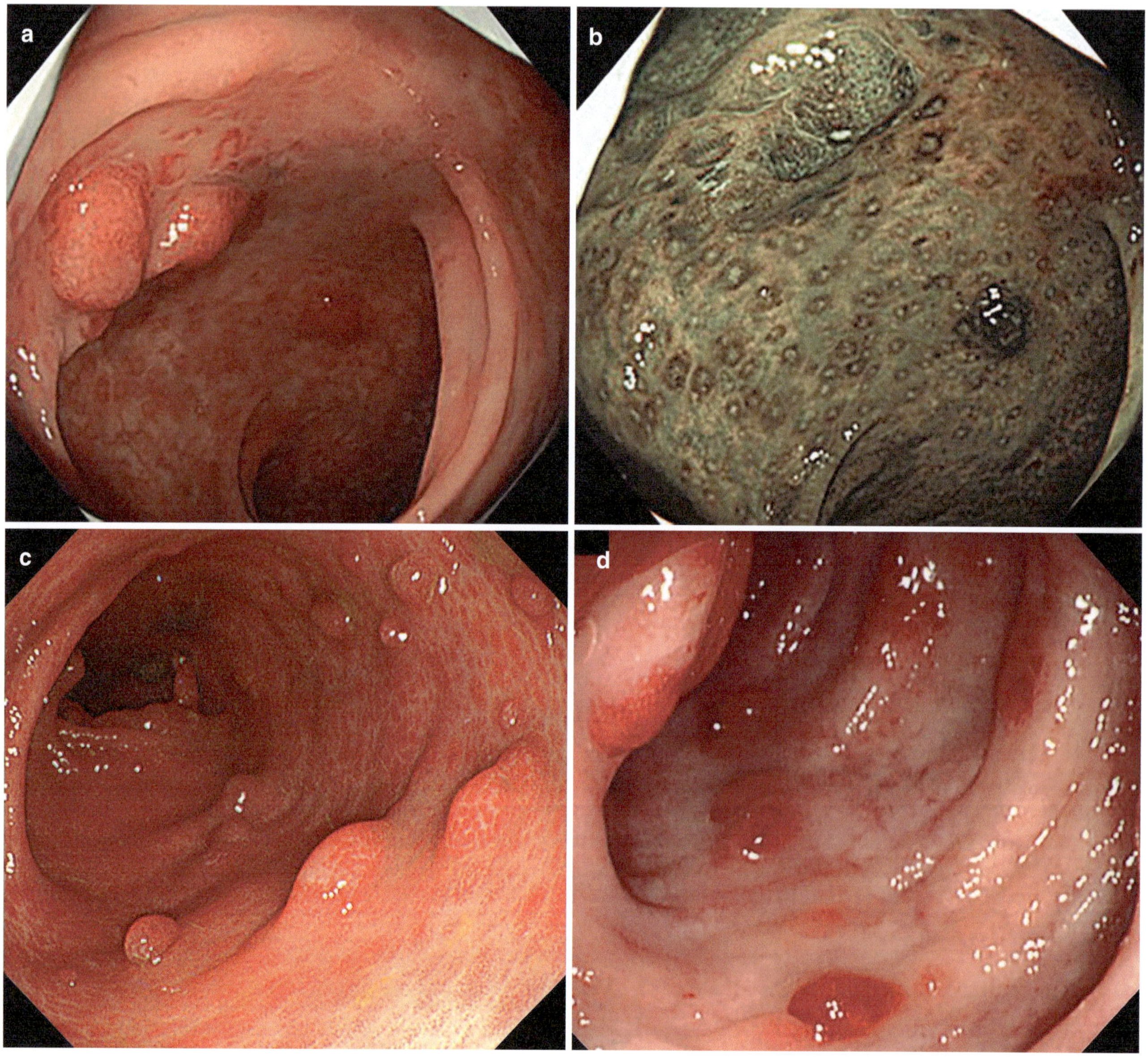

Fig. 7 (**a**), (**b**) Small, erythematous, and mild edematous polyps were observed. The intervening mucosa had multiple erythematous patchy mucosa with a central white spot, which were more clearly visible under NBI observation (**b**). (**c**) Small to medium-sized polyps. Polyp arrangement is irregular. White mucosa is present around glands of slightly elevated erythematous mucosa. The intervening mucosa is diffusely erythematous. (**d**) Medium to small polyps. Longitudinal arrangement of severely erythematous polyps. The intervening mucosa is edematous, and vascular pattern is decreased. (**e**) Medium to small polyps. Erythematous and edematous polyps are scattered circumferentially. The intervening mucosa is edematous. (**f**) Medium-sized polyps. Erythematous and erosive polyps are scattered circumferentially. The intervening mucosa is coarse and edematous

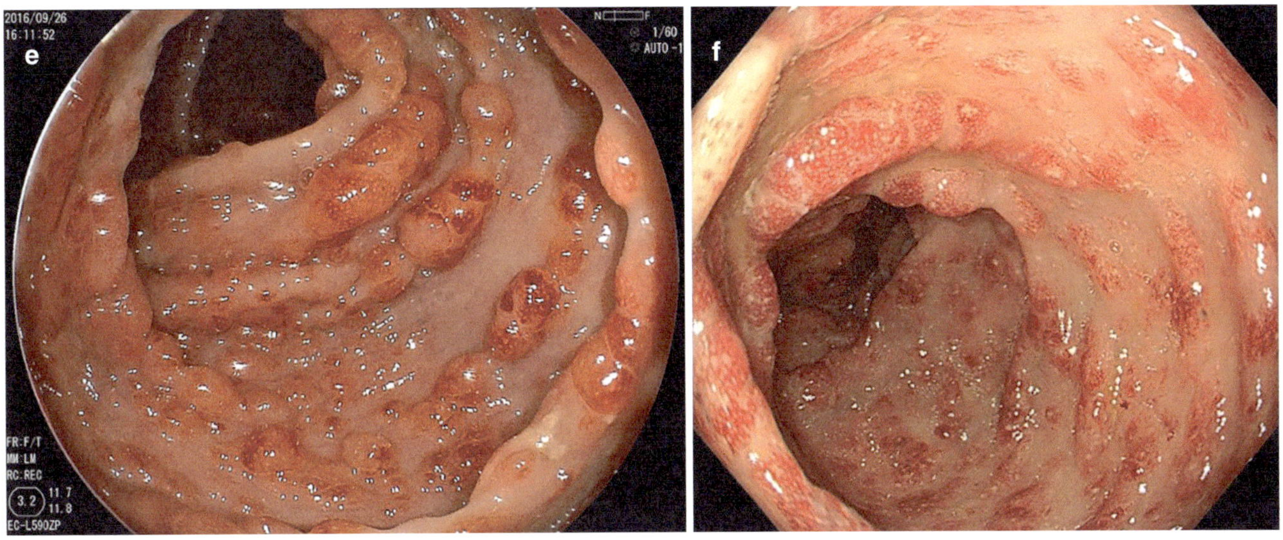

Fig. 7 (continued)

2.4 Confluent subtype: Thickening type (A-2-2) (Fig. 8)

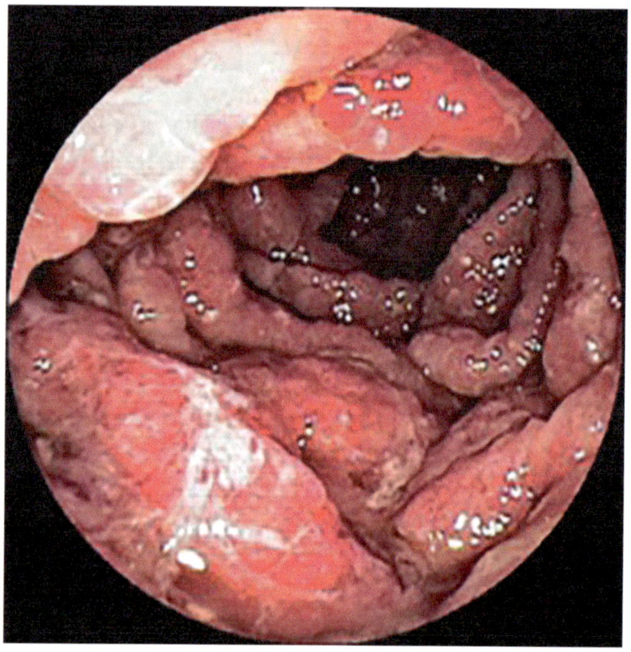

Fig. 8 The mucosa is edematous and erythematous, and the lumen is narrowed. There are no elevated polypoid lesions

3 Other Polyps

[Esophageal polyps]

Usually, no abnormal findings are observed in the esophagus under white light observation, and if polyps are present, they are small and scattered, papilloma-like polyps. In rare cases, multiple whitish SMTs instead of polyps are detected.

Although multiple polyps may be observed at the esophagogastric junction, most are gastric polyps arising from the gastric mucosal side. Therefore, polyposis disease other than CCS should be considered when dense polyps are observed in the esophagus (Fig. 9).

[Duodenal polyps]

Edematous and white villi are often observed. The polyps are often small and sparse, and histological study shows non-neoplastic polyps with edematous changes and inflammatory cell infiltration, as in other sites (Fig. 10).

[Jejunal and ileal polyps]

As in the duodenum, edematous and white villi and scattered small polyps are often observed. Physiologically, the form of villi in small intestine is different depending on the location. The majority of the villi in the jejunum and ileum are finger-like, but in the terminal ileum, there is a change to lobular (lingual) and ridge-like villi. Thus, it is important to take into account the location of small intestine before estimating disease activity. Although less common than in other sites, cases of adenoma have also been reported (Fig. 11).

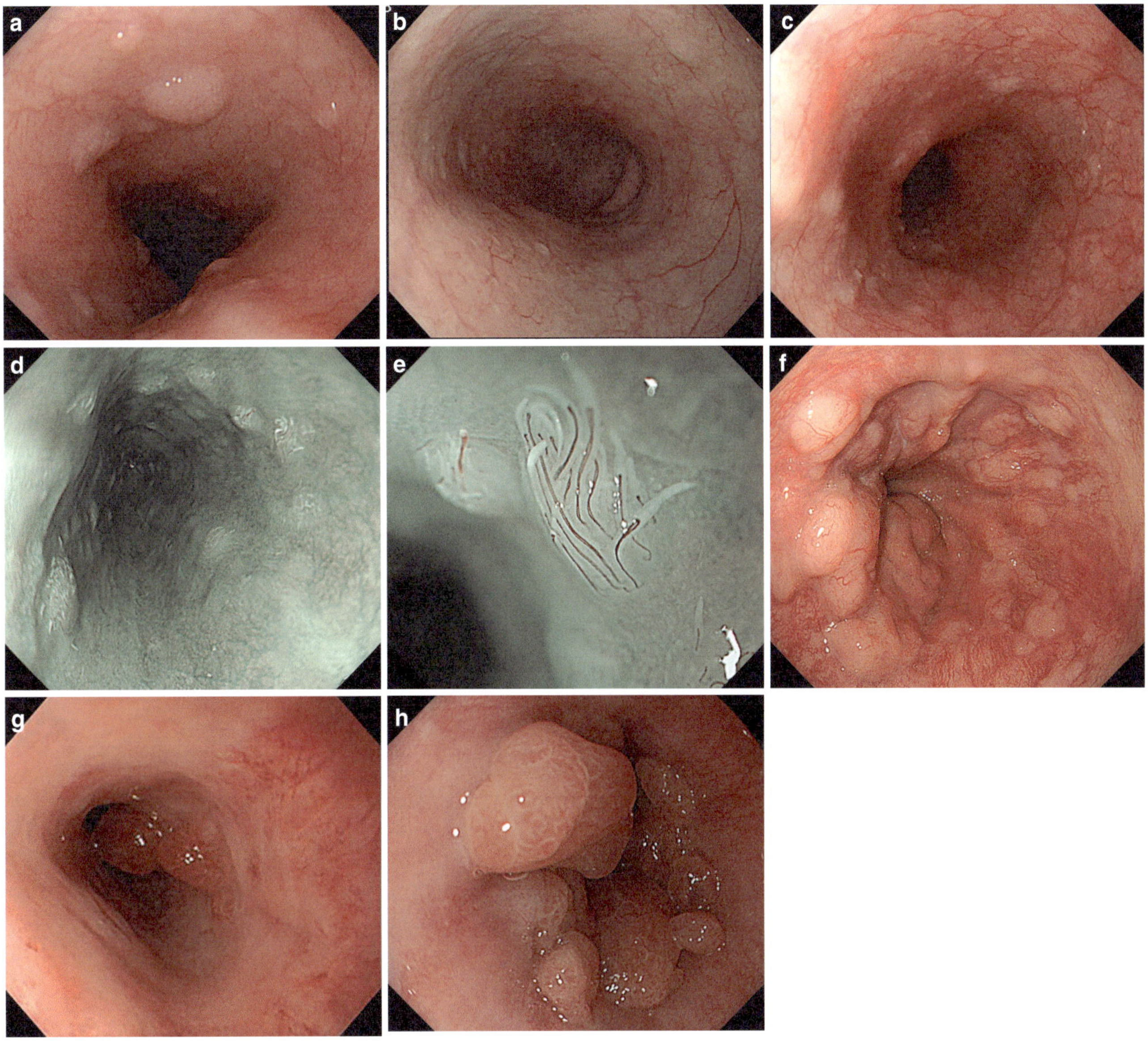

Fig. 9 (**a**)–(**c**) White scattered polyps. (**d**) Small size. Papillomatous polyps. Distant view by NBI. (**e**) Magnified observation of (**d**). (**f**) Whitish SMT. (**g**) Dense polyps at the esophagogastric junction. Distant view. (**h**) Close view of (**g**)

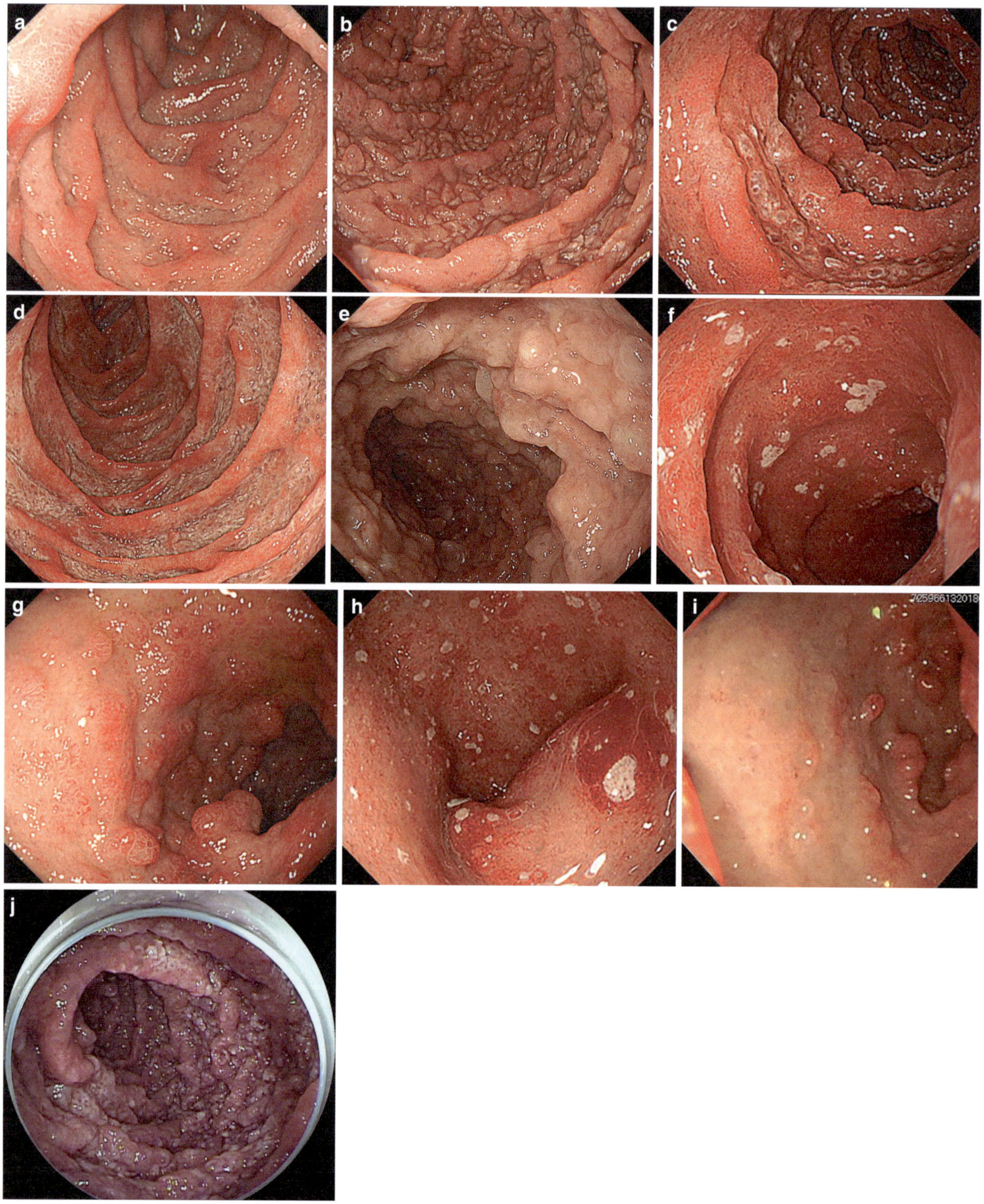

Fig. 10 **Duodenal polyps** (**a**) Fold thickening type with erythematous mucosa. (**b**) Fold thickening type with confluent polyps. (**c**) Fold thickening type with erythematous mucosa and white villi. (**d**) Fold thickening type with erythematous mucosa and white villi. (**e**) Confluent type. Small, edematous polyps with white villi. (**f**) Fold thickening type with erythematous and erosive mucosa. (**g**) Sparse type. Small, erythematous polyps. (**h**) Fold thickening type with erythematous mucosa and white villi. (**i**) Sparse type. Small, erythematous polyps. (**j**) Fold thickening type with erythematous mucosa and white villi

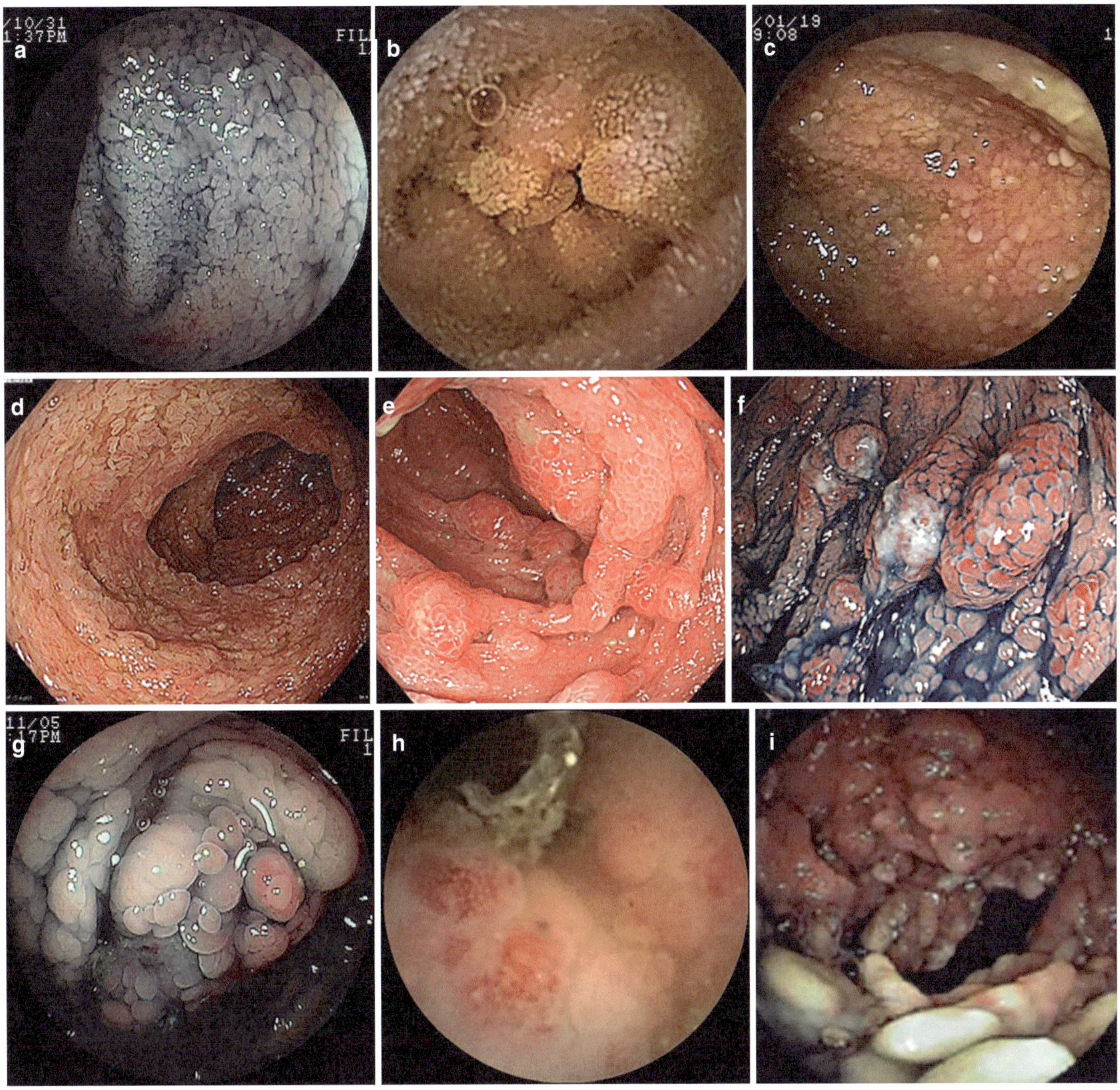

Fig. 11 Jejunal and ileal polyps (**a**) Flattened villi. (**b**) White villi. (**c**) Flattened and white villi. (**d**) Swollen villi. (**e**) Flattened, erythematous, and swollen villi, fold thickening. (**f**) Erythematous and swollen villi. (**g**) Flattened, swollen villi. (**h**) Erythematous and swollen villi. (**i**) Swollen and while villi, and an SMT-like elevation

Endoscopic Images of Small Bowel Capsule Endoscopy, Balloon-Assisted Enteroscopy, and Image-Enhanced Endoscopy

Ryota Hokari, Tadakazu Hisamatsu, and Masaaki Higashiyama

1 Balloon-Assisted Enteroscopy (BAE) and Small Bowel Capsule Endoscopy (SBCE)

The development of BAE (Fig. 1a, b) and SBCE (Fig. 1c, d) in the 2000s made it much easier to observe entire small bowel compared with previous small bowel endoscopy. This increased the number of CCS cases whose small bowels were observed endoscopically. SBCE is noninvasive and simple, while BAE has the advantage of dye spreading, biopsy, image-enhancement, and magnification for more detailed evaluation.

2 Chromoendoscope

There are many various-sized polyps in CCS, especially in confluent type cases, in which the exact shape of the polyps is difficult to identify and the boundaries between the polyps and the intervening mucosa become unclear. Thus, it is difficult to obtain accurate endoscopic findings using only white light. The contrast method using indigocarmine dyeing is highly recommended because it facilitates the clarification of these findings (Fig. 2).

3 Image-Enhanced Endoscopy, Magnifying Endoscopy

Magnifying endoscopy using Narrow Band Imaging (NBI) and Blue Light Imaging (BLI) is used for detailed examination of neoplastic lesions. Even in apparently normal intervening mucosa by white light observation, deformations of glandular structures and capillaries have been reported under higher magnification observation (Fig. 3).

R. Hokari (✉) · M. Higashiyama
Department of Internal Medicine, National Defense Medical College, Tokorozawa, Saitama, Japan
e-mail: ryota@ndmc.ac.jp; masaakih@ndmc.ac.jp

T. Hisamatsu
Department of Gastroenterology and Hepatology, Kyorin University School of Medicine, Mitaka, Tokyo, Japan

R. Hokari, T. Hisamatsu (eds.), *Atlas of Cronkhite-Canada Syndrome*, https://doi.org/10.1007/978-981-19-0652-7_3

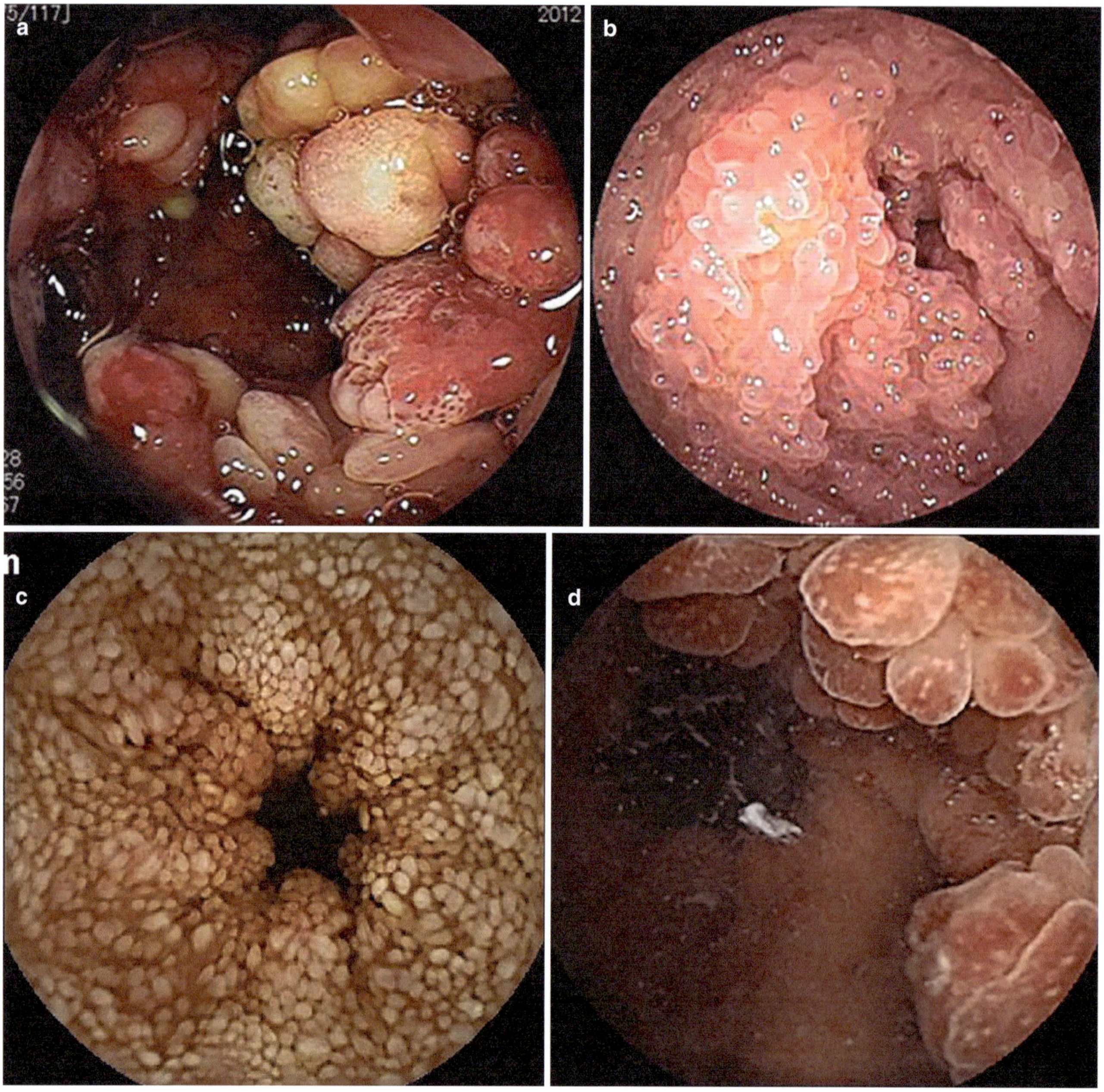

Fig. 1 (**a**), (**b**) BAE. (**c**), (**d**) SBCE. (**a**) White polyps, mixed with erythematous polyps. (**b**) Swollen villi and an SMT-like elevation. (**c**) White villi. (**d**) Small polyps with white spot

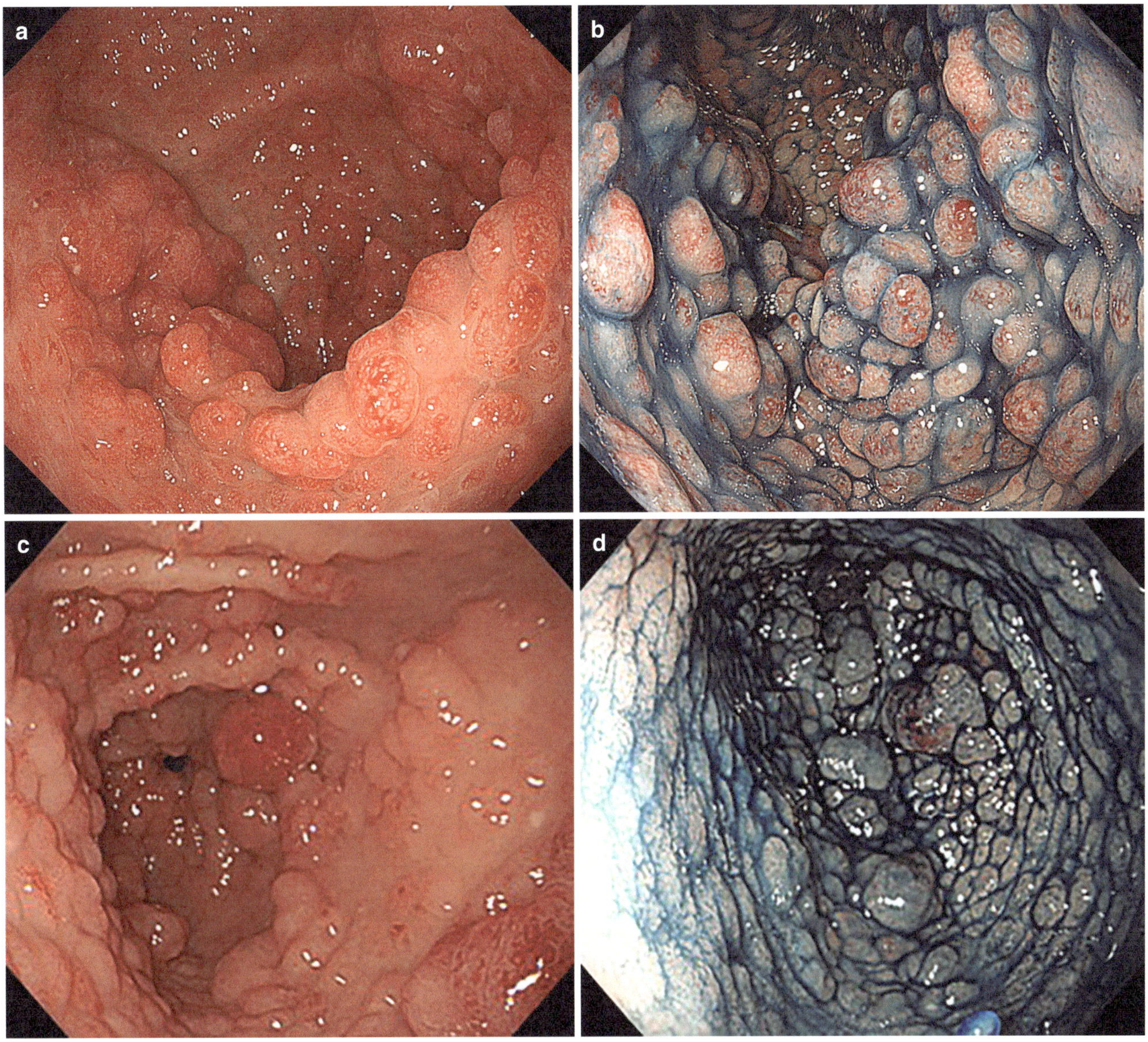

Fig. 2 Chromoendoscope. (**a**), (**c**) White light observations. (**b**), (**d**) Indigocarmine dyeing of (**a**), (**c**)

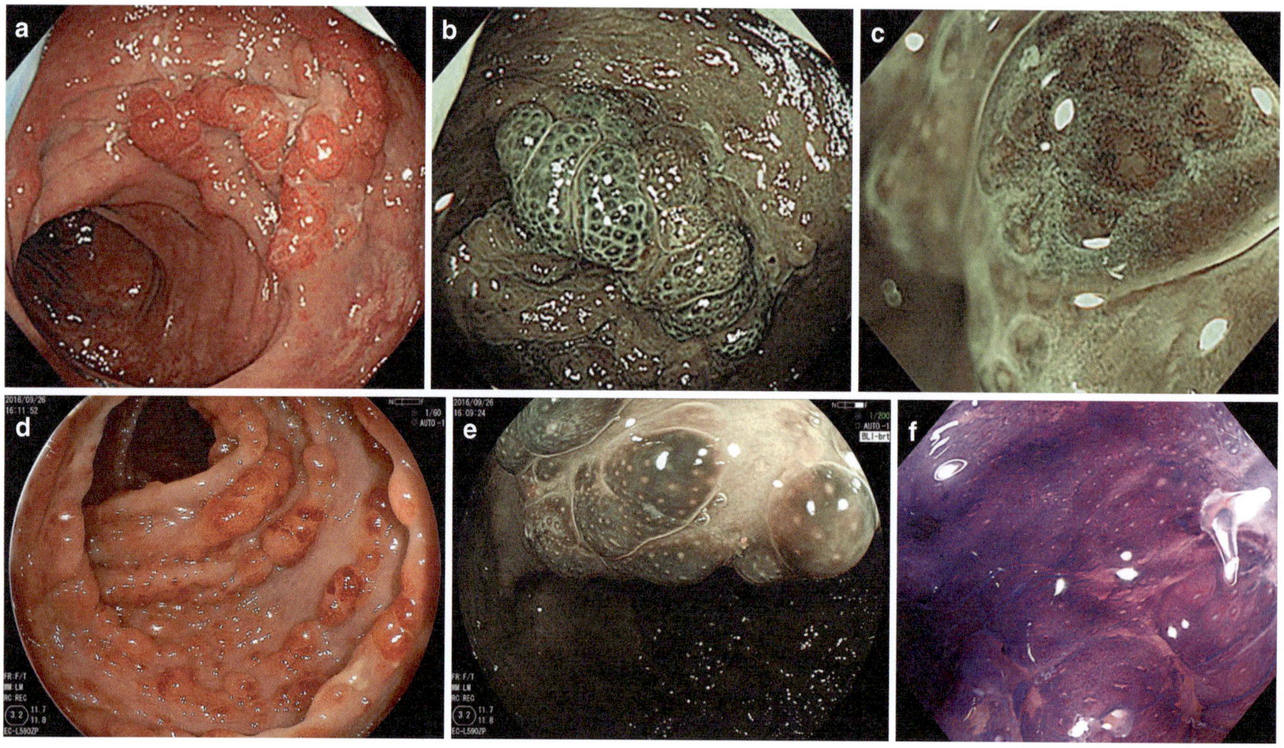

Fig. 3 Colonic inflammatory hyperplastic polyps observed by NBI/BLI or magnified endoscopy after crystal violet staining. (**a**) Colon: Confluent type. Erythematous, strawberry-like polyps. (**b**) NBI observation. (**c**) Magnified observation of (**b**). The pits corresponding to strawberry seeds are pale, and the area surrounding pits is brownish. The distances between pits are broadened. The interstitium surrounding the brownish area is light blue colored. (**d**) Colon: Severely erythematous polyps are observed. (**e**) Magnified BLI observation. The polyps are brownish in color, the pits are open and pale, and the distances between pits are broadened. (**f**) Magnified observation after crystal violet staining. Polyps are heterogeneously stained. The number of pit is markedly decreased, and the distances between pits are broadened. This is a non-neoplastic pattern corresponding to type II open pit pattern (Figs. 4, 5, 6, and 7)

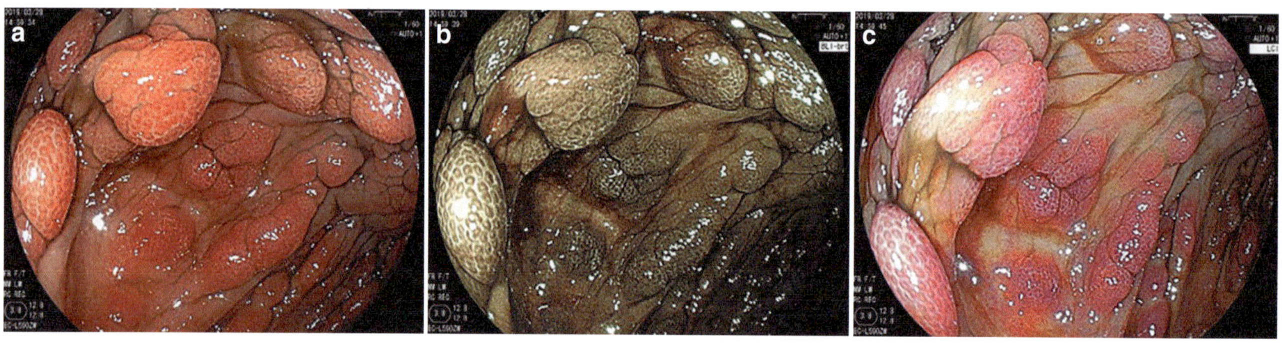

Fig. 4 BLI and Linked Color Imaging (LCI) observations of colonic inflammatory hyperplastic polyps. (**a**) Colon: Strawberry-like polyps. (**b**) BLI observation of (**a**). Polyps are brownish in color, and the pits are observed as white in the same way as NBI observation. (**c**) LCI observation of (**a**). Polyps are identified with magenta tone enhancement. Inflamed and non-inflamed areas are easily distinguished, and the presence of non-inflammed intervening mucosa is clear

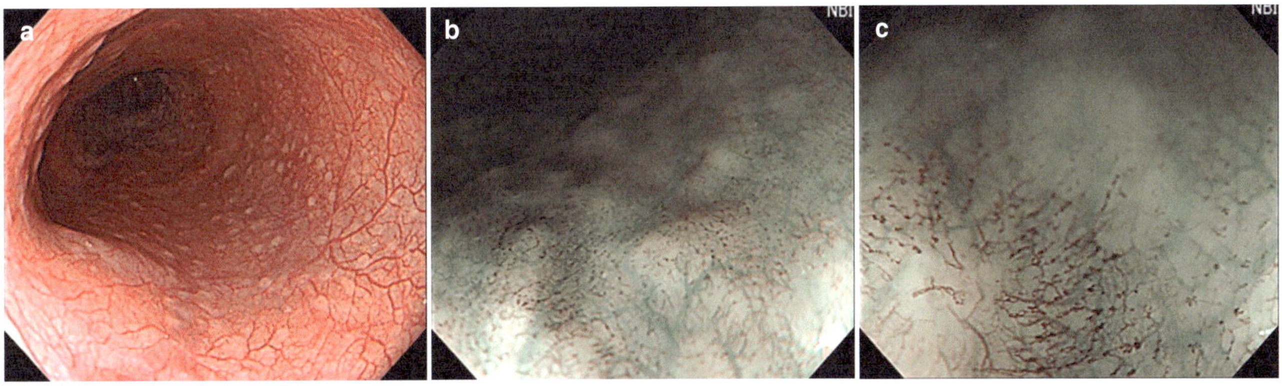

Fig. 5 Magnified NBI observation of multiple small esophageal polyps. (**a**) Multiple small white polyps are observed in the esophagus. (**b**) Low magnified NBI observation of (**a**). Brown dots are distributed independently of the small polyps. (**c**) High magnified NBI observation of (**a**). The vessel is mildly dilated, but there is no evidence of tortuosity, caliber irregularity, or heterogeneity in shape, classified to type A vessel (classification by the Japan Esophageal Society), which is diagnosed as non-neoplastic

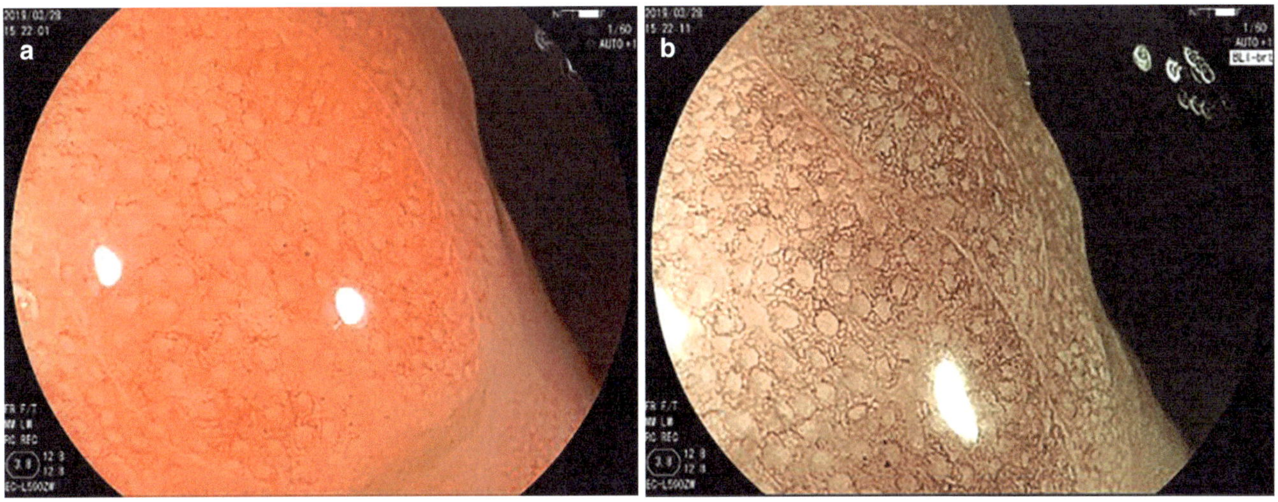

Fig. 6 Magnified observation of mildly inflamed intervening mucosa of the colon under white light or NBI. (**a**) Magnified observation. Mildly erythematous and edematous intervening mucosa of the colon with slightly dilated pits. (**b**) Magnified NBI observation of (**a**). Mildly brownish coloration is observed, and capillaries around the pits are increased

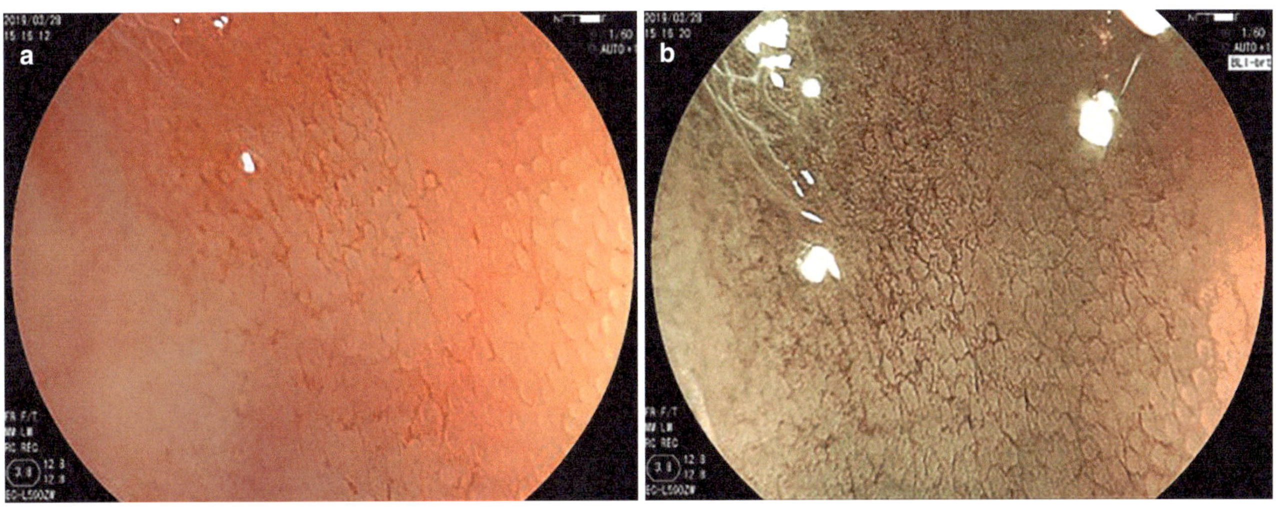

Fig. 7 Magnified observation of almost normal intervening mucosa of the colon under white light or NBI. (**a**) Magnified observation. (**b**) Magnified BLI observation of (**a**). The capillaries surrounding the pits have proliferated linearly or reticularly with slight disruption of honeycomb-like arrangement of glands. The interpit distances are normal

Endoscopic Images of Coincident Carcinoma and Adenoma to Differentiate from Non-neoplastic Polyps

Ryota Hokari, Tadakazu Hisamatsu, and Masaaki Higashiyama

Coincident carcinoma and adenoma are not rare in CCS. Thus, it is very important to pick up them from multiple polyps. NBI and BLI, although using different wavelengths of light respectively, are both techniques that allow detailed observation of glandular and microvascular structures. Case reports using NBI have shown that many inflammatory hyperplastic polyps do not have abnormal microvasculature on their surface, whereas adenomas have dilated, tortuous microvasculature of variable diameter, making it possible to diagnose endoscopically. In addition, the usages of indigocarmine and crystal violet dyeing are also considered to be useful tools in the diagnosis of neoplastic lesions. However, in the presence of inflammatory hyperplastic polyps, diagnosis before corticosteroid treatment is not easy. Most tumors are detected after the inflammatory hyperplastic polyps have diminished after the initial treatment (Figs. 1, 2, and 3).

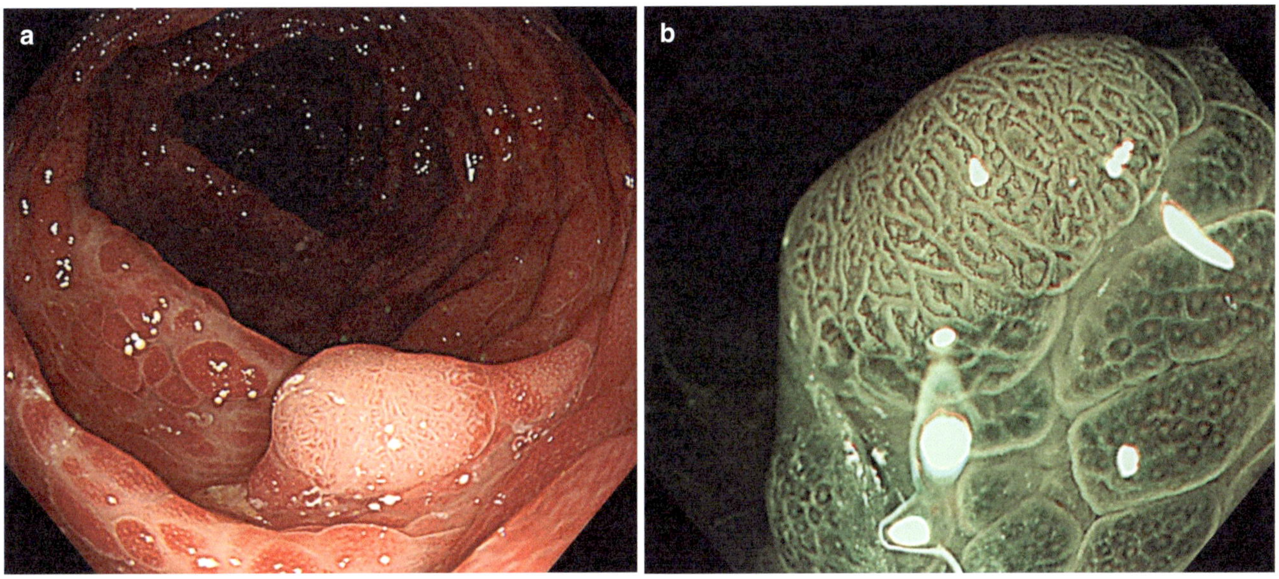

Fig. 1 Colorectal carcinoma before corticosteroid treatments: Tubular adenocarcinoma, well differentiated (tub 1). (**a**) Multiple small erythematous polyps are detected in the sigmoid colon, and the tumor (Is polyp) is recognized from the surrounding area as a medium-sized mass lesion with mild erythema. (**b**) Magnified NBI observation of (**a**). Slight irregularity in microvascular structures is detected and diagnosed as JNET 2B. The color of inflamed (non-neoplastic) mucosa surrounding the tumor is deeper than that of tumor

R. Hokari (✉) · M. Higashiyama
Department of Internal Medicine, National Defense Medical College, Tokorozawa, Saitama, Japan
e-mail: ryota@ndmc.ac.jp; masaakih@ndmc.ac.jp

T. Hisamatsu
Department of Gastroenterology and Hepatology, Kyorin University School of Medicine, Mitaka, Tokyo, Japan

R. Hokari, T. Hisamatsu (eds.), *Atlas of Cronkhite-Canada Syndrome*, https://doi.org/10.1007/978-981-19-0652-7_4

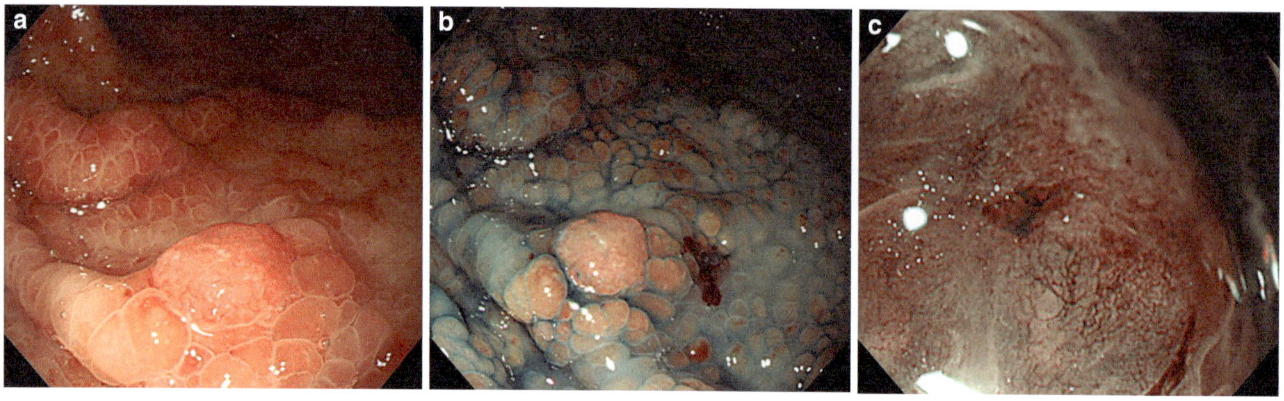

Fig. 2 Gastric carcinoma after corticosteroid treatments. (**a**) Small, confluent polyps are flattened and shiny. There is a slightly larger, less shiny, elevated lesion in the center (well-differentiated adenocarcinoma). (**b**) Acetic acid and indigocarmine mixture dyeing of (**a**). The elevated lesions are observed in an erythematous tone, but some confluently surrounding small polyps are also erythematous, and the boundary is difficult to distinguish. (**c**) Magnified NBI observation of (**a**). The elevated lesion has microvascular structures which are positive of irregular microvascular pattern, and shows dendritic or heterogeneously distributed vessels. However, the non-tumor area also has a high vascular density, and the demarcation line is indistinct

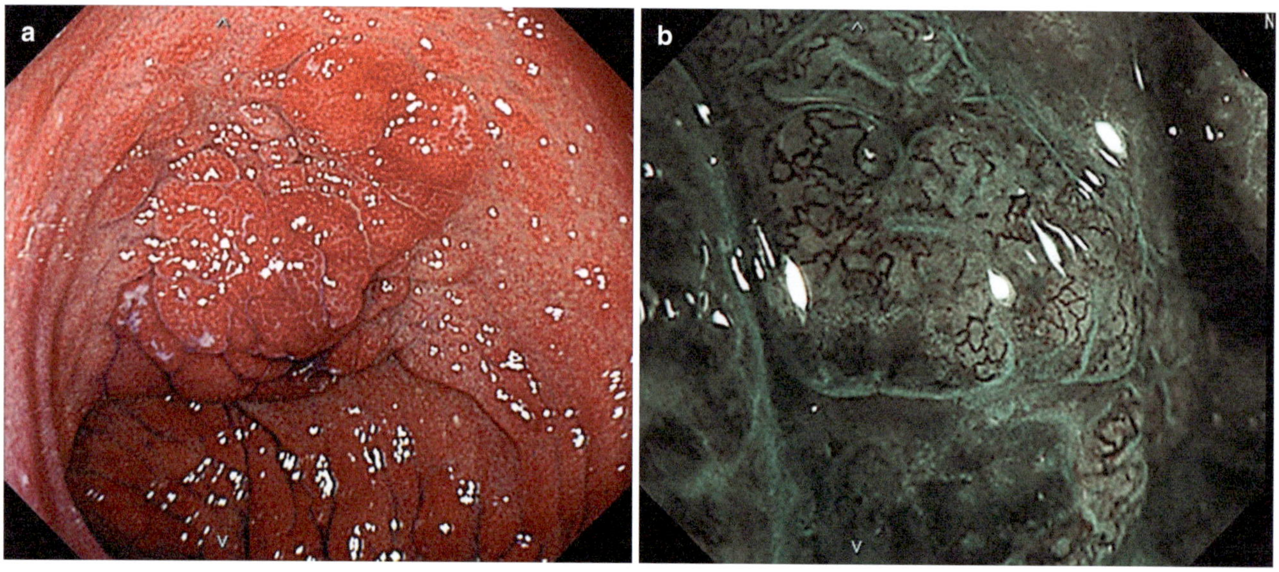

Fig. 3 Hyperplastic and inflammatory changes in the sigmoid colon before corticosteroid treatments. (**a**) Large, erythematous, flat polyps. (**b**) NBI observation of (**a**). The polyp is mainly recognized as dark green, but there are some discolored areas (weak brownish) with a slightly dilated microvascular structure. The diameter of the vasculature is irregular and the vessel density is uneven

Comparison of Pathological and Endoscopic Images (per Organ)

Ryota Hokari, Tadakazu Hisamatsu, and Masaaki Higashiyama

Polyps observed in CCS are classified as non-neoplastic. The glandular ducts are unequally sized, irregularly branched, and dilated, and may show the appearance of serrated changes. In cases with endoscopically white mucus adhered appearance, there is often an accumulation of eosinophilic exudate in the dilated glandular ducts. In the interstitium, edematous changes, telangiectasias, and inflammatory cell infiltrates: eosinophils, neutrophils, lymphocytes, and plasma cells are observed. Edematous changes are accompanied by decreased density of glandular ducts. Dilatation of lymphatic vessels is often mild, even if present. In this chapter, pathological images (a in each figure) with pathological evaluations and corresponding endoscopic images (b in each figure) are shown.

1 Stomach

Pathological image of whitish mucus adhered polyps.
Interstitial edema: 3+
Inflammatory cell infiltration: 2+
Glandular duct hyperplastic changes: 2+
Dilation of glandular duct: 2+
Serrated changes: –
(Fig. 1)

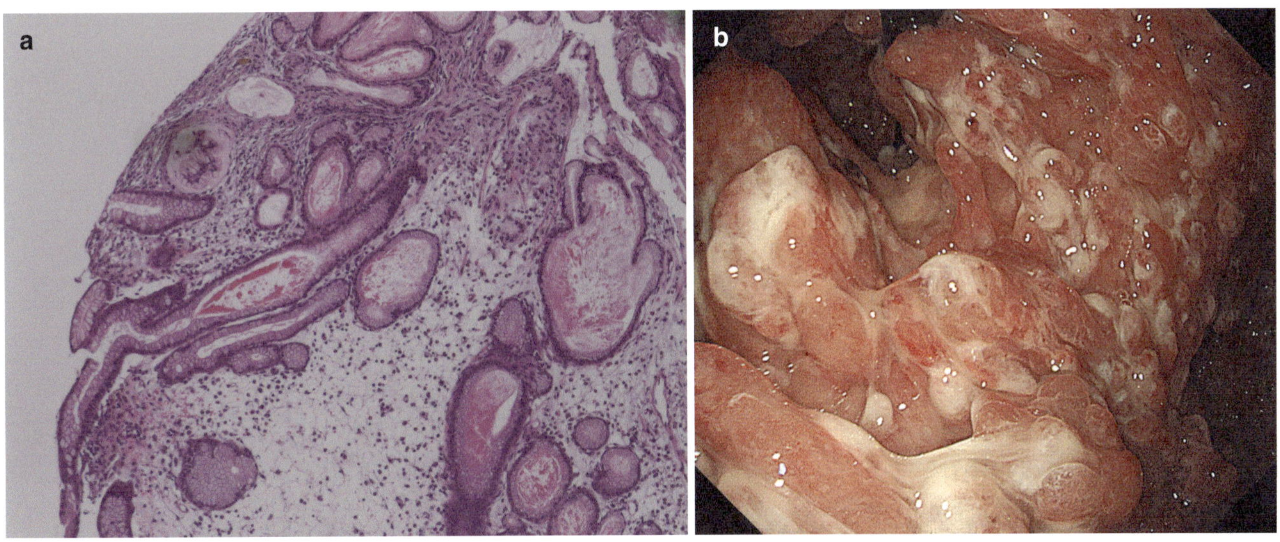

Fig. 1 Pathological image of whitish mucus adhered polyps. The interstitium shows marked edematous changes and heterogeneous infiltration of lymphocytes, plasma cells, and eosinophils. The dilated glandular ducts are filled with eosinophilic exudate. Areas of intense inflammatory cell infiltration do not always coincide with edematous changes

R. Hokari (✉) · M. Higashiyama
Department of Internal Medicine, National Defense Medical College, Tokorozawa, Saitama, Japan
e-mail: ryota@ndmc.ac.jp; masaakih@ndmc.ac.jp

T. Hisamatsu
Department of Gastroenterology and Hepatology, Kyorin University School of Medicine, Mitaka, Tokyo, Japan

R. Hokari, T. Hisamatsu (eds.), *Atlas of Cronkhite-Canada Syndrome*, https://doi.org/10.1007/978-981-19-0652-7_5

Pathological image of small, "red cavir like" polyps.
Interstitial edema: –
Inflammatory cell infiltration: 2+
Glandular duct hyperplastic changes: 2+
Dilation of the glandular duct: +
Serrated changes: +
(Fig. 2)

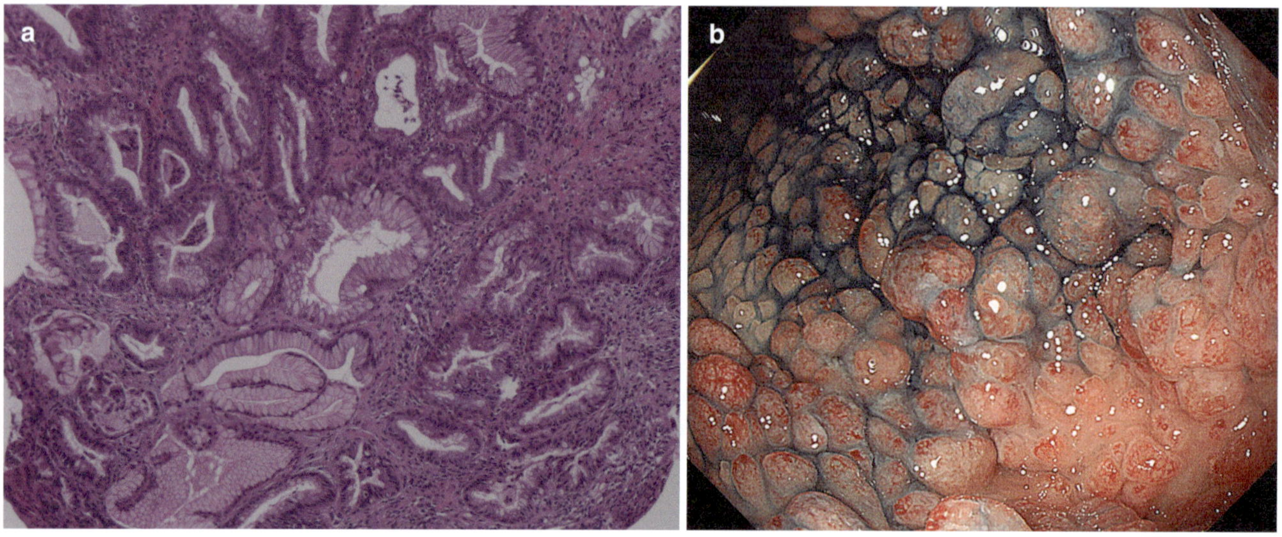

Fig. 2 Pathological image of small, "red cavir like" polyps. The foveolar epithelium shows hyperplastic changes with some serrated protrusion into the mildly dilated crypt. Edematous changes in the interstitum are unremarkable, and there is a moderate lymphocyte and plasma cell infiltrate with eosinophils and neutrophils

Pathological image of medium-sized polyps with strong edematous changes.
Interstitial edema: 3+
Inflammatory cell infiltration: +
Glandular ductal hyperplastic change: +
Dilation of glandular ducts: –
Serrated changes: –
(Fig. 3)

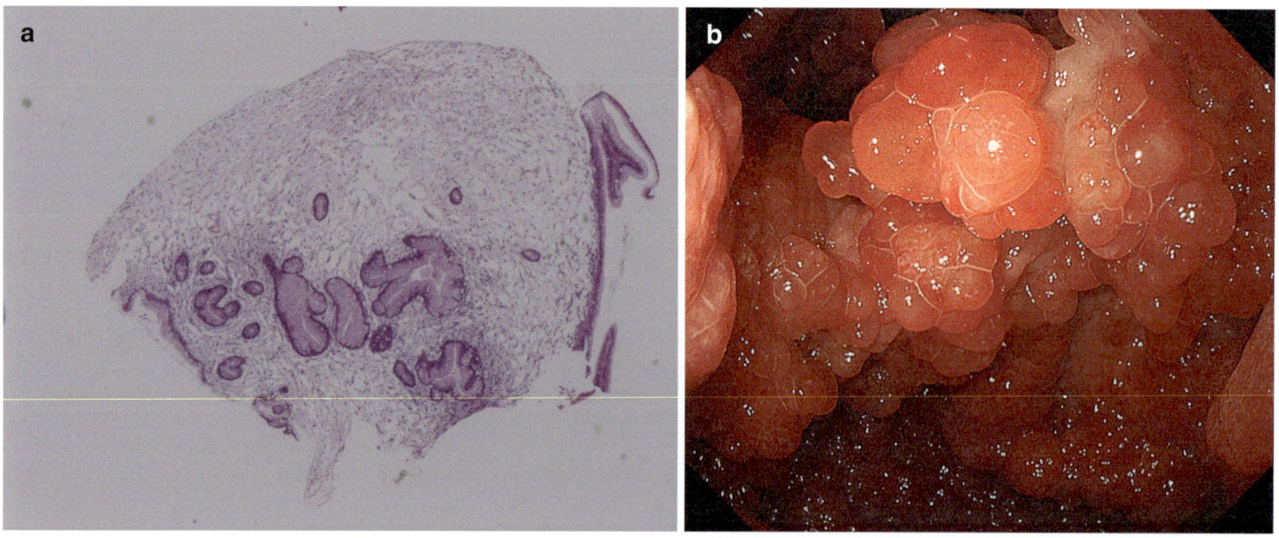

Fig. 3 Pathological image of medium-sized polyps with strong edematous changes. There are regenerating glandular ducts of unequal size and irregular branching, equivalent to non-neoplastic polyps. The interstitium is extremely edematous with only a mild eosinophilic, lymphocytic, and plasma cell infiltrate

2 Colon

Pathological image of sparse small polyps.
Interstitial edema: +
Inflammatory cell infiltration: 2+
Glandular duct hyperplastic changes: 2+
Dilation of the glandular duct: +
Serrated changes: –
(Fig. 4)

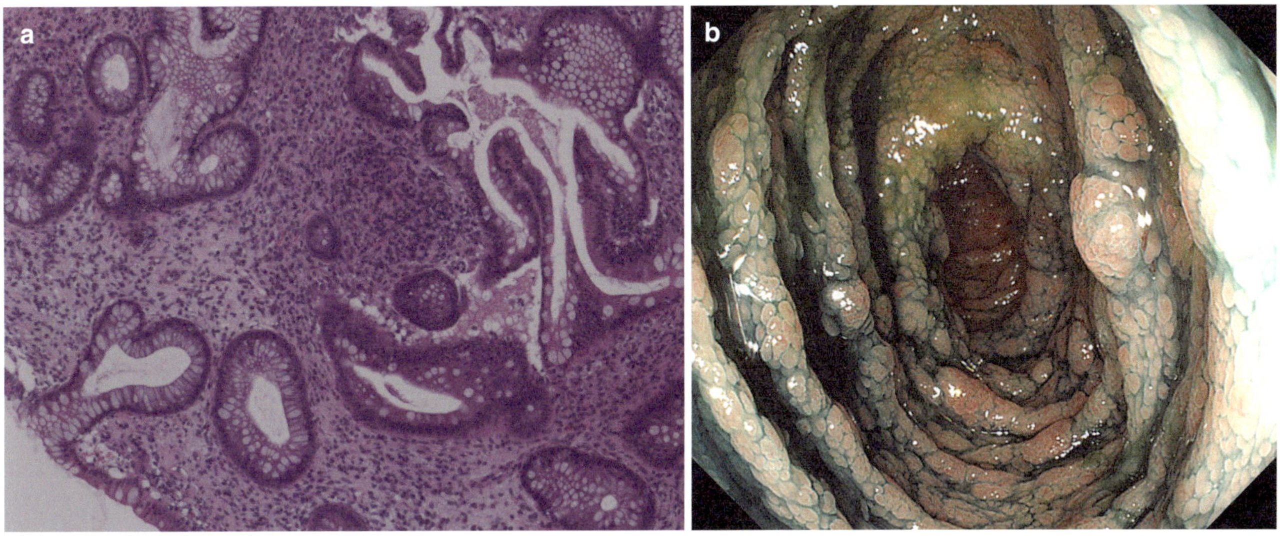

Fig. 4 Pathological image of sparse small polyps. Regenerating, unequally sized and dilated glandular ducts with irregular branching are observed. Accumulation of eosinophilic exudate is shown in dilated glandular ducts. Edematous changes in the interstitium are mild, and there is a moderate infiltration of lymphocytes, plasma cells, and eosinophils

Pathological image of confluent small polyps.
Interstitial edema: –
Inflammatory cell infiltration: 3+
Glandular ductal hyperplastic change: +
Dilation of glandular duct: 3+
Serrated changes: –
(Fig. 5)

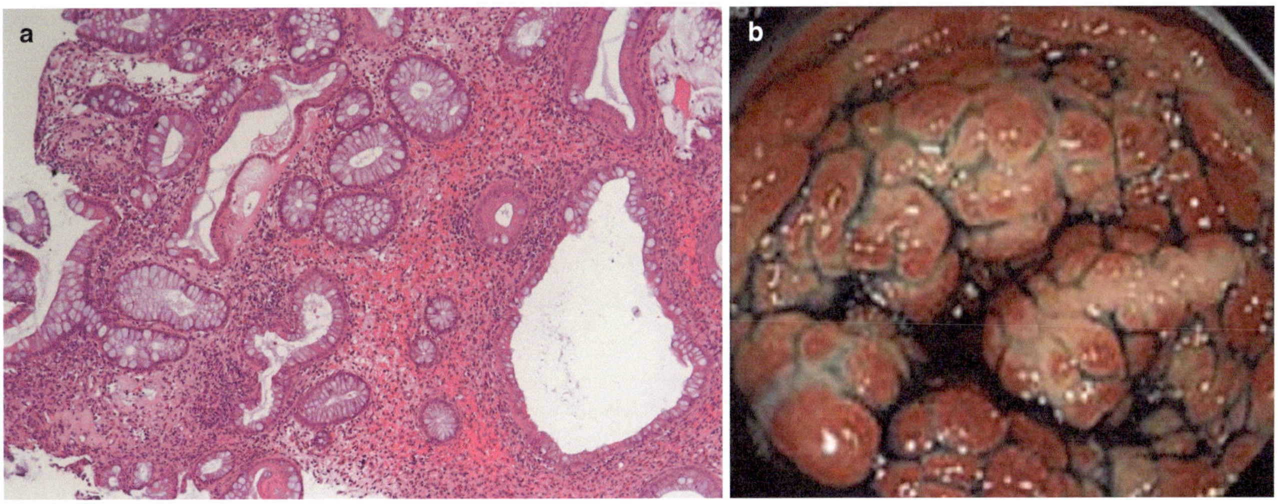

Fig. 5 Pathological image of confluent small polyps. There are cystic dilatations of the glandular ducts and intense eosinophilic infiltration of the lamina propria. Edematous changes in the interstitium are not evident

Pathological image of large sparse polyps with intense erythematous changes.
Interstitial edema: 3+
Inflammatory cell infiltration: 2+
Glandular duct hyperplastic change: –
Dilation of glandular ducts: –
Serrated changes: –
(Fig. 6)

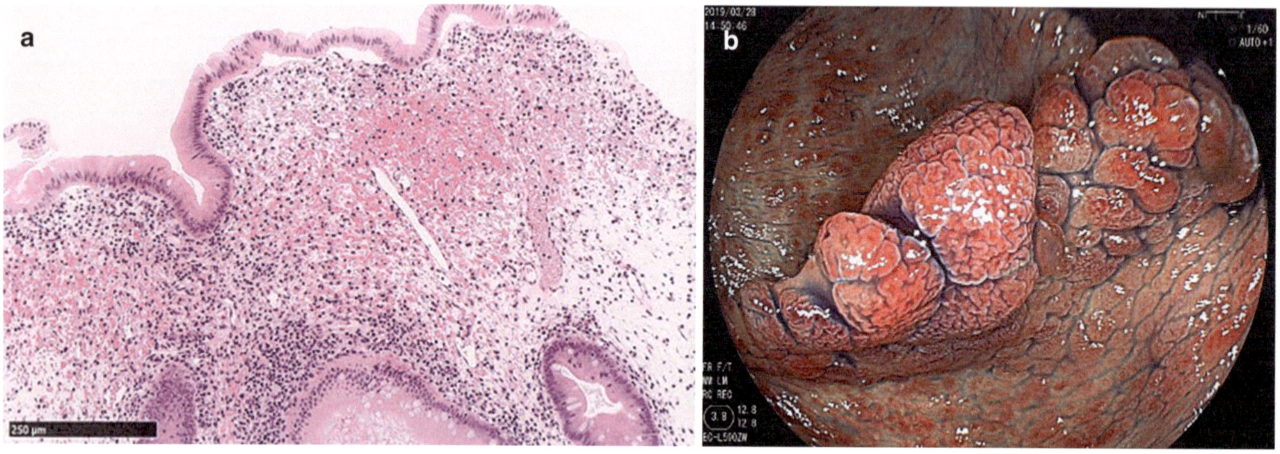

Fig. 6 Pathological image of large sparse polyps with intense erythematous changes. Strong edematous changes and inflammatory cell infiltration of the interstitium are present. Dilation of the glandular ducts is not evident

Pathological image of sparse medium-sized polyps with intense erythematous changes.
Interstitial edema: 3+
Inflammatory cell infiltration: +
Glandular duct hyperplastic change: –
Dilation of glandular ducts: –
Serrated changes: –
(Fig. 7)

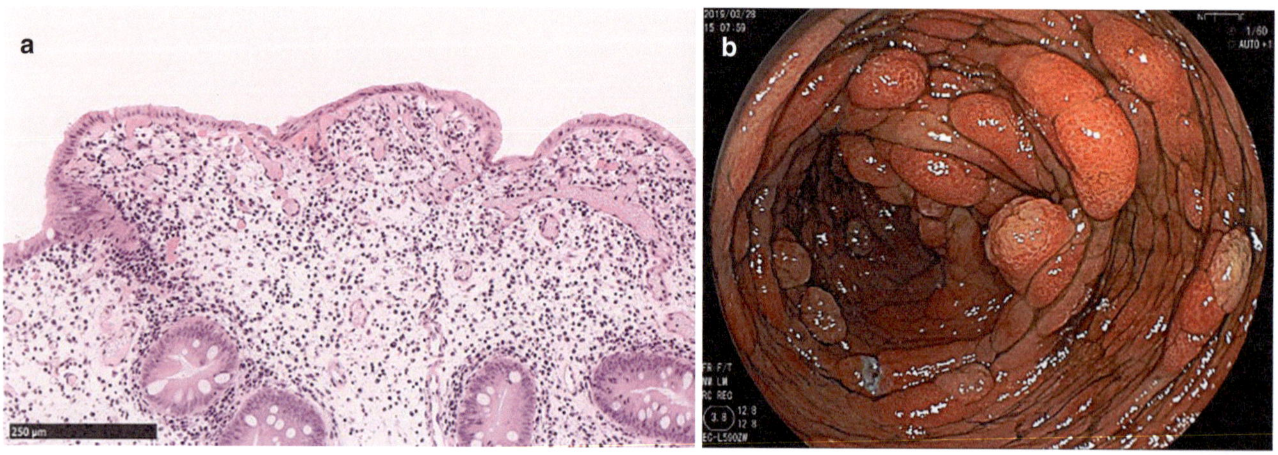

Fig. 7 Pathological image of sparse medium-sized polyps with intense erythematous changes. There are strong edematous changes in the interstitium and vasodilatation just below the epithelium. Dilation of the glandular ducts is not evident

3 Duodenum

Pathological image of edematous and enlarged white villi.
Interstitial edema: 2+
Inflammatory cell infiltration: +
Glandular duct hyperplastic changes: 3+
Dilation of glandular duct: 3+
(Fig. 8)

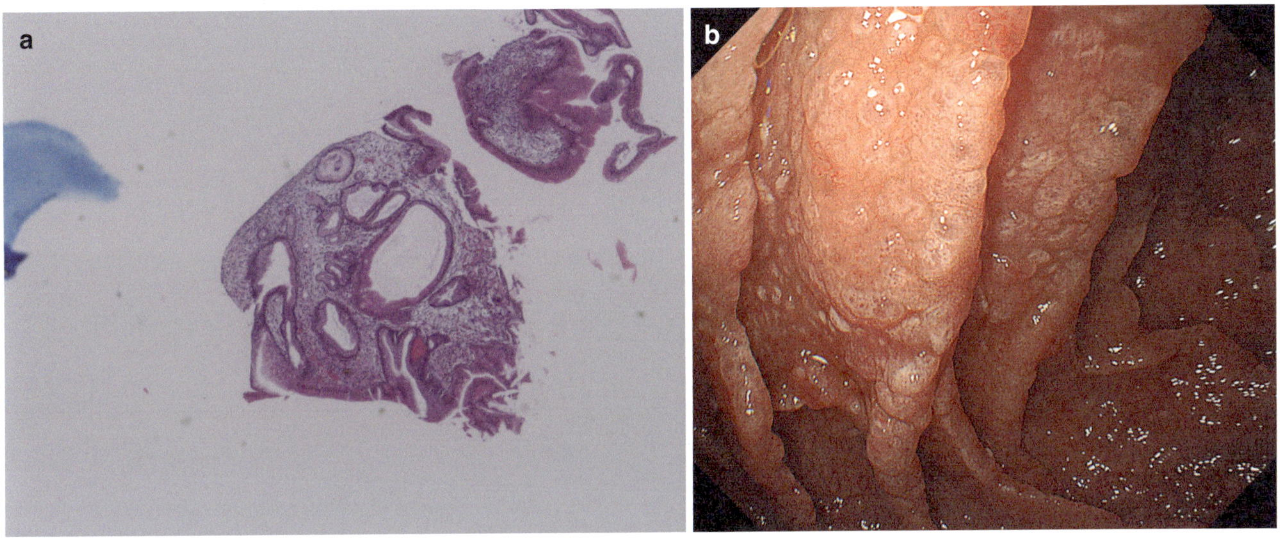

Fig. 8 Pathological image of edematous and enlarged white villi. Markedly dilated, regenerating glandular ducts of unequal size and irregular branching are observed, and the interstitum is edematous, equivalent to a hamartomatous polyp

Pathological image of edematous enlarged villi.
Interstitial edema: +
Inflammatory cell infiltration: 2+
Glandular duct hyperplastic changes: 2+
Dilation of glandular duct: 3+
(Fig. 9)

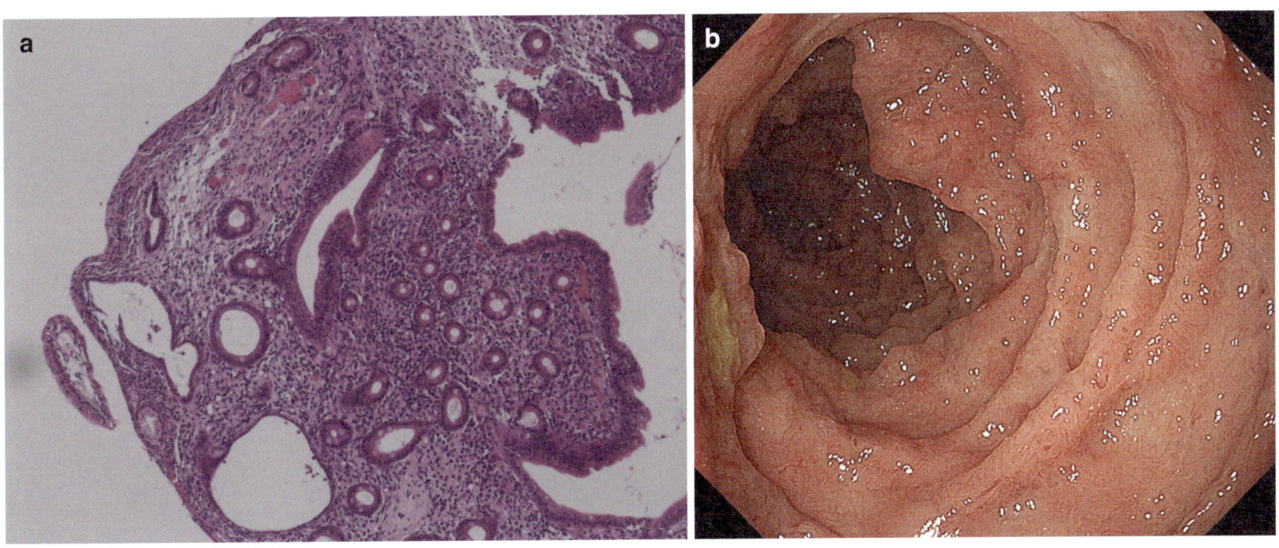

Fig. 9 Pathological image of edematous enlarged villi. The glandular ducts are dilated. The interstitum is mildly edematous with moderate lymphocytic, plasma cell, and eosinophilic infiltrates

Pathological image of an SMT-like elevation with remarkably edematous mucosa and white villi.
Interstitial edema: +
Inflammatory cell infiltration: 2+
Glandular duct hyperplastic changes: 3+
Dilation of glandular duct: 3+
(Fig. 10)

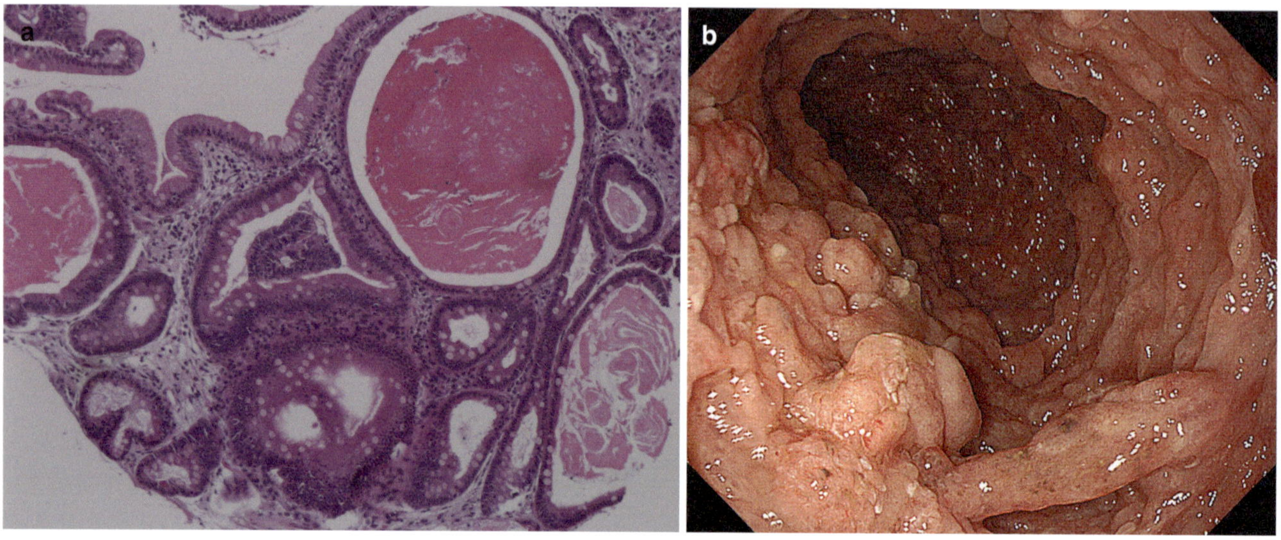

Fig. 10 Pathological image of an SMT-like elevation with remarkably edematous mucosa and white villi. The epithelium shows hyperplastic changes, and there is marked cystic dilatation of the glandular ducts in some areas. The crypts contain an eosinophilic mucus-like substance or exudate. The interstitium is mildly edematous and partially hemorrhagic, with a moderate lymphocytic and plasma cell infiltrate mixed with eosinophils and neutrophils

Pathological image of remarkably edematous changes and thickened white villi.
Interstitial edema: 3+
Inflammatory cell infiltration: 2+
Glandular duct hyperplastic changes: 2+
Dilation of glandular duct: 2+
(Fig. 11)

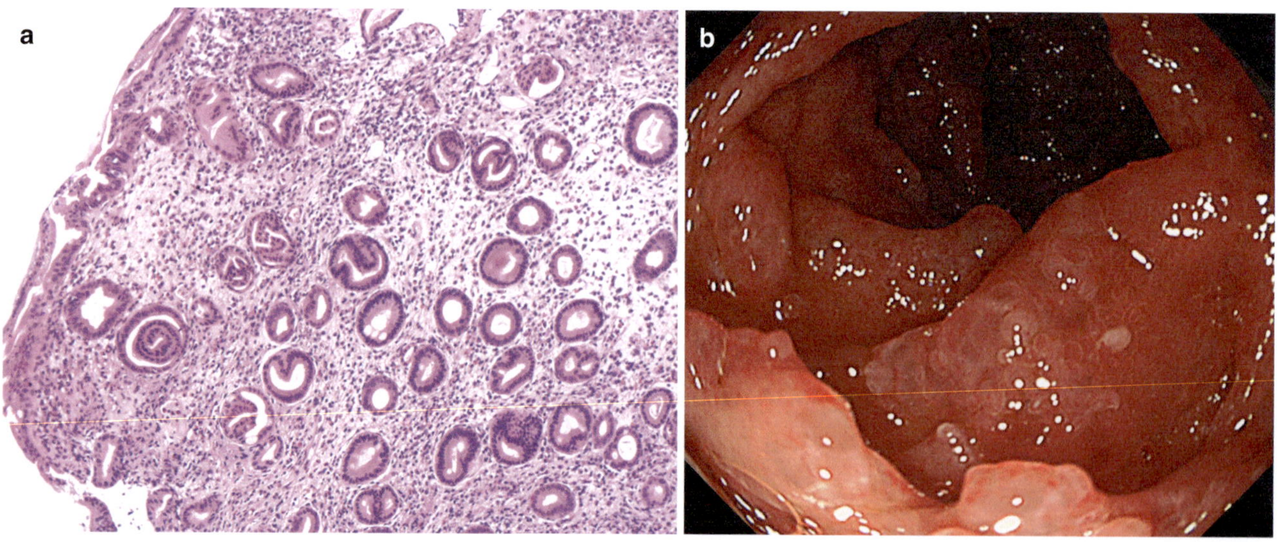

Fig. 11 Pathological image of remarkably edematous changes and thickened white villi. The hyperplastic glandular epithelium is dilated and proliferates in a tortuous fashion. The crypts are cystic, dilated, and filled with mucus. The interstitium shows a high degree of edema and inflammatory cell infiltration

4 Jejunum and Ileum

Pathological image of edematous villi with white plaque.
Interstitial edema: +
Inflammatory cell infiltration: +
Glandular duct hyperplastic change: –
Dilation of glandular ducts: –
(Fig. 12)

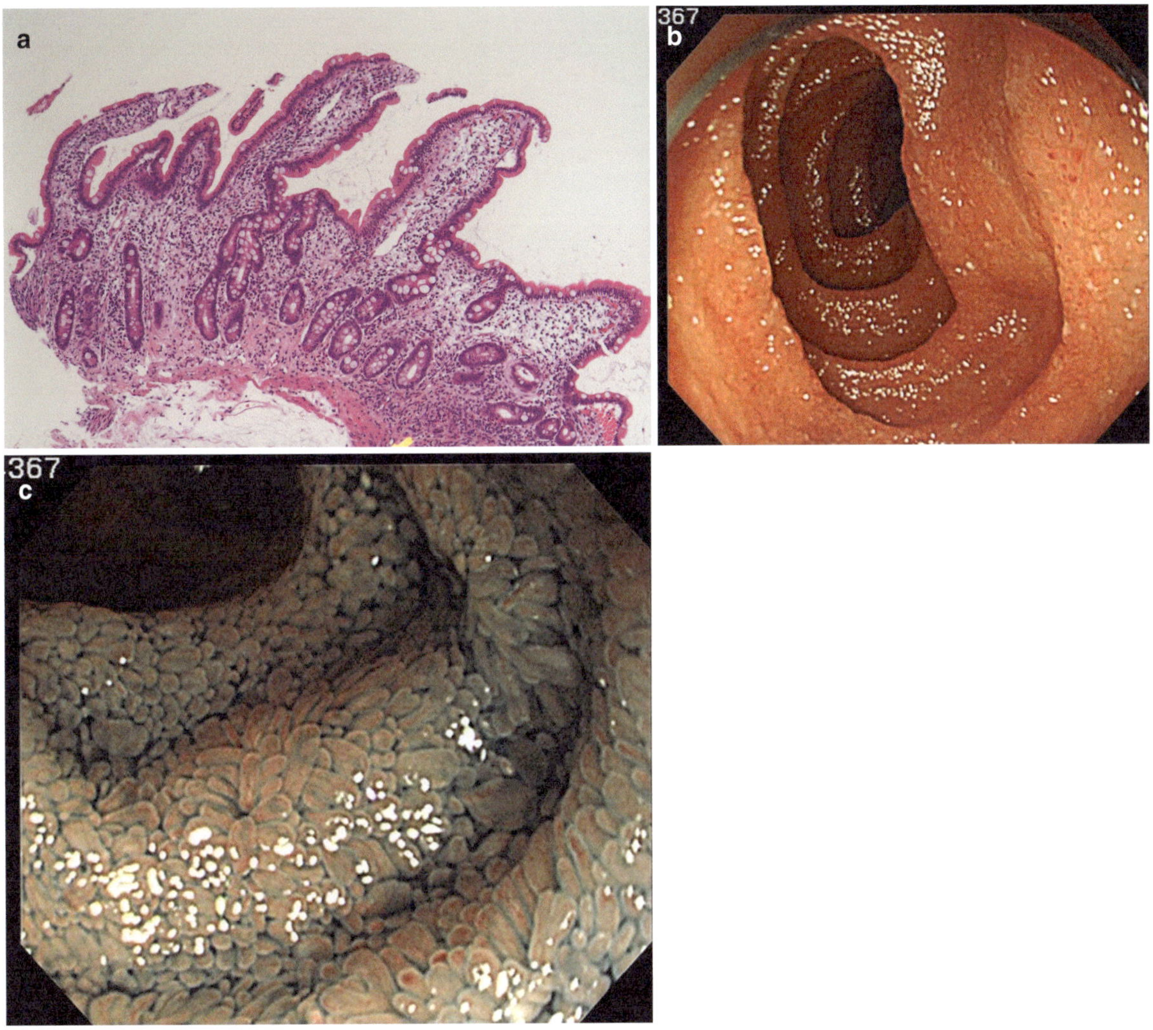

Fig. 12 Pathological image of edematous villi with white plaque. Edematous changes in the villi and mild dilation of the lymphatic vessels are observed. (**c**) Indigocarmine dyeing and close view of (**b**)

Pathological image of edematous and erythematous villi.
Interstitial edema: +
Inflammatory cell infiltration: +
Glandular duct hyperplastic change: –
Dilation of the glandular duct: +
(Fig. 13)

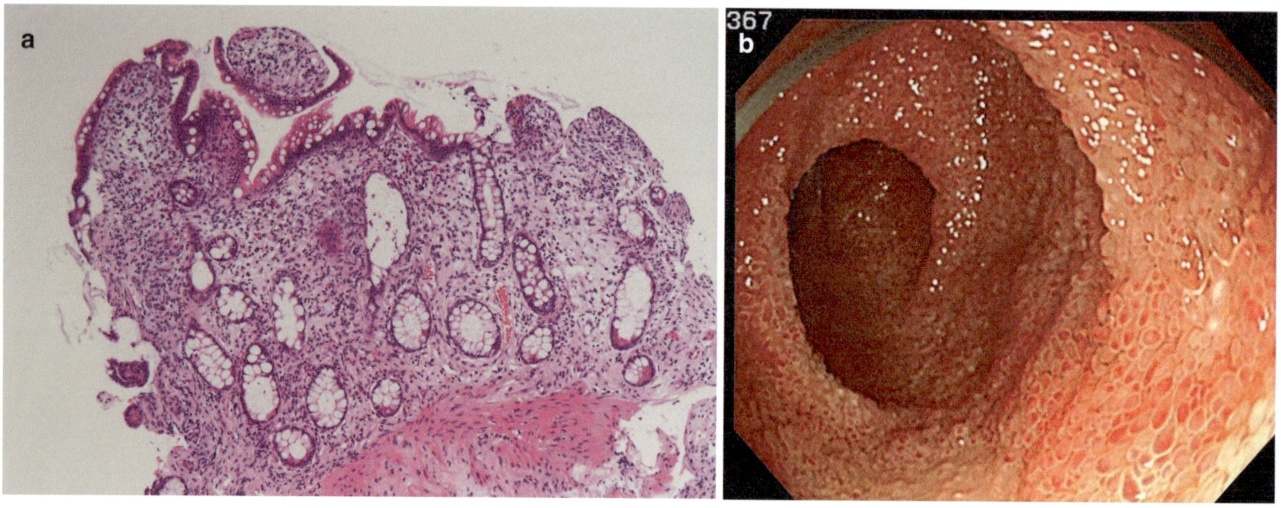

Fig. 13 Pathological image of edematous and erythematous villi. Strong edematous changes, enlargement, and hyperemia of the villi are observed

Pathological image of small polyp-like changes.
Interstitial edema: 2+
Inflammatory cell infiltration: 2+
Glandular duct hyperplastic changes: 2+
Dilation of glandular duct: 2+
(Fig. 14)

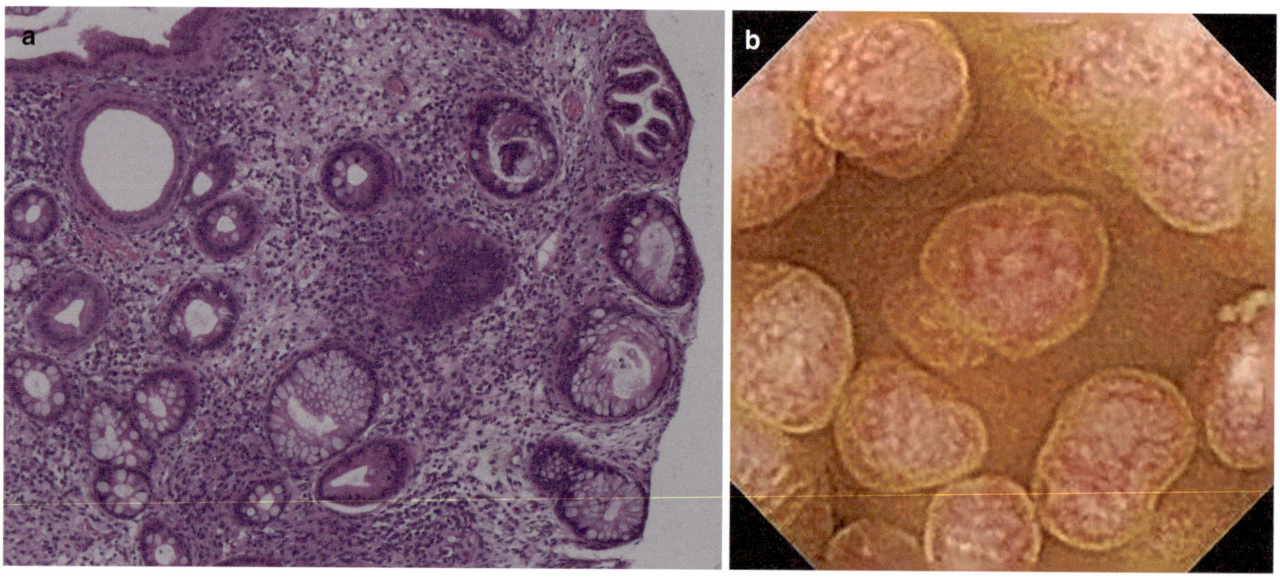

Fig. 14 Pathological image of small polyp-like changes. Regenerating, unequally sized and dilated glandular ducts with irregular branching are observed. The interstitum is edematous with moderate infiltration of eosinophils, lymphocytes, and plasma cells

Pathological image of fold thickening (Kerckring's fold).
Interstitial edema: 3+
Inflammatory cell infiltration: +
Glandular duct hyperplastic changes: 2+
Dilation of glandular duct: 2+
(Fig. 15)

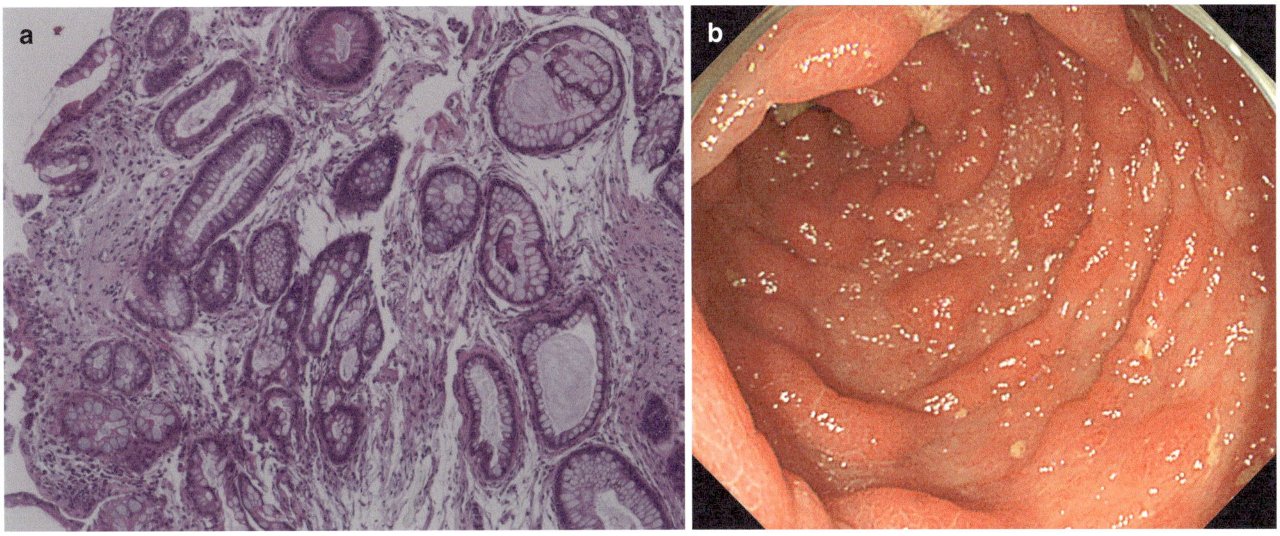

Fig. 15 Pathological image of fold thickening (Kerckring's fold). The structure of villi has disappeared overall, and serrated, bifurcated, and dilated crypts are observed in the background of edematous inflammatory interstitium

Case-Based Images: First Attack Case

Ryota Hokari, Tadakazu Hisamatsu, and Masaaki Higashiyama

1 Selection Criteria for Cases and Key Points of Image Description

After approval by the Ethics Committee, images of cases from all 35 institutions in Japan were collected and reviewed by endoscopists to select images for inclusion in this atlas. Pictures were preferentially selected from the cases with definite diagnosis and those whose therapeutic effects were comparable before and after treatments.

The case descriptions are presented in the following order: age, sex, chief complaints, clinical findings, various test results, presenting images, clinical course and treatment details. The order of presentation of the images was arranged so that the characteristics of the endoscopic images of the syndrome and the changes after treatment could be compared.

R. Hokari (✉) · M. Higashiyama
Department of Internal Medicine, National Defense Medical College, Tokorozawa, Saitama, Japan
e-mail: ryota@ndmc.ac.jp; masaakih@ndmc.ac.jp

T. Hisamatsu
Department of Gastroenterology and Hepatology, Kyorin University School of Medicine, Mitaka, Tokyo, Japan

R. Hokari, T. Hisamatsu (eds.), *Atlas of Cronkhite-Canada Syndrome*, https://doi.org/10.1007/978-981-19-0652-7_6

2 Case-Based Images: First Attack Case

2.1 Endoscopic Remission Cases

Case 1: A typical case who responded markedly to corticosteroids and achieved steroid-free endoscopic remission

Provided by Makoto Ooi and Yuzo Kodama

[Patient]

A 56-year-old woman. Chief complaints (CC): Lower extremity edema, dysgeusia, alopecia, nausea, hyperpigmentation of hands.

[Clinical findings]

Alopecia (+), onychodystrophy (+), hyperpigmentation (+), dysgeusia (+), defecation: 5 times/day, mild edema.

[Laboratory findings]

Alb 3.1 mg/dL, CRP 0.23 mg/dL, Hb 16.0 g/dL.

[Endoscopic images 1] (Fig. 1a–f)

[Clinical course]

First attack type.

Initial treatment: PSL 40 mg for 2 weeks.

Clinical response: 1 week.

Clinical remission: 8 weeks.

Maintenance dose: PSL 0 mg.

[Endoscopic images 2] (Fig. 2a–d)

EGD and CS during remission.

In all lesions, the inflamed mucosa improved and the polyps almost disappeared with only a few residual scattered polyps.

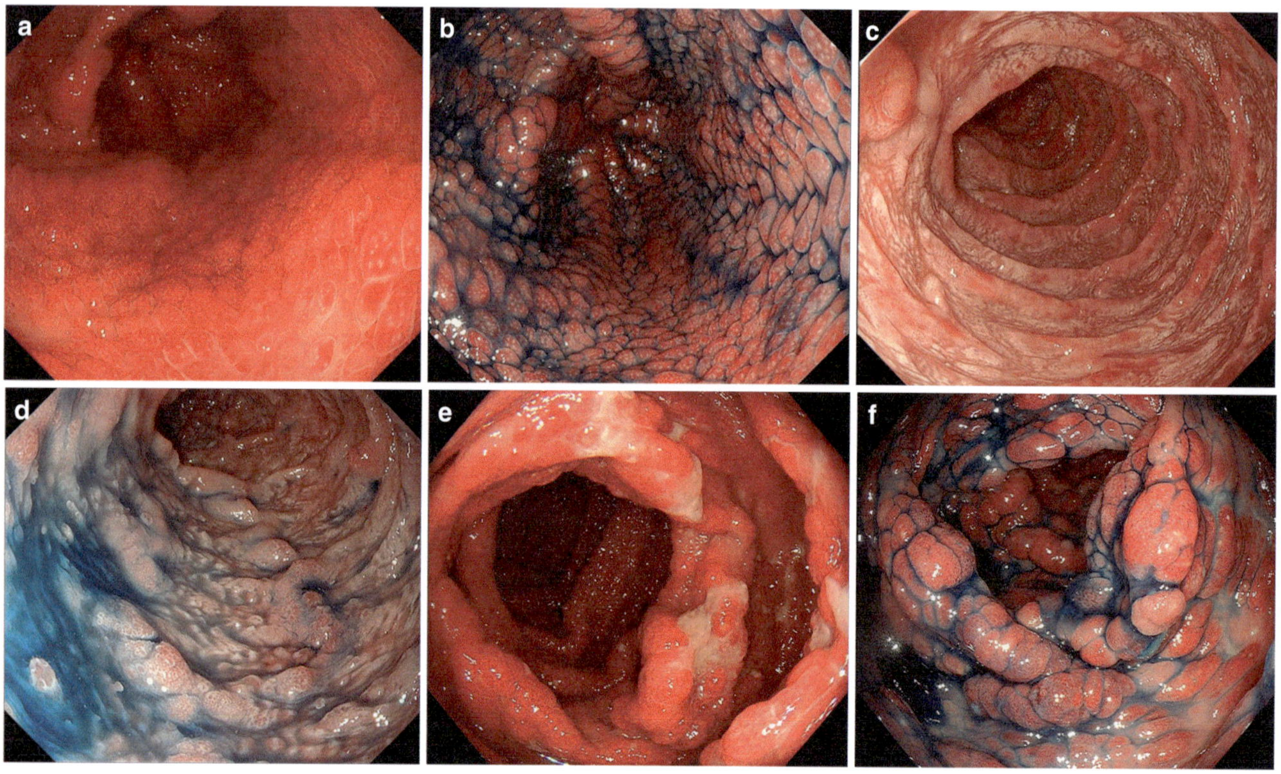

Fig. 1 (**a**), (**b**) Stomach: Confluent type. Small, edematous, and erythematous polyps. Defined edematous intervening mucosa. (**c**), (**d**) Duodenum: Confluent type. Small, edematous polyps with white villi. (**e**), (**f**) Colon: Confluent type. Medium, edematous, erythematous, and whitish mucus adhered polyps. (**b**), (**d**), (**f**) Indigocarmine dyeing of (**a**), (**c**), (**e**), respectively

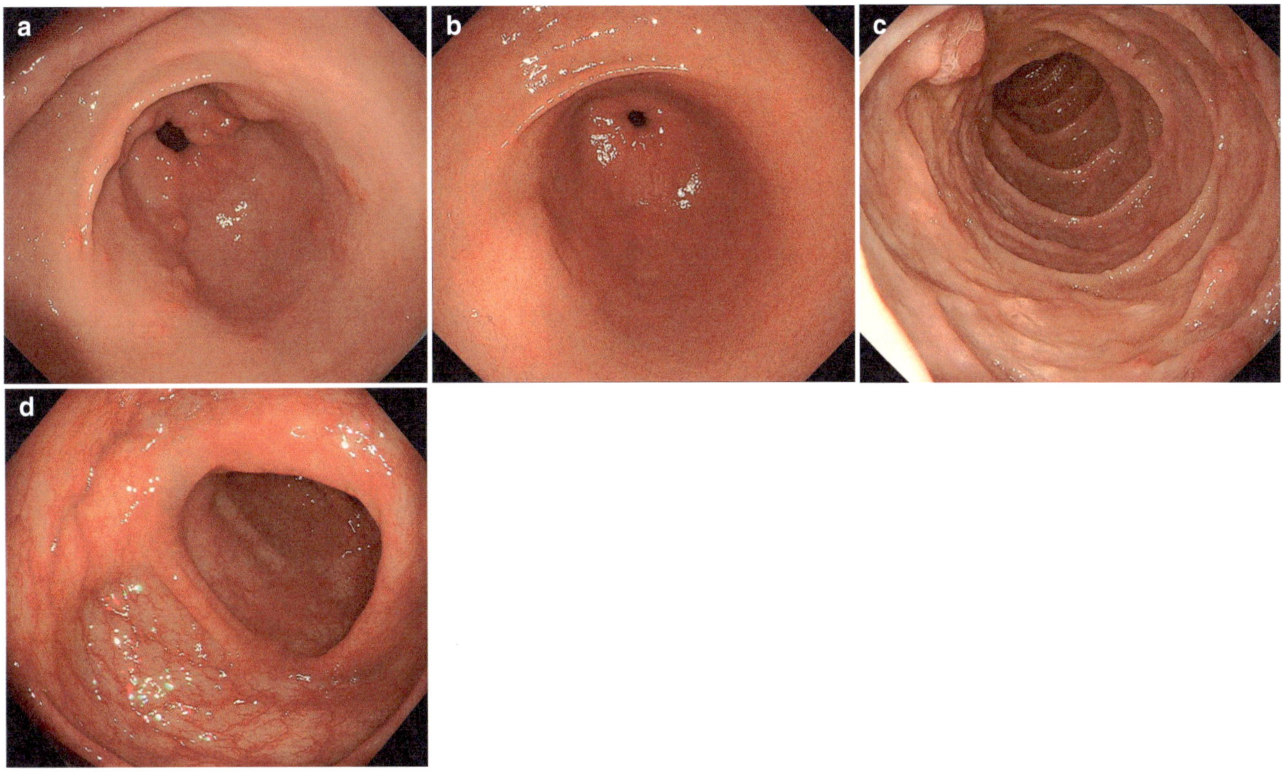

Fig. 2 (**a**) Stomach (9 months after the diagnosis). (**b**) Stomach (4 years after the diagnosis). (**c**) Duodenum (9 months after the diagnosis). (**d**) Colon (11 months after the diagnosis)

Case 2: A typical case who responded markedly to corticosteroids and achieved steroid-free endoscopic remission

Provided by Mari Hayashida

[Patient]

A 70-year-old male. CC: Anorexia, dysgeusia, diarrhea.

[Clinical findings]

Alopecia (+), onychodystrophy (+), hyperpigmentation (+), dysgeusia (+), defecation: 8 times/day

[Laboratory findings]

Alb 3.2 mg/dL, CRP 7.4 mg/dL, Hb 15.8 g/dL.

99mTc-human serum albumin scintigraphy: Abnormal leakage from the ileum and splenic flexure of the colon.

Fecal alpha-antitrypsin clearance: 88.9 mL/day.

[Endoscopic images 1] (Fig. 3a–e)

[Clinical course]

First attack type.

Initial treatment: PSL 40 mg for 2 weeks.

Clinical response: 1 week.

Clinical remission: 3 weeks.

Maintenance dose: PSL 0 mg.

[Endoscopic images 2] (Fig. 4a–d)

EGD (1 year after the diagnosis) and CS (3 years after the diagnosis) during remission.

In all the lesions, the endoscopic findings improved to remission.

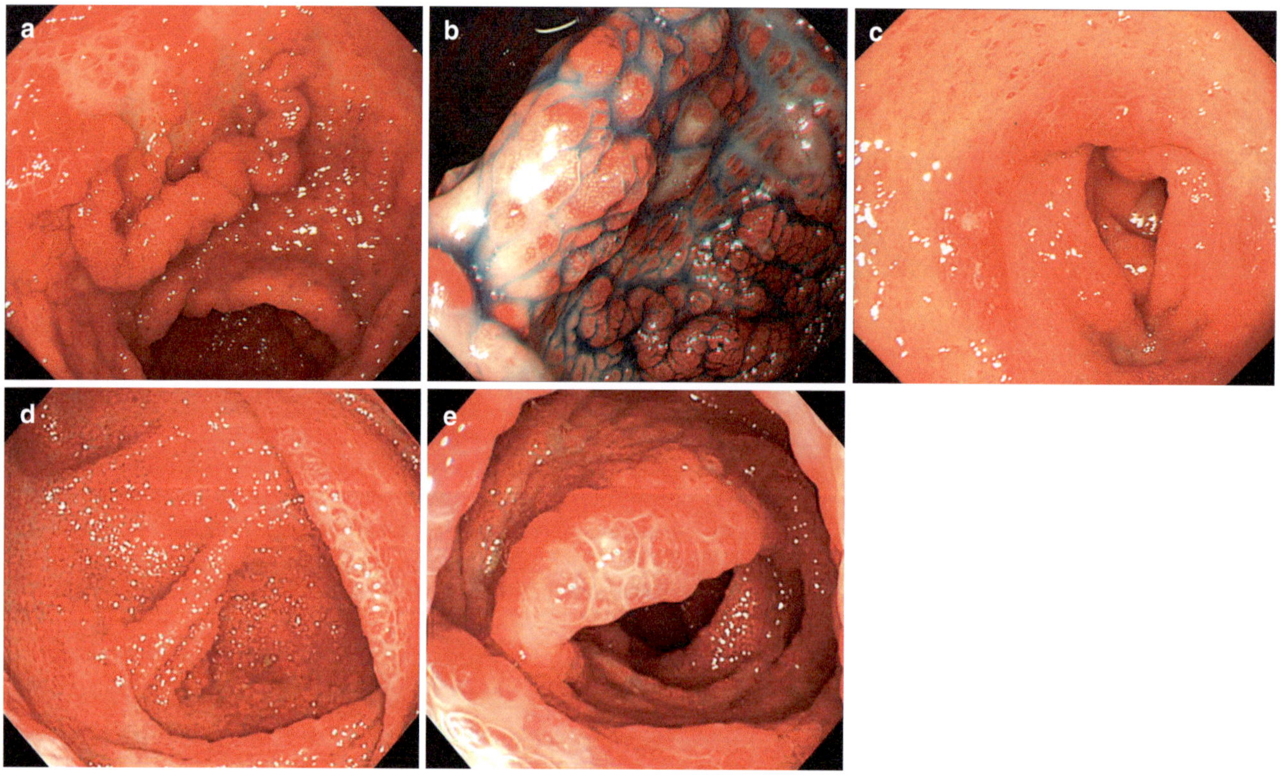

Fig. 3 (**a**) Stomach: Confluent type. Small, edematous, erythematous, and whitish mucus adhered. (**b**) Indigocarmine dyeing of (**a**). (**c**) Duodenum: Fold thickening type with edematous and erythematous mucosa with unclear villi. (**d**), (**e**) Colon: Confluent type. Small to medium, edematous, and erythematous polyps

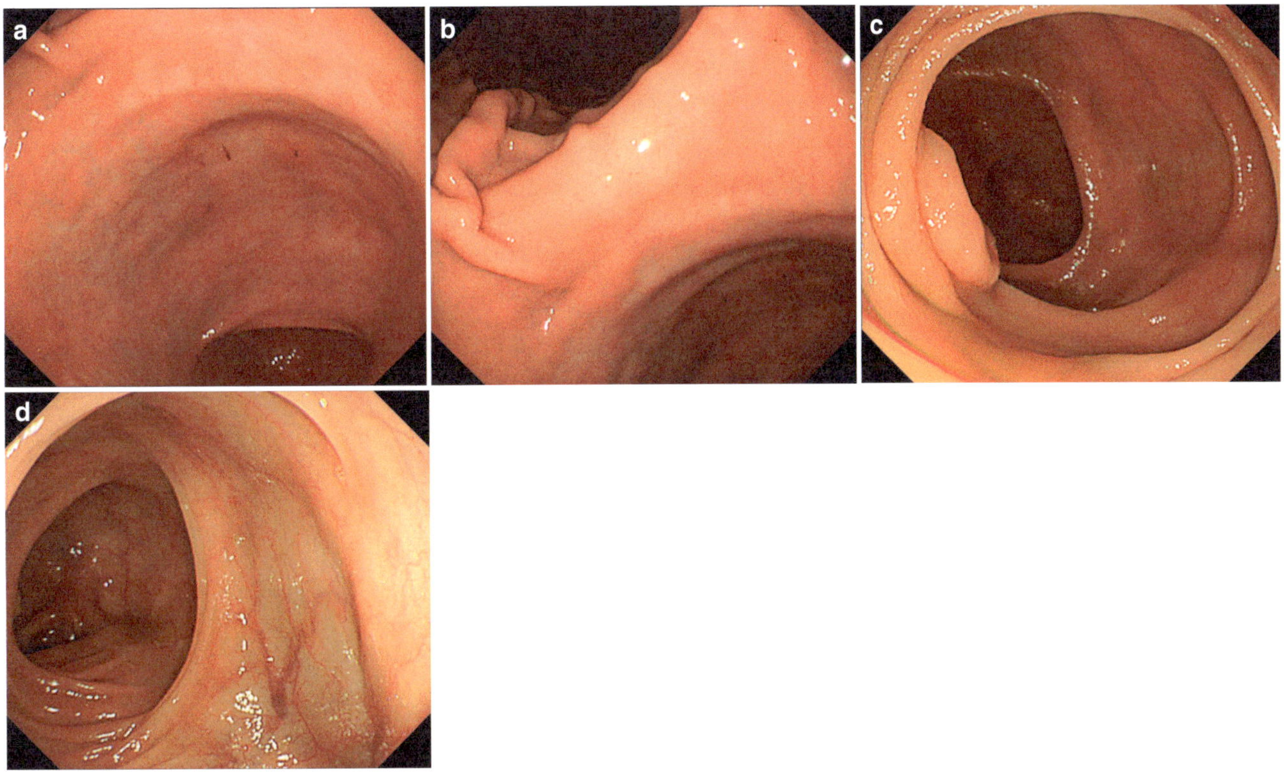

Fig. 4 (**a**), (**b**) Stomach. (**c**), (**d**) Colon

Case 3: A typical case who responded markedly to corticosteroids and achieved steroid-free endoscopic remission

Provided by Masakazu Nagahori

[Patient]

A 44-year-old female. CC: Epigastralgia, diarrhea, dysgeusia, alopecia, and cutaneous manifestation.

[Clinical findings]

Alopecia (+), onychodystrophy (+), hyperpigmentation (+), dysgeusia (+), defecation: 10 times/day, mild edema.

[Laboratory findings]

Alb 2.4 mg/dL, CRP 0.06 mg/dL, Hb 14.2 g/dL.

[Endoscopic images 1] (Fig. 5a–d)

[Clinical course]

First attack type.

Initial treatment: PSL 30 mg for 4 weeks.

Clinical response: 4 weeks.

Clinical remission: 24 weeks.

Maintenance dose: PSL 0 mg.

[Endoscopic images 2] (Fig. 6)

EGD 1 year after the diagnosis.

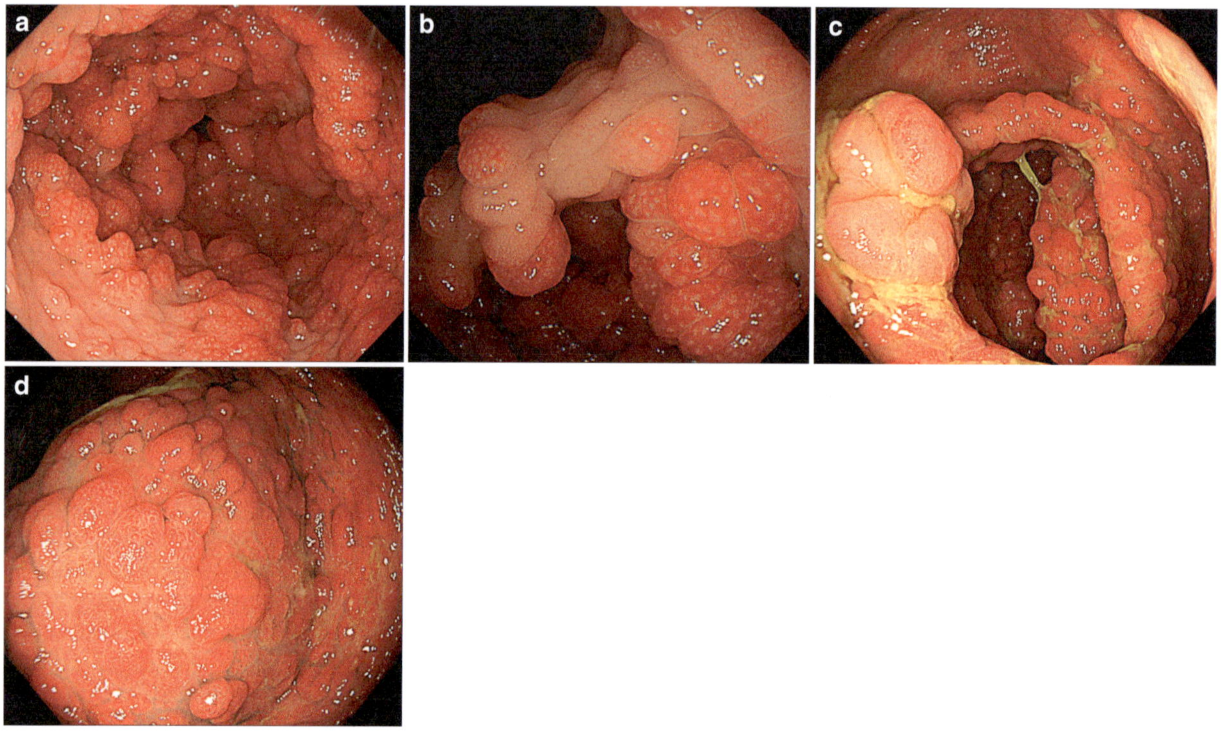

Fig. 5 (**a**), (**b**) Stomach: Confluent type. Large, edematous, and erythematous polyps. (**c**), (**d**) Colon: Confluent type. Small to medium, edematous, erythematous, and erosive polyps

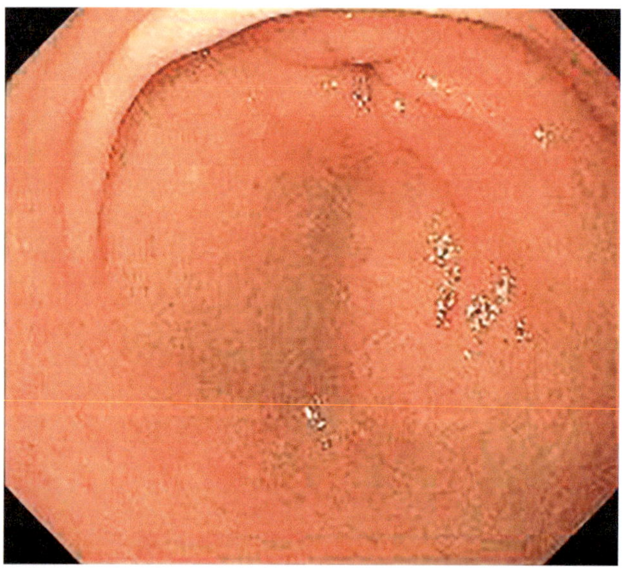

Fig. 6 The polyps and inflammatory findings in the gastric antrum disappeared

Case 4: A typical case who responded markedly to corticosteroids and achieved steroid-free endoscopic remission

Provided by Kazuki Kakimoto and Kazuhide Higuchi

[Patient]

61 years old. CC: Diarrhea, abdominal pain, bloody stool.

[Clinical findings]

Alopecia (+), onychodystrophy (+), hyperpigmentation (+), dysgeusia (+), defecation: 15 times/day

[Laboratory findings]

TP 5.8 mg/dL, Alb 3.4 mg/dL, CRP 1.83 mg/dL, Hb 14.6 g/dL.

[Clinical course]

First attack type.

Initial treatment: PSL 40 mg for 1 week

Clinical response: 1 week.

Endoscopic response: 0.5 months.

Endoscopic remission: 20 months.

Maintenance dose: PSL 0 mg.

[Endoscopic images 1] (Fig. 7a–e)

[Endoscopic images 2] (Fig. 8a–e)

EGD and CS 1 year after the diagnosis.

In all lesions, the polyps disappeared.

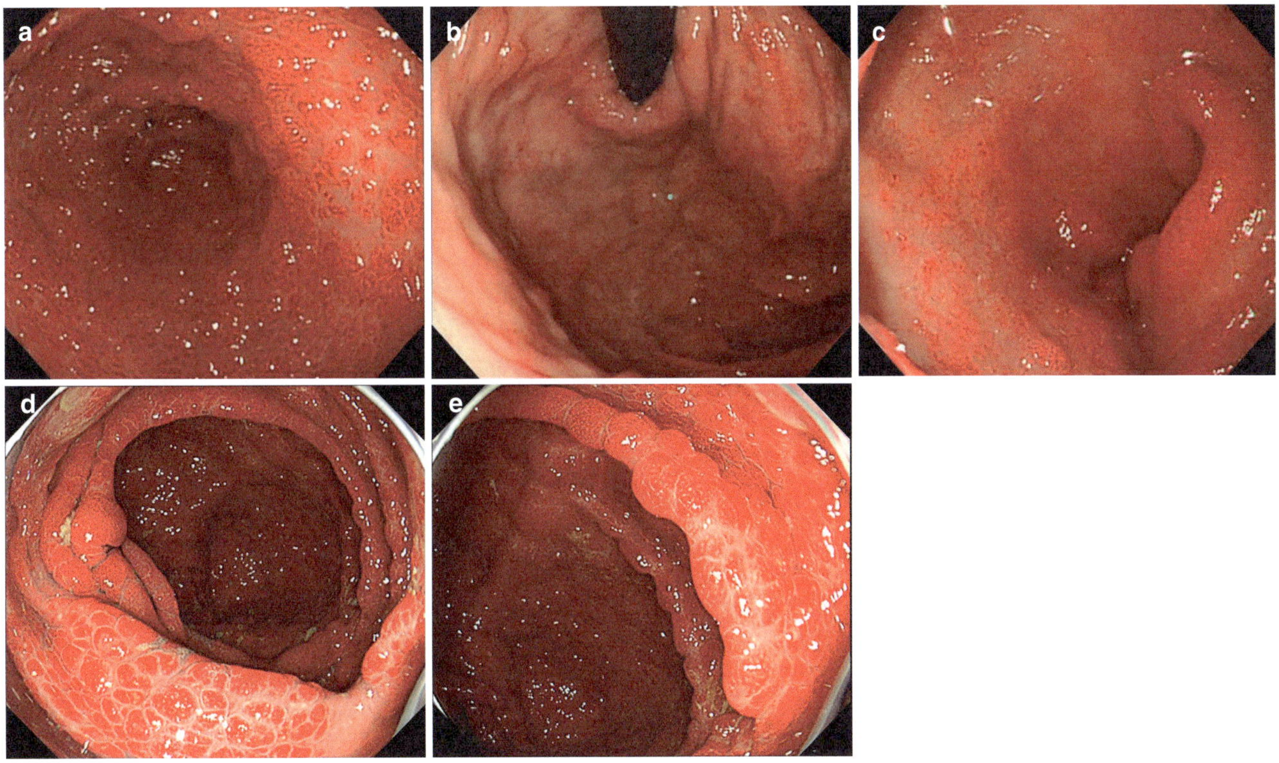

Fig. 7 (**a**) Gastric antrum: Confluent type. Small, erythematous polyps. (**b**) Gastric cardia: Edematous mucosa without polyps. (**c**) Duodenal bulb: Sparse type. Small, erythematous polyps. (**d**) Cecum: Confluent type. Small, erythematous polyps. (**e**) Ascending colon: Confluent type. Small, erythematous polyps

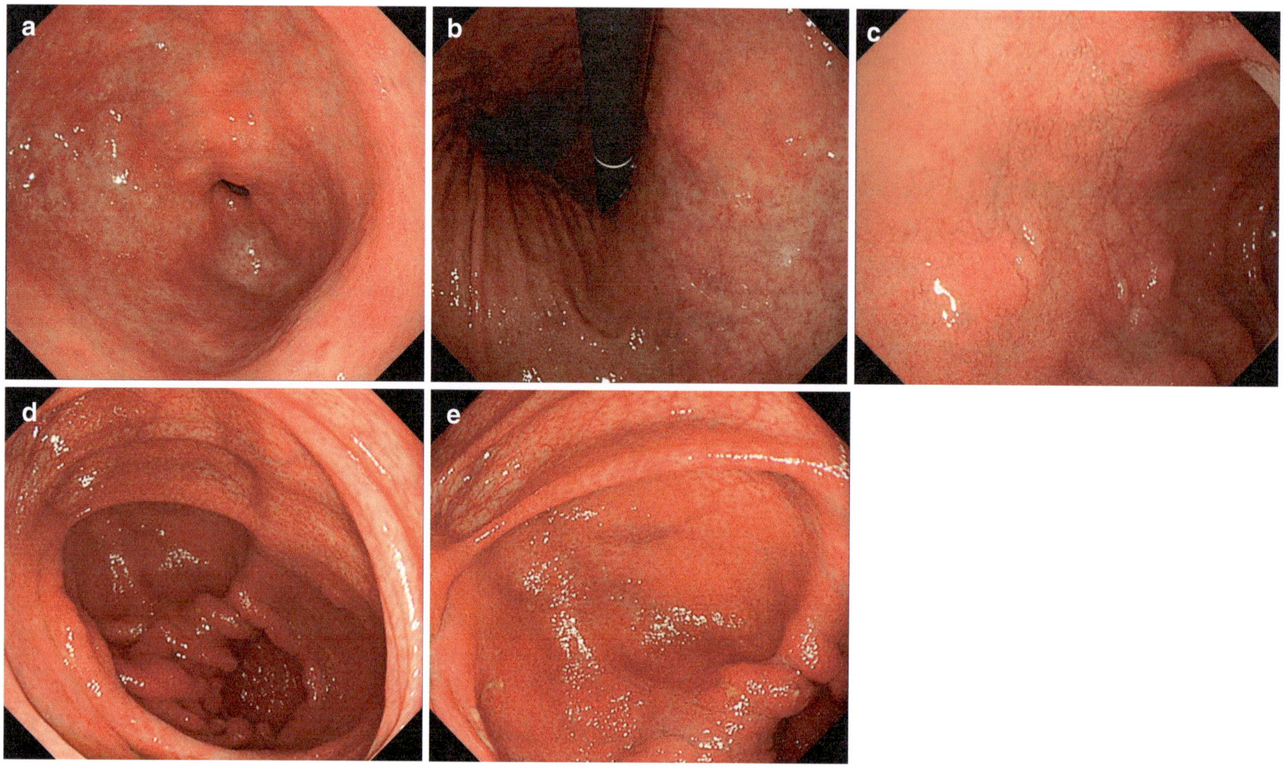

Fig. 8 (**a**) Gastric antrum. (**b**) Gastric body. (**c**) Duodenal bulb. (**d**) Cecum. (**e**) Ascending colon

Case 5: A typical case who responded markedly to corticosteroids and achieved steroid-free endoscopic remission

Provided by Shunji Ishihara

[Patient]

A 69-year-old male. CC: Dysgeusia, diarrhea.

[Clinical findings]

Alopecia (+), onychodystrophy (+), hyperpigmentation (−), dysgeusia (+), defecation: 5 times/day, mild edema.

[Laboratory findings]

Alb 3.4 mg/dL, CRP 0.79 mg/dL, Hb 12.3 g/dL.

[Cutaneous manifestations and endoscopic images 1] (Fig. 9a–d)

[Clinical course]

First attack type.

Initial treatment: PSL 40 mg for 1 week.

Clinical response: 1 week.

Clinical remission: 1 week.

Maintenance dose: 0 mg.

[Cutaneous manifestations and endoscopic images 2] (Fig. 10a–d)

Post-treatment.

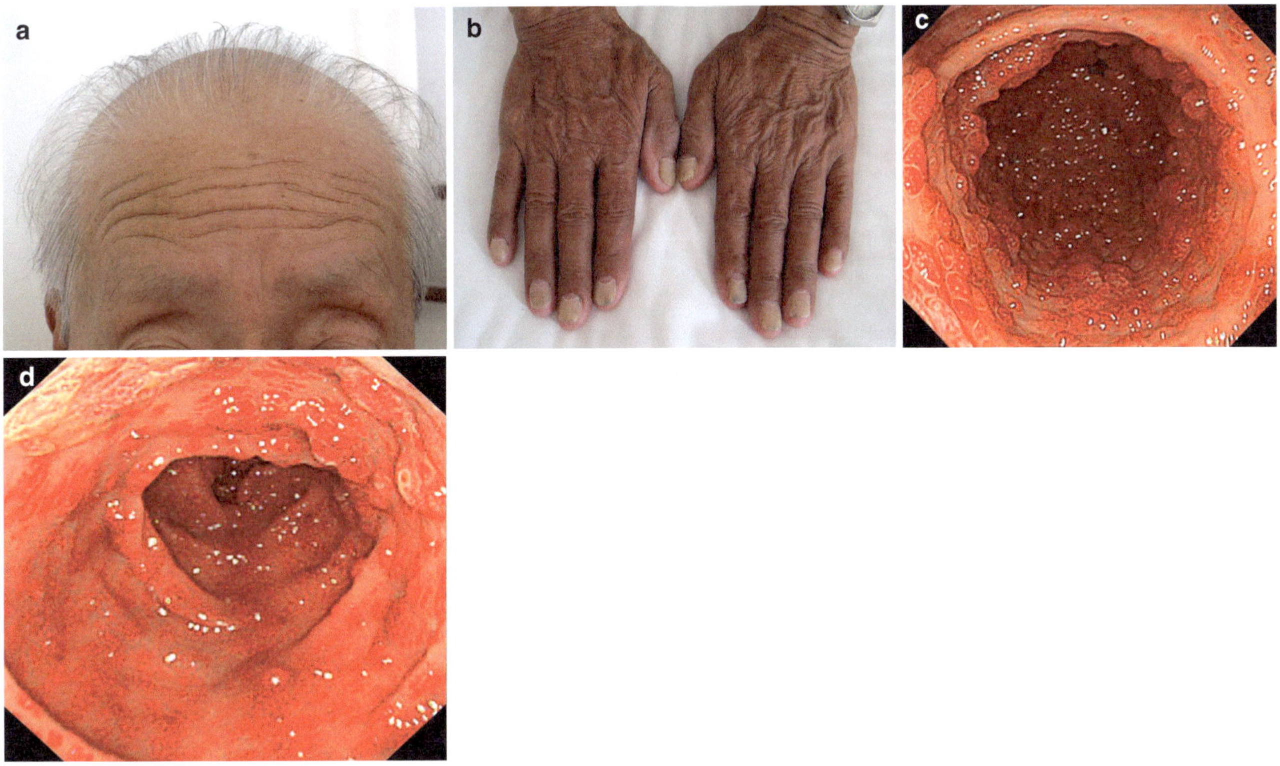

Fig. 9 (**a**) Head: Alopecia. (**b**) Fingers: Onychodystrophy. (**c**) Stomach: Confluent type. Medium, erythematous polyps. Edematous intervening mucosa. (**d**) Colon: Semi-confluent type. Medium, erythematous polyps

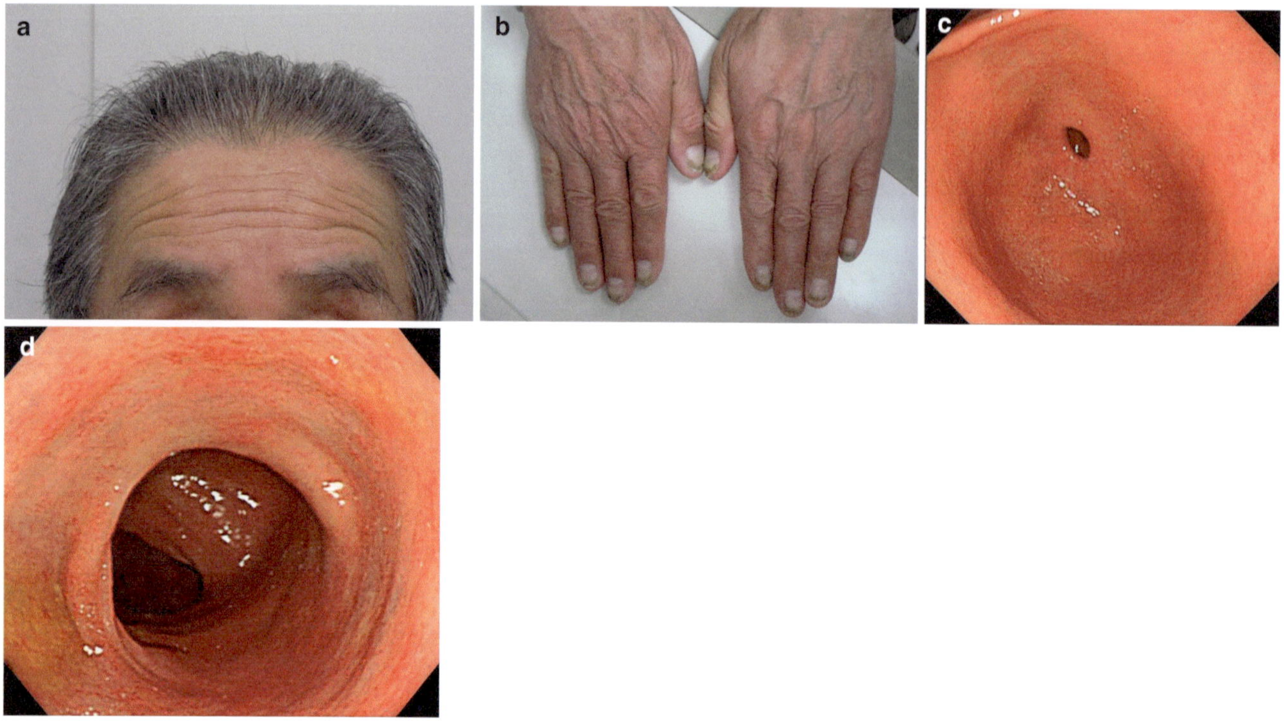

Fig. 10 (**a**) Head. (**b**) Fingers. (**c**) Stomach. (**d**) Descending colon

2.2 Clinical Remission Cases

Case 6: A typical case except poor cutaneous manifestations, who responded markedly to corticosteroids and achieved clinical remission maintained by PSL 1 mg

Provided by Takehiro Torisu and Junji Umeno

[Patient]

A 76-year-old man. CC: Onychodystrophy, dysgeusia, weight loss (−5 kg/year).

[Clinical findings]

Alopecia (−), onychodystrophy (+), hyperpigmentation (−), defecation: 10 times/day

[Laboratory findings]

Alb 4.0 mg/dL, CRP 0.58 mg/dL, Hb 14.6 g/dL.

[Endoscopic images] (Fig. 11)

[Clinical course]

First attack type.

Initial treatment: PSL 30 mg for 2 weeks.

Clinical response: 8 weeks.

Clinical remission: 12 weeks.

Maintenance dose: PSL 5 mg.

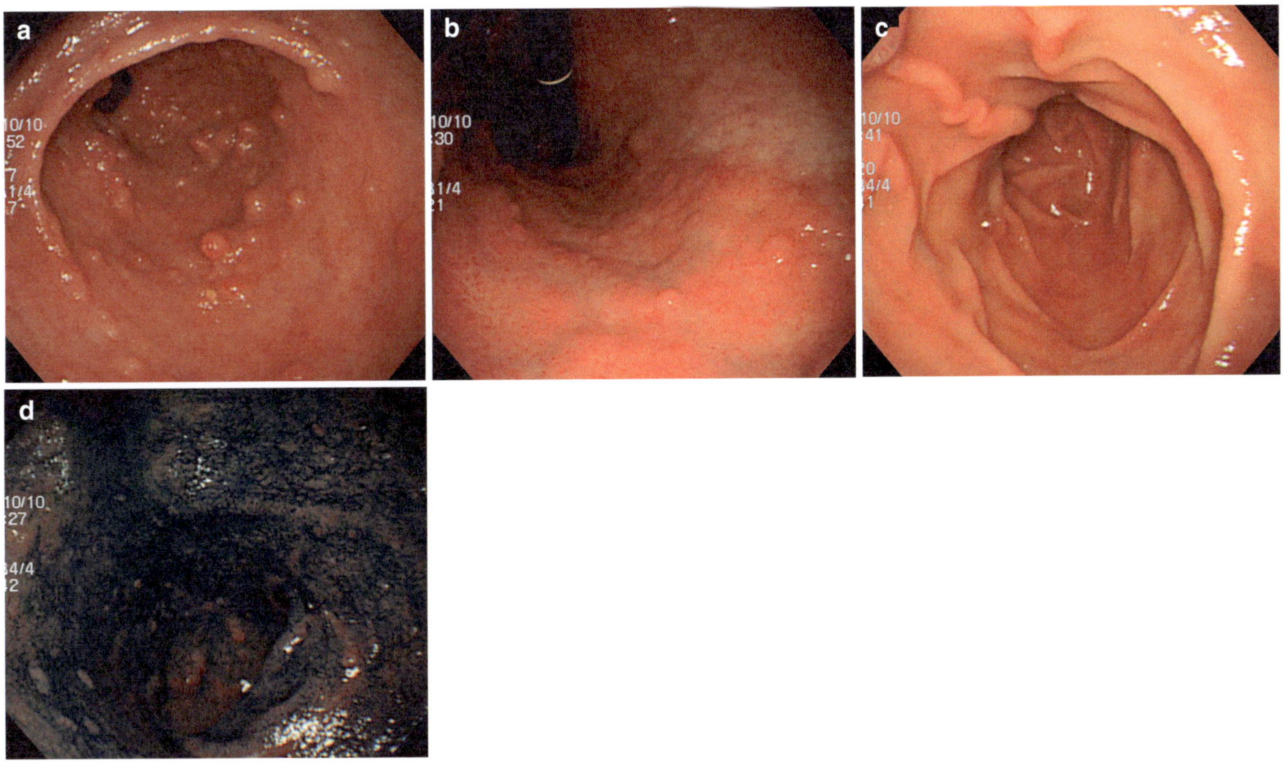

Fig. 11 (**a**), (**b**) Stomach: Semi-confluent type. Medium, edematous polyps. (**c**) Duodenum: Sparse type. Small polyps. (**d**) Indigocarmine dyeing of (**c**)

Case 7: A typical case except poor cutaneous manifestations, who responded markedly to corticosteroids and achieved clinical remission maintained by PSL 1 mg

Provided by Takehiro Torisu and Junji Umeno

[Patient]

A 55-year-old man. CC: Onychodystrophy, diarrhea.

[Clinical findings]

Alopecia (−), onychodystrophy (+), hyperpigmentation (−), defecation: 10 times/day, mild edema.

[Laboratory findings]

Alb 1.8 mg/dL, CRP 0.11 mg/dL, Hb 12.0 g/dL.

[Endoscopic images] (Fig. 12)

[Clinical course]

First attack type.

Initial treatment: PSL 50 mg for 2 weeks.

Clinical response: 2 weeks.

Clinical remission: 12 weeks.

Maintenance dose: PSL 5 mg

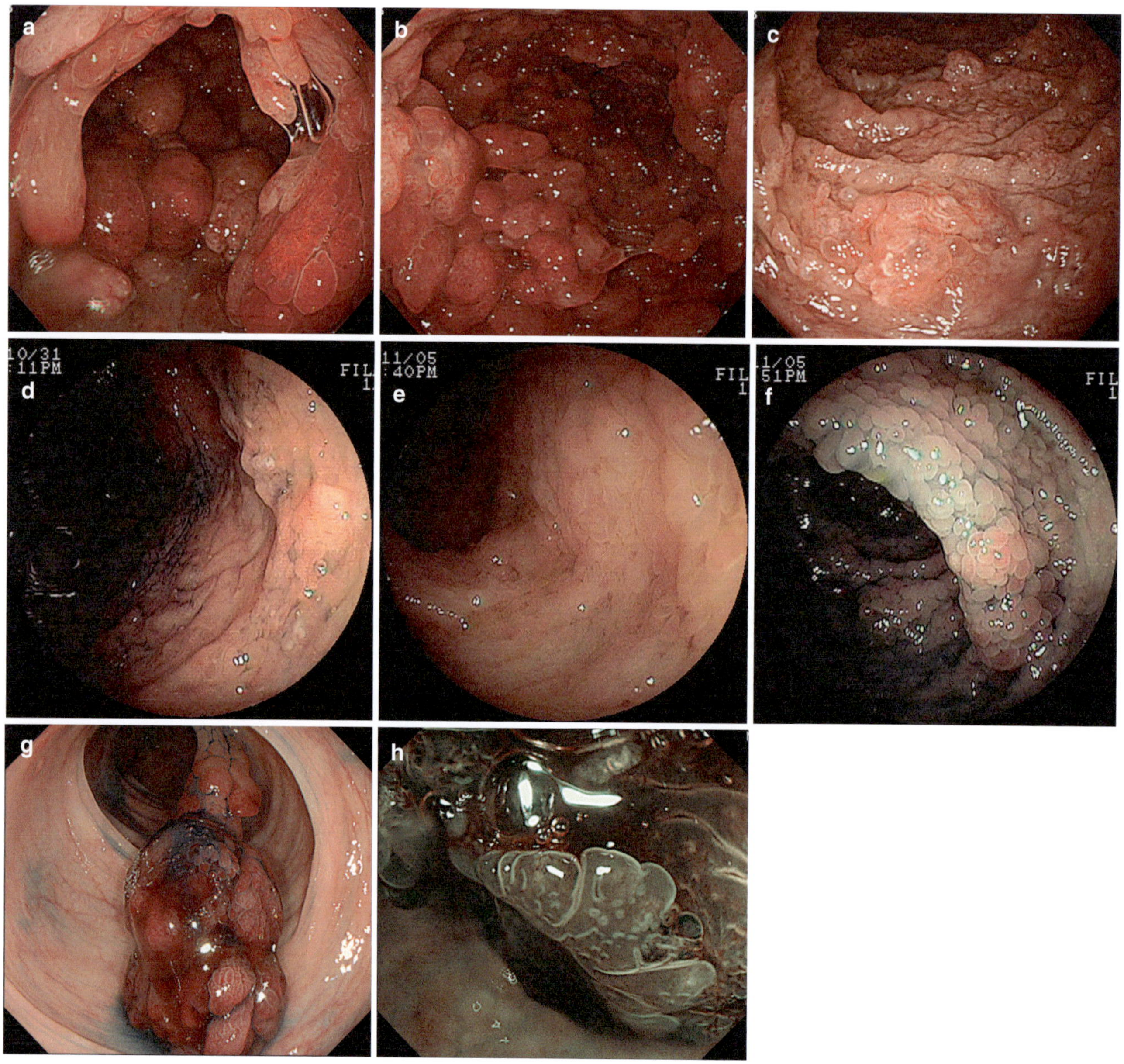

Fig. 12 (**a**), (**b**) Stomach: Confluent type. Medium, edematous, and whitish mucus adhered polyps. (**c**) Duodenum: Confluent type. Small, edematous polyps. (**d**) Jejunum (BAE): Fold thickening type with white villi. (**e**) Ileum (BAE): Fold thickening type with swollen villi. (**f**) Indigocarmine dyeing of (**e**). (**g**) Colon: Sparse type. Large, edematous, and hemorrhagic polyps. (**h**) Magnified NBI observation of (**g**)

Case 8: A typical case who responded markedly to corticosteroids and achieved clinical remission maintained by PSL 5 mg

Provided by Takehiro Torisu and Junji Umeno

[Patient]

A 72-year-old man. CC: Diarrhea

[Clinical findings]

Alopecia (+), onychodystrophy (+), hyperpigmentation (+), defecation: 10 times/day

[Laboratory findings]

Alb 2.9 mg/dL, CRP 0.55 mg/dL, Hb 14.3 g/dL.

[Cutaneous manifestations and endoscopic images] (Fig. 13)

[Clinical course]

First attack type.

Initial treatment: PSL 50 mg for less than 1 week.

Clinical response: 1 week.

Clinical remission: 4 weeks.

Maintenance dose: PSL 5 mg.

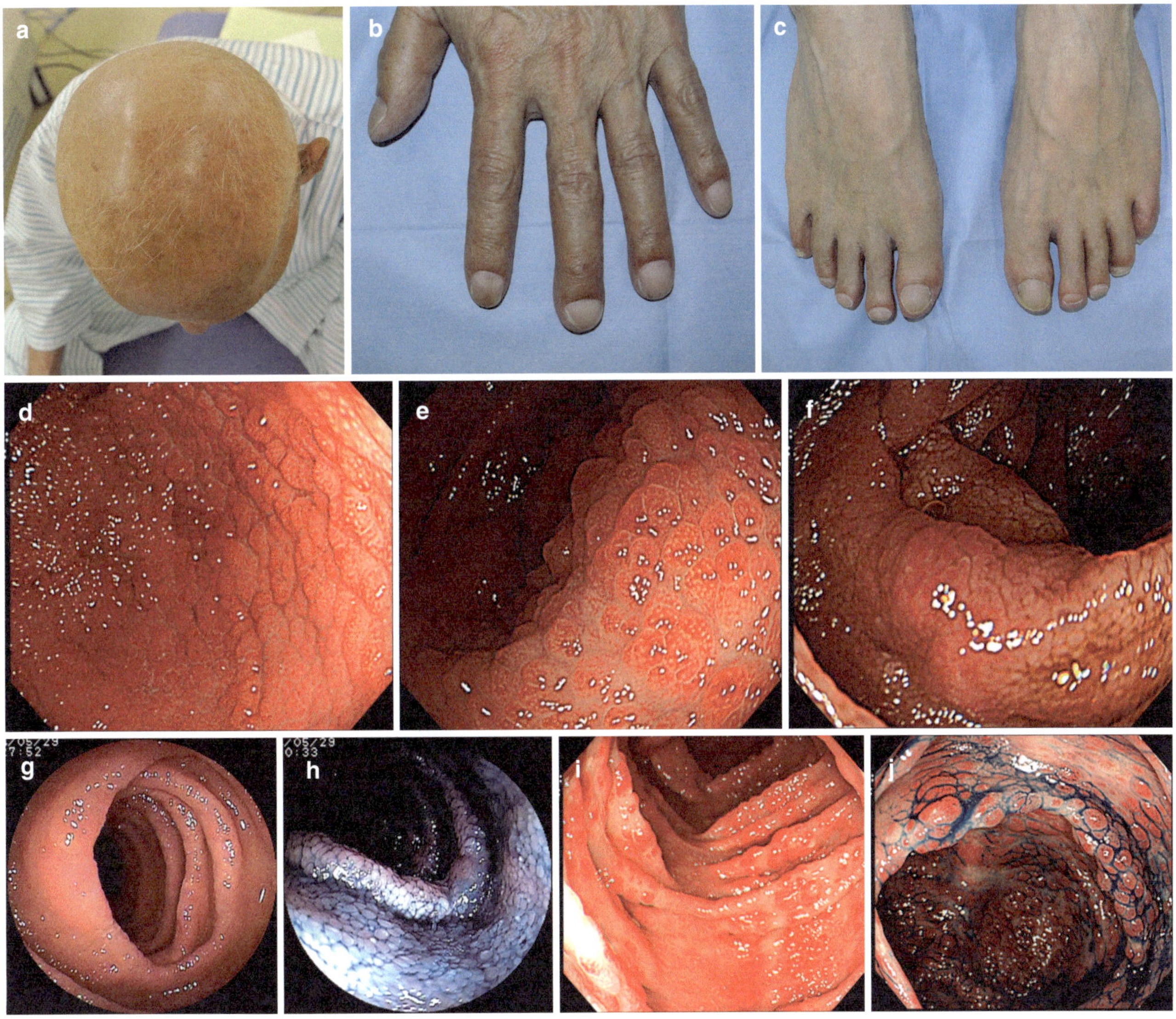

Fig. 13 (**a**) Head: Alopecia. (**b**) Hand: Onychodystrophy and hyperpigmentation. (**c**) Feet: Onychodystrophy. (**d**), (**e**) Stomach: Confluent type. Small, edematous, and erythematous polyps. (**f**) Duodenum: Fold thickening type. (**g**) Jejunum: Fold thickening type. (**h**) Indigocarmine dyeing of (**g**). (**i**), (**j**) Colon: Confluent type. Small, edematous, and hemorrhagic polyps. Indigocarmine dyeing in (**j**)

Case 9: A typical case who responded markedly to corticosteroids and achieved clinical remission maintained by PSL 1 mg

Provided by Takehiro Torisu and Junji Umeno

[Patient]

A 56-year-old male. CC: Diarrhea, dysgeusia, and alopecia appearing about 1 month after the common cold symptoms.

[Clinical findings]

Alopecia (+), onychodystrophy (+), hyperpigmentation (+), dysgeusia (+), defecation: 7 times/day.

[Laboratory findings]

Alb 3.3 mg/dL, CRP 0.13 mg/dL, Hb 14.0 g/dL.

Fecal alpha1 antitrypsin clearance: 2 mL/day

[Endoscopic images] (Fig. 14)

[Clinical course]

First attack type.

Initial treatment: PSL 30 mg for 2 weeks.

Clinical response: 2 weeks.

Clinical remission: 8 weeks.

Maintenance dose: PSL 1 mg

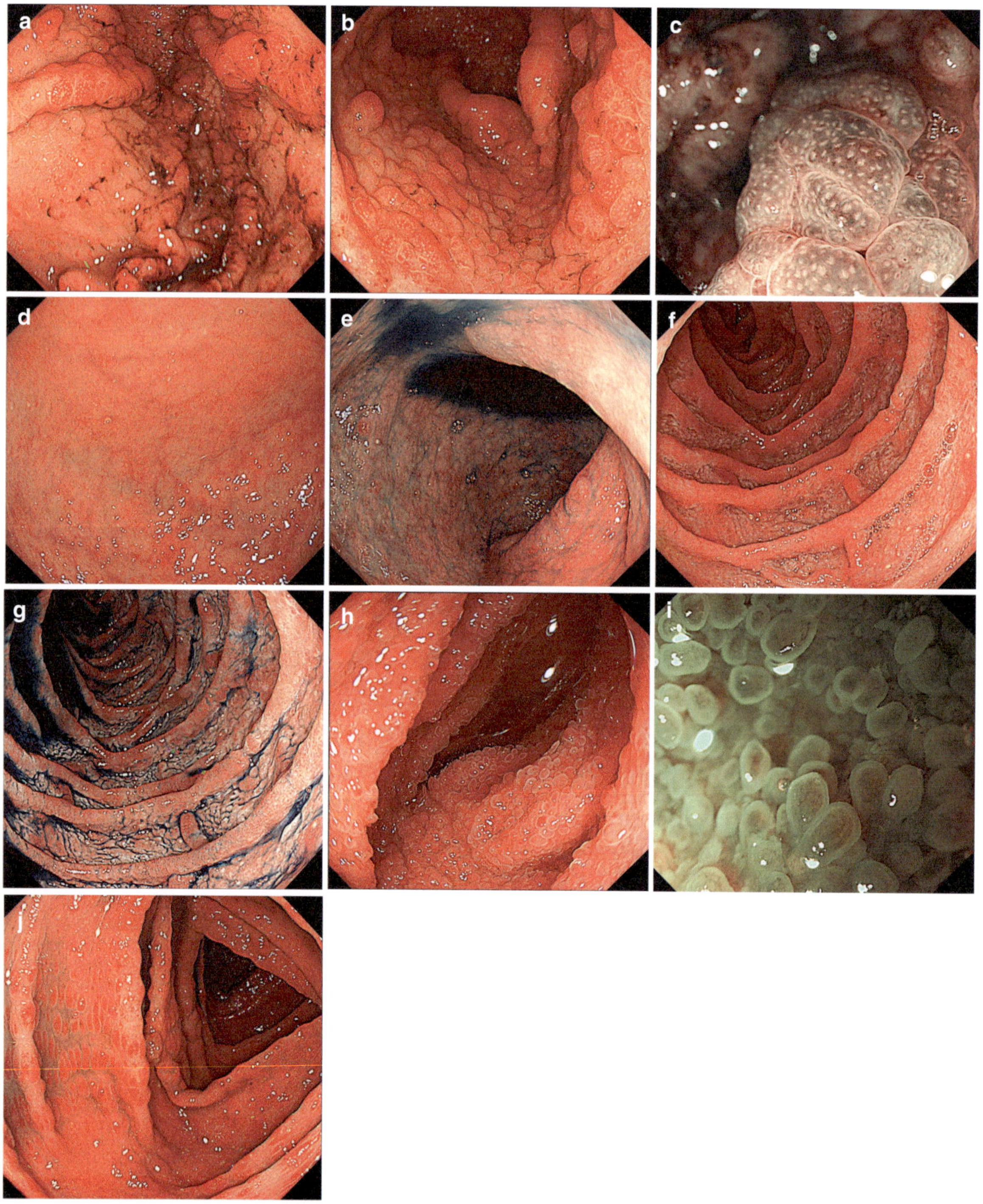

Fig. 14 (**a**), (**b**) Stomach: Confluent type. Small, edematous, and hemorrhagic polyps. (**c**) Indigocarmine dyeing of (**b**). (**d**), (**f**) Duodenum: Fold thickening type with white villi. (**e**), (**g**) Indigocarmine dyeing of (**d**), (**f**), respectively. (**h**) Ileum: Diffusely swollen villi. (**i**) Magnified NBI observation of (**h**). (**j**) Colon: Semi-confluent type. Small, edematous, and erythematous polyps

Case 10: A mostly typical case who responded markedly to corticosteroids and achieved steroid-free clinical remission

Provided by Yuji Naito and Ken Inoue

[Patient]

A 58-year-old female. CC: Alopecia, hyperpigmentation.

[Clinical findings]

Alopecia (+), onychodystrophy (+), hyperpigmentation (−), dysgeusia (+), defecation: 5 times/day, mild edema.

[Laboratory findings]

Alb 3.4 mg/dL, CRP 0.79 mg/dL, Hb 12.3 g/dL.

[Endoscopic images] (Fig. 15)

[Clinical course]

First attack type.

Initial treatment: PSL 40 mg for 1 week.

Clinical response: 1 week.

Clinical remission: 1 week.

Maintenance dose: PSL 0 mg.

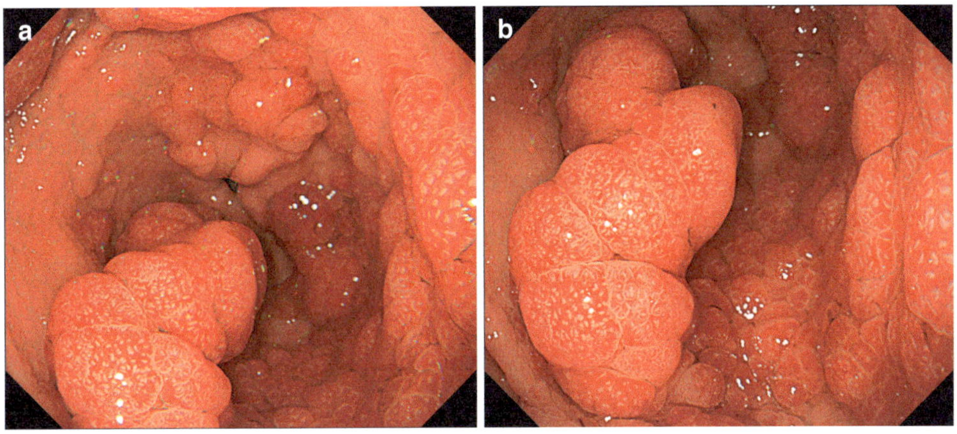

Fig. 15 (**a**), (**b**) Stomach: Semi-confluent type. Medium, erythematous polyps. Edematous intervening mucosa

Case 11: A typical case except poor cutaneous manifestations, who responded markedly to corticosteroids and achieved steroid-free clinical remission

Provided by Yuji Naito and Ken Inoue

[Patient]

A 74-year-old man. CC: Dysgeusia, diarrhea.

[Clinical findings]

Alopecia (+), onychodystrophy (+), hyperpigmentation (+), dysgeusia (+), defecation: 15 times/day, mild edema.

[Laboratory findings]

Alb 3.4 mg/dL, CRP 0.79 mg/dL, Hb 12.3 g/dL.

[Endoscopic images] (Fig. 16)

[Clinical course]

First attack type.

Initial treatment: PSL 40 mg for 1 week.

Clinical response: 1 week.

Clinical remission: 1 week.

Maintenance dose: PSL 0 mg.

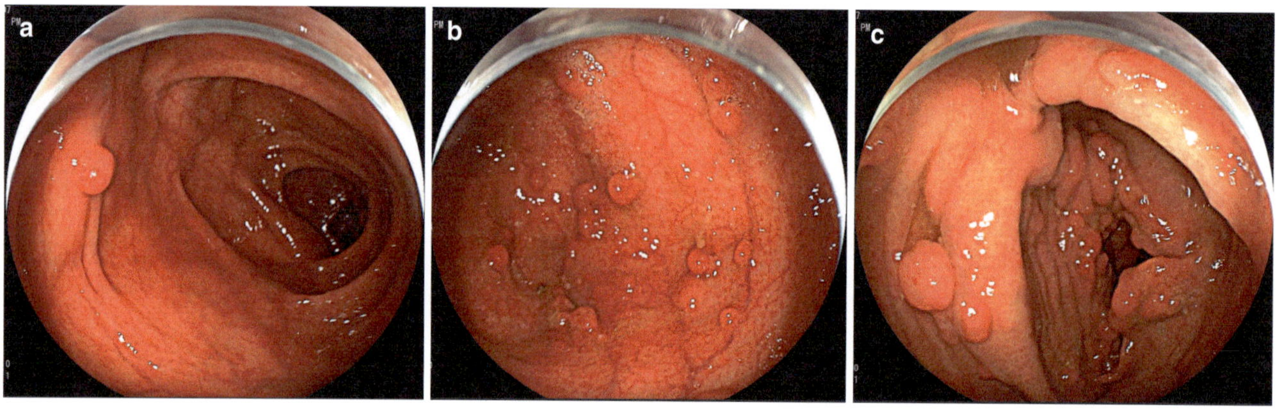

Fig. 16 (**a**), (**b**), (**c**) Colon: Sparse type. Medium, erythematous polyps

Case 12: A typical case who responded markedly to corticosteroids and achieved steroid-free clinical remission

Provided by Naoki Hosoe and Takanori Kanai

[Patient]

A 55-year-old man. CC: Diarrhea, alopecia, nail abnormality.

[Clinical findings]

Alopecia (+), onychodystrophy (+), hyperpigmentation (+), dysgeusia (+), mild edema.

[Laboratory findings]

Alb 2.7 mg/dL, CRP 0.01 mg/dL, Hb 7.5 g/dL.

[Endoscopic images] (Fig. 17)

[Clinical course]

First attack type.

Initial treatment: PSL 30 mg for 4 weeks.

Clinical response: 1 week.

Clinical remission: 8 weeks.

Maintenance dose: PSL 0 mg.

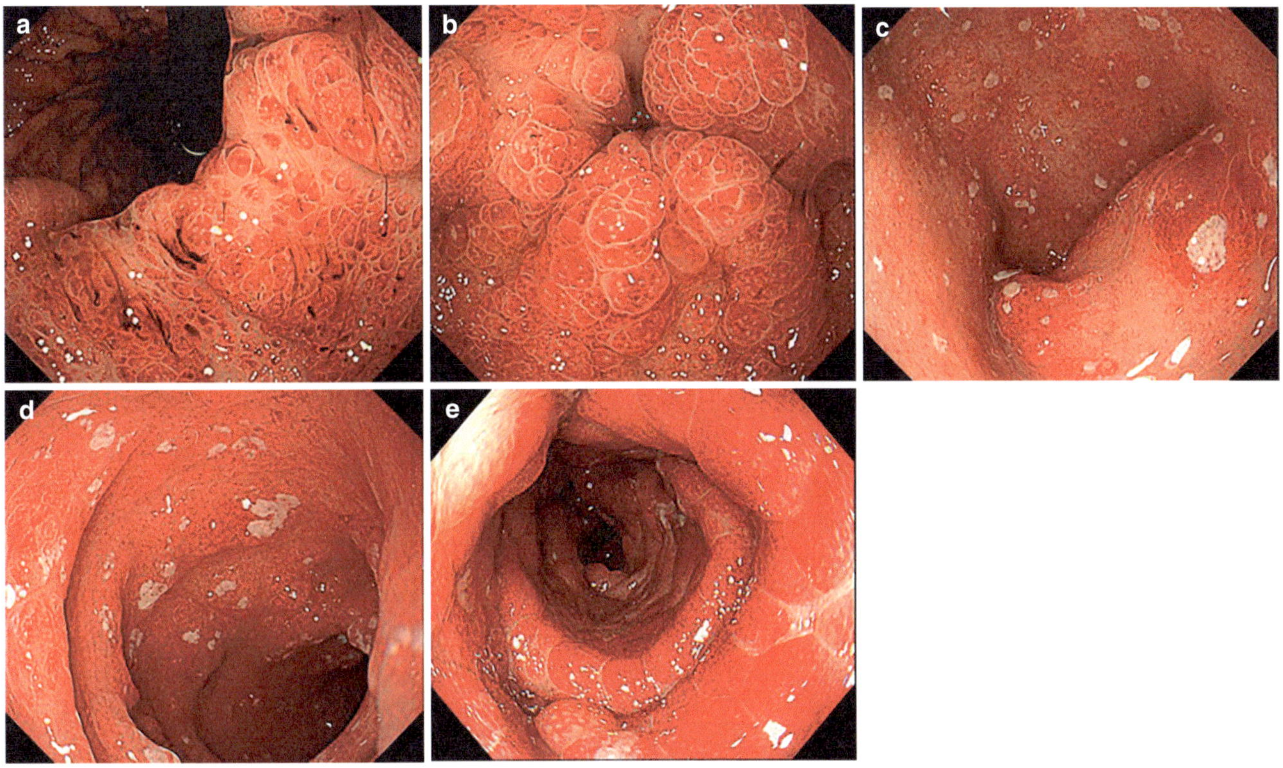

Fig. 17 (**a**), (**b**) Stomach: Confluent type. Large, erythematous, and hemorrhagic polyps. (**c**), (**d**) Duodenum: Sparse type. Small, erosive, and erythematous polyps with swollen villi. (**e**) Colon: Thickening type. Erythematous mucosa

Case 13: A rapidly developing case suffering from diarrhea, dysgeusia, and alopecia after a medical checkup, who responded markedly to corticosteroids and achieved steroid-free clinical remission

Provided by Kan Uchiyama

[Patient]

A 70-year-old male. He received the following exams for medical checkup just before the onset.

[Barium X-ray radiography of the stomach] (Fig. 18a–c)

[Barium enema] (Fig. 19a, b)

Two days after these exams, he began to suffer from diarrhea and dysgeusia, and visited a doctor. Then, alopecia and weight loss appeared, and the patient was referred to the hospital.

[Clinical findings]

Alopecia (+), onychodystrophy (+), hyperpigmentation (−), dysgeusia (+), defecation: 6 times/day, mild edema.

[Laboratory findings]

Alb 3.0 mg/dL, CRP 0.10 mg/dL, Hb 12.4 g/dL.

[Endoscopic images] (Fig. 20a–f)

[Clinical course]

First attack type.

Initial treatment: PSL 20 mg for 4 weeks.

Clinical response: 4 weeks.

Maintenance dose: PSL 0 mg.

The dose of PSL was tapered from 20 mg to 15 mg after 4 weeks.

His diarrhea and dysgeusia improved, and his weight increased. However, insomnia and malaise appeared while he was taking 15 mg, and he reduced the dose from 15 to 5 mg at his own discretion. Then, PSL was discontinued by the doctor.

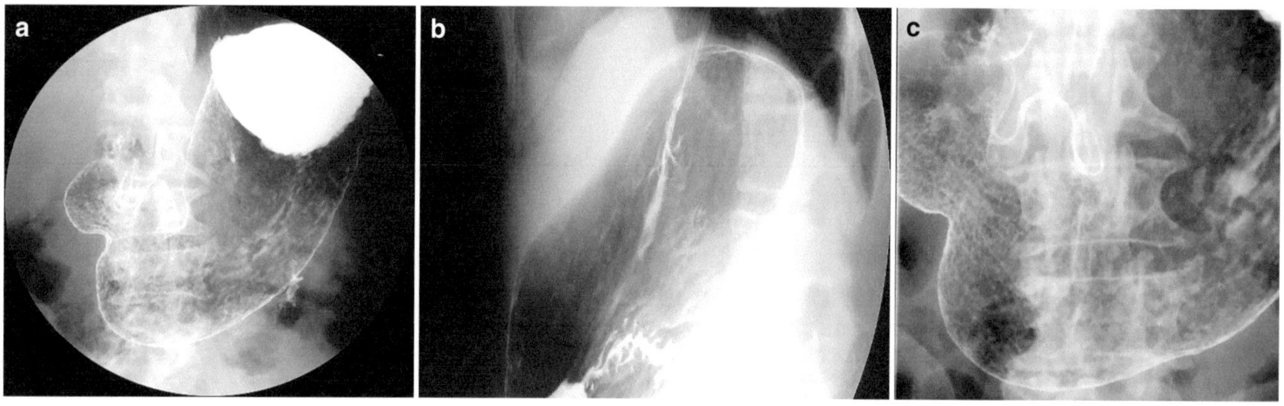

Fig. 18 (**a**) Full view of the stomach. (**b**) Gastric fornix. No abnormal findings. (**c**) Gastric antrum: Small granular mucosa in antrum and uneven barium adherence in body. No obvious polyps

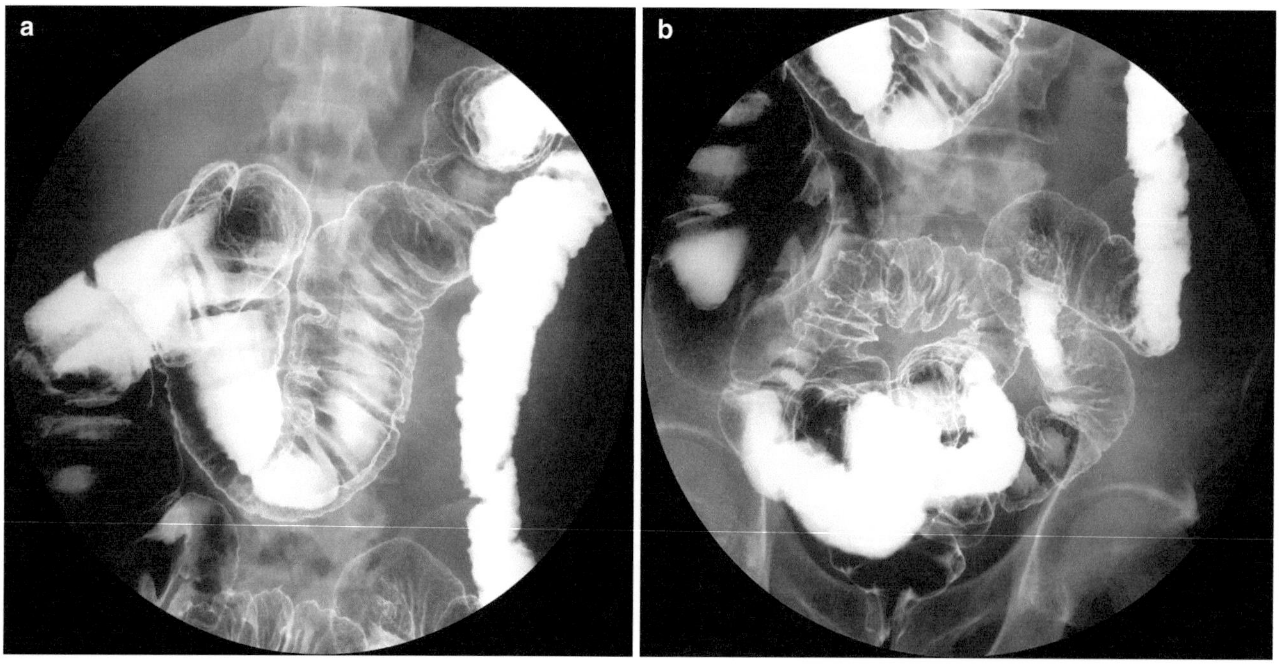

Fig. 19 (**a**), (**b**) Only a few scattered small polyps were detected

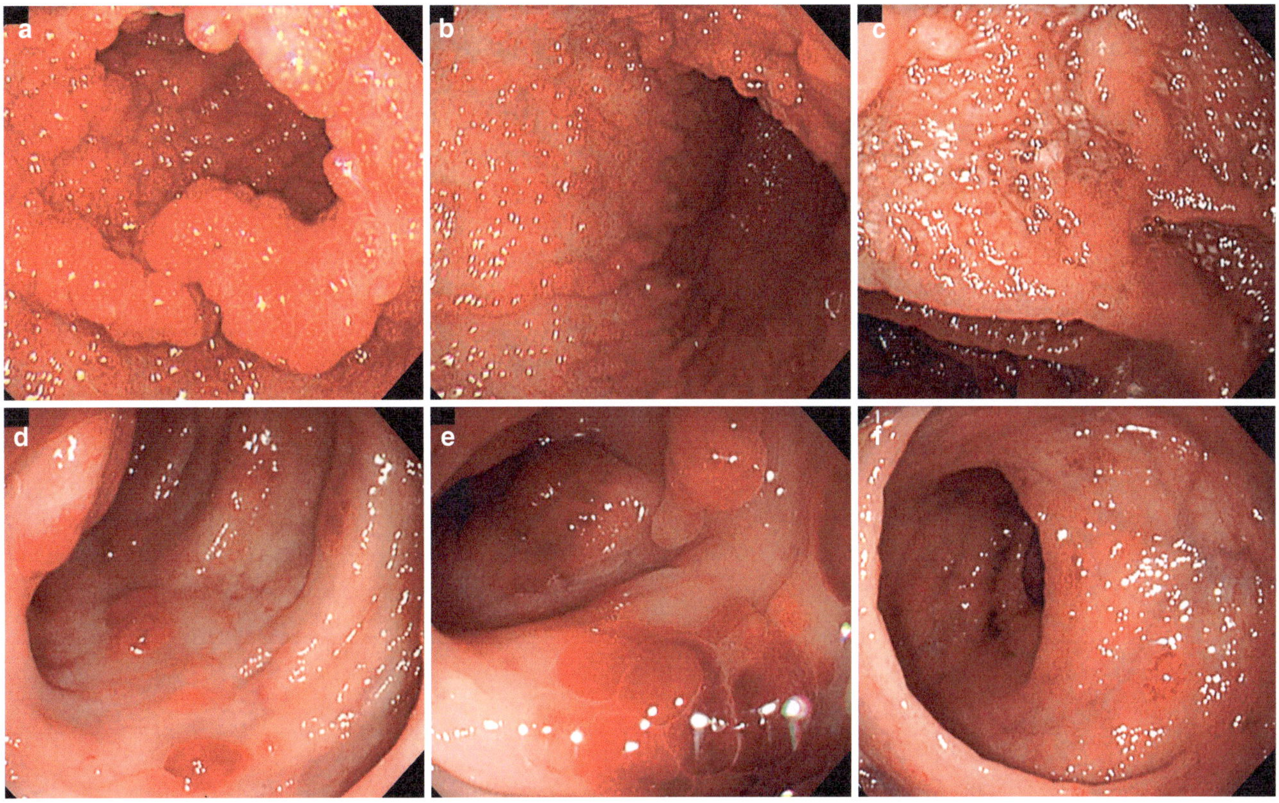

Fig. 20 (**a**), (**b**) Stomach: Confluent type. Small, erythematous, and edematous polyps. (**c**) Duodenum: Fold thickening type with white villi. (**d**), (**e**), (**f**) Colon: Sparse type. Medium, erythematous, and edematous polyps

Case 14: A mostly typical case who responded markedly to corticosteroids and achieved steroid-free clinical remission

Provided by Masakazu Nagahori

[Patient]

A 66-year-old man. CC: Alopecia, hyperpigmentation of extremities.

[Clinical findings]

Alopecia (+), onychodystrophy (−), hyperpigmentation (+), dysgeusia (+), defecation: 4 times/day, mild edema.

[Laboratory findings]

Alb 2.9 mg/dL, CRP 0.28 mg/dL, Hb 14.4 g/dL.

[Endoscopic images] (Fig. 21)

[Clinical course]

First attack type.

Initial treatment: PSL 30 mg for 4 weeks.

Clinical response: 2 weeks.

Clinical remission: 8 weeks.

Maintenance dose: PSL 0 mg.

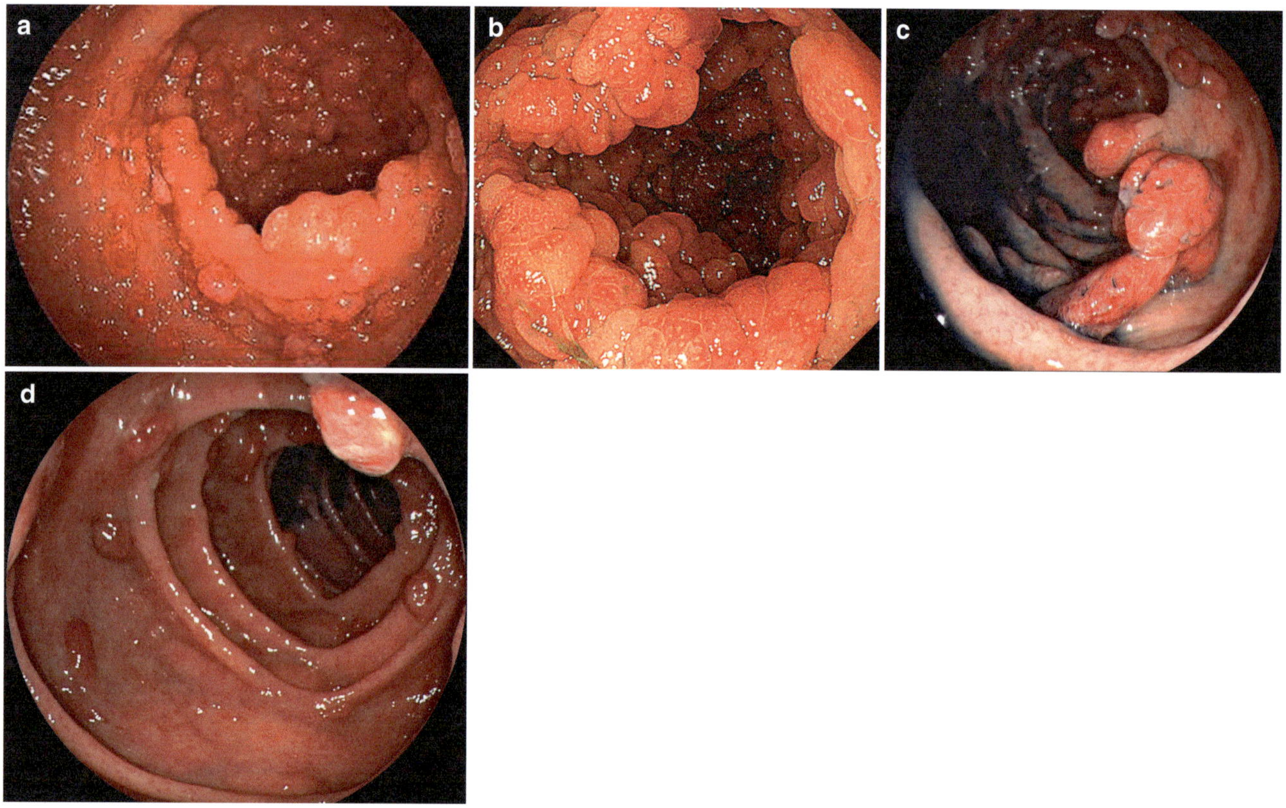

Fig. 21 (**a**) Stomach: Confluent type. Large, edematous, and erythematous polyps. (**b**) Colon: Confluent type. Large, edematous, and erythematous polyps. (**c**), (**d**) Colon (BAE): After treatments, polyps decreased and inflammation improved. Some stalked polyps were identified. (**a**), (**b**): Before treatments. (**c**), (**d**): After treatments

Case 15: A mostly typical case who responded markedly to corticosteroids and achieved clinical remission

Provided by Naoki Ohmiya

[Patient]

A 52-year-old man. CC: Dysgeusia, glossodynia, lower abdominal pain, diarrhea, weight loss, alopecia, onychalgia.

[Clinical findings]

Alopecia (+), onychodystrophy (−), hyperpigmentation (+), dysgeusia (+), defecation: 16 times/day, mild edema.

[Laboratory findings]

Alb 2.7 mg/dL, CRP 0.9 mg/dL.

99mTc-human serum albumin scintigraphy: Abnormal leakage from the entire colon.

Fecal alpha1-antitrypsin clearance: 229 mL/day.

[Endoscopic images] (Fig. 22)

[Clinical course]

First attack type.

Initial treatment: PSL 40 mg for 3 weeks

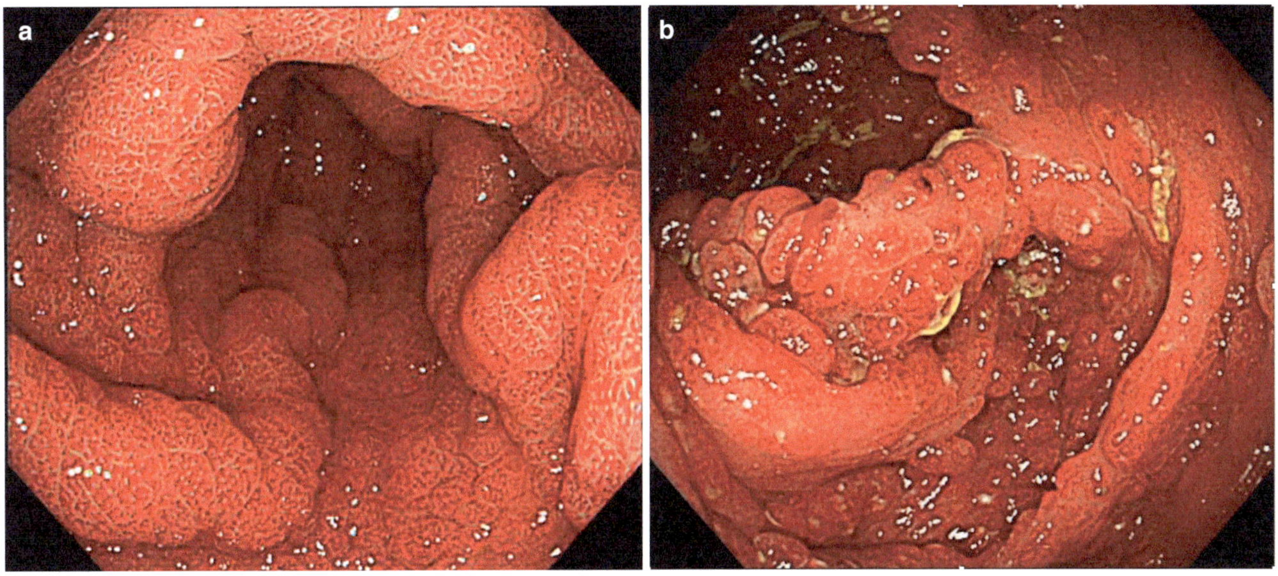

Fig. 22 (**a**) Stomach: Thickening type. Mucosa became more edematous and erythematous as it got closer to the distal stomach in the body. Normal pits were observed between the folds. The gastric angle and antrum were the most severely affected areas with diffusely edematous mucosa. (**b**) Colon: Semi-confluent type. Medium, erythematous polyps. Erythematous inflammatory polyps were distributed through the entire colon. There are many polyps, especially in the cecum, ascending, transverse, and descending colon. The polyps tend to be aligned longitudinally and intervening mucosa between polyps showed atrophic discolored mucosa. The rectum had a large area of atrophic mucosa

2.3 Endoscopic Non-remission Cases

Case 16: A case who responded to corticosteroids clinically but did not endoscopically

Provided by Tsukasa Yamakawa and Hiroshi Nakase

[Patient]

A 77-year-old man. CC: Dysgeusia, diarrhea.

[Clinical findings]

Alopecia (−), onychodystrophy (+), hyperpigmentation (−), defecation: 4–6 times, mild edema.

[Laboratory findings]

Alb 4.4 mg/dL, CRP 0.24 mg/dL, Hb 13.1 g/dL.

[Endoscopic images] (Fig. 23a–h)

[Clinical course]

First attack type.

Initial treatment: PSL 50 mg for 2 weeks.

Clinical response: 2 weeks.

Maintenance dose: PSL 0 mg.

[Endoscopic images 2] (Fig. 24a–d)

EGD and CS 5 years after the diagnosis.

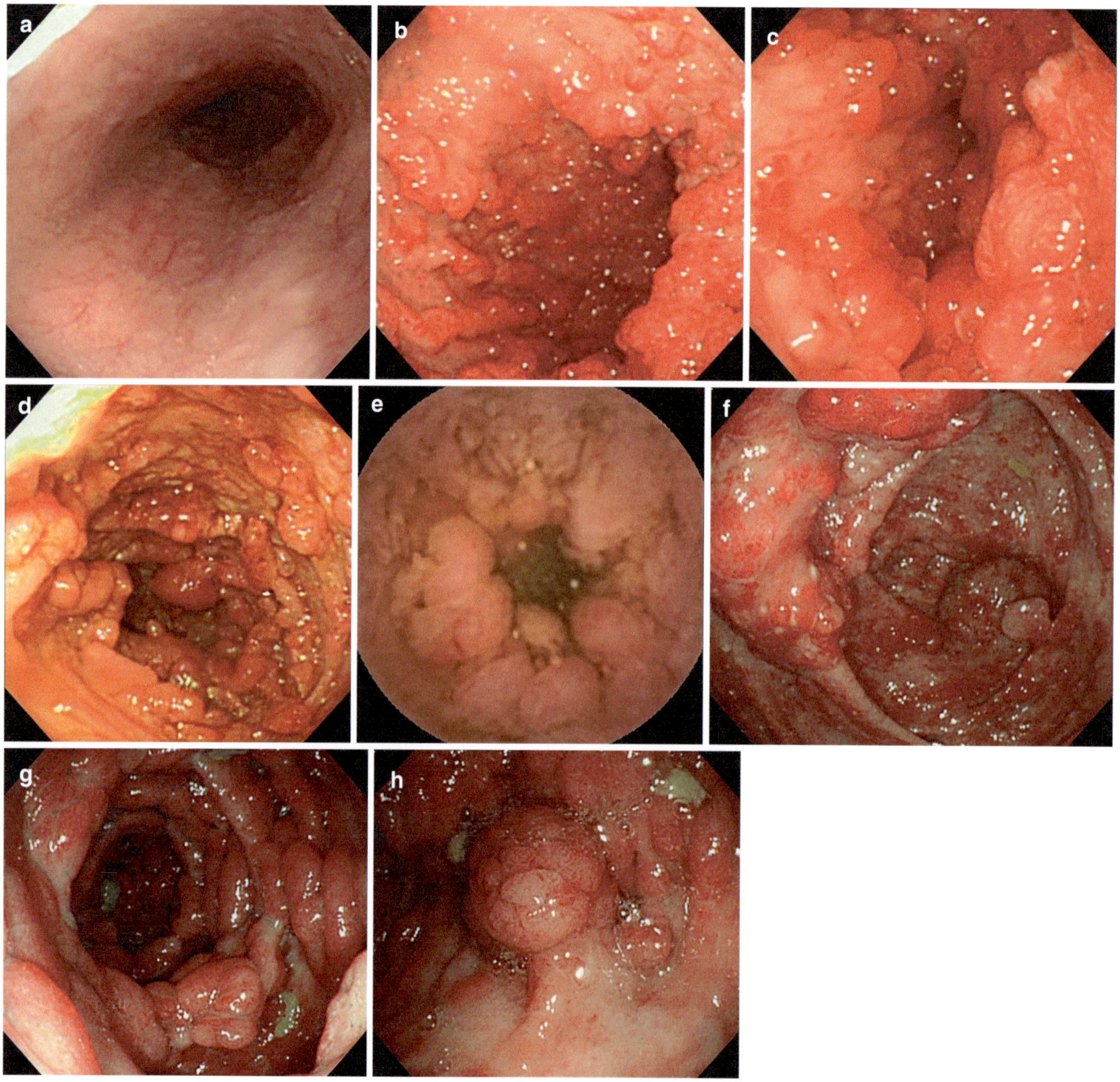

Fig. 23 (**a**) Esophagus: normal. (**b**), (**c**) Stomach: Confluent type. Medium, erythematous, and edematous polyps. Edematous intervening mucosa with ill-defined margin from polyps. (**d**) Duodenum: Confluent type. Medium polyps. (**e**) Small intestine (SBCE): Sparse type. Small polyps. (**f**), (**g**), (**h**) Colon: Semi-confluent type. Medium to large, edematous, and erythematous polyps. Edematous and erythematous intervening mucosa

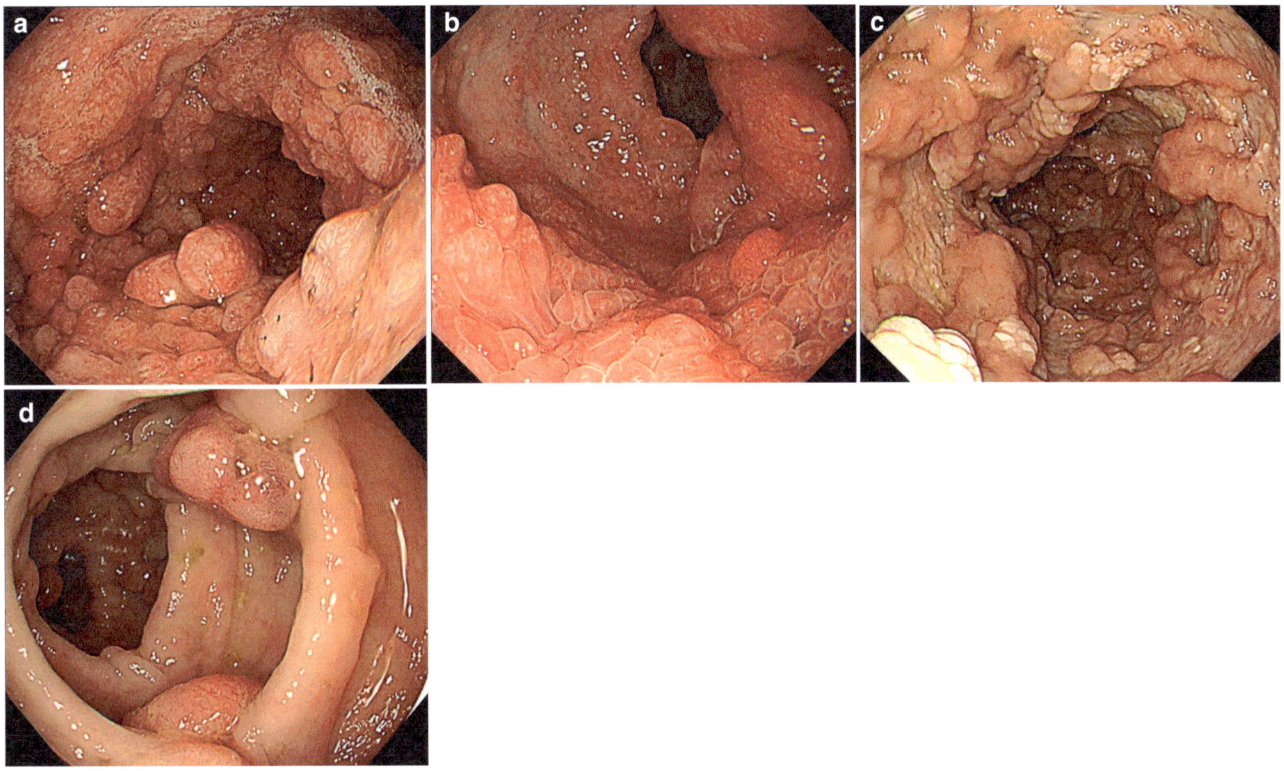

Fig. 24 (**a**), (**b**) Stomach: Confluent type. Medium, flat to hemispherical polyps. Slightly less erythematous than first appearance. (**c**) Duodenum: Confluent type. Small, flat to hemispherical polyps with white villi. (**d**) Colon: Sparse type. Almost normal intervening mucosa

Case 17: A case who achieved clinical remission by corticosteroids, whose gastric and colonic lesions improved endoscopically, but the duodenal lesion exacerbated paradoxically

Provided by Kazuki Kakimoto and Kazuhide Higuchi

[Patient]

64 years old. CC: Dysgeusia, anorexia, diarrhea, bloody stool, alopecia, onychodystrophy.

[Clinical findings]

Alopecia (+), onychodystrophy (+), hyperpigmentation (−), dysgeusia (+), defecation: 3 times/day.

[Laboratory findings]

TP 5.9 mg/dL, Alb 3.5 mg/dL, CRP 0.68 mg/dL, Hb 14.7 g/dL.

[Endoscopic images 1] (Fig. 25a–e)

[Clinical course]

First attack type.

Initial treatment: PSL 30 mg for 4 weeks.

Clinical response: 2 weeks.

Clinical remission: 4 weeks.

Endoscopic response: 4 months.

Endoscopic remission: 7 months.

Maintenance dose: PSL 0 mg.

[Endoscopic images 2] (Fig. 26a–e)

EGD and CS 1 year after the treatment.

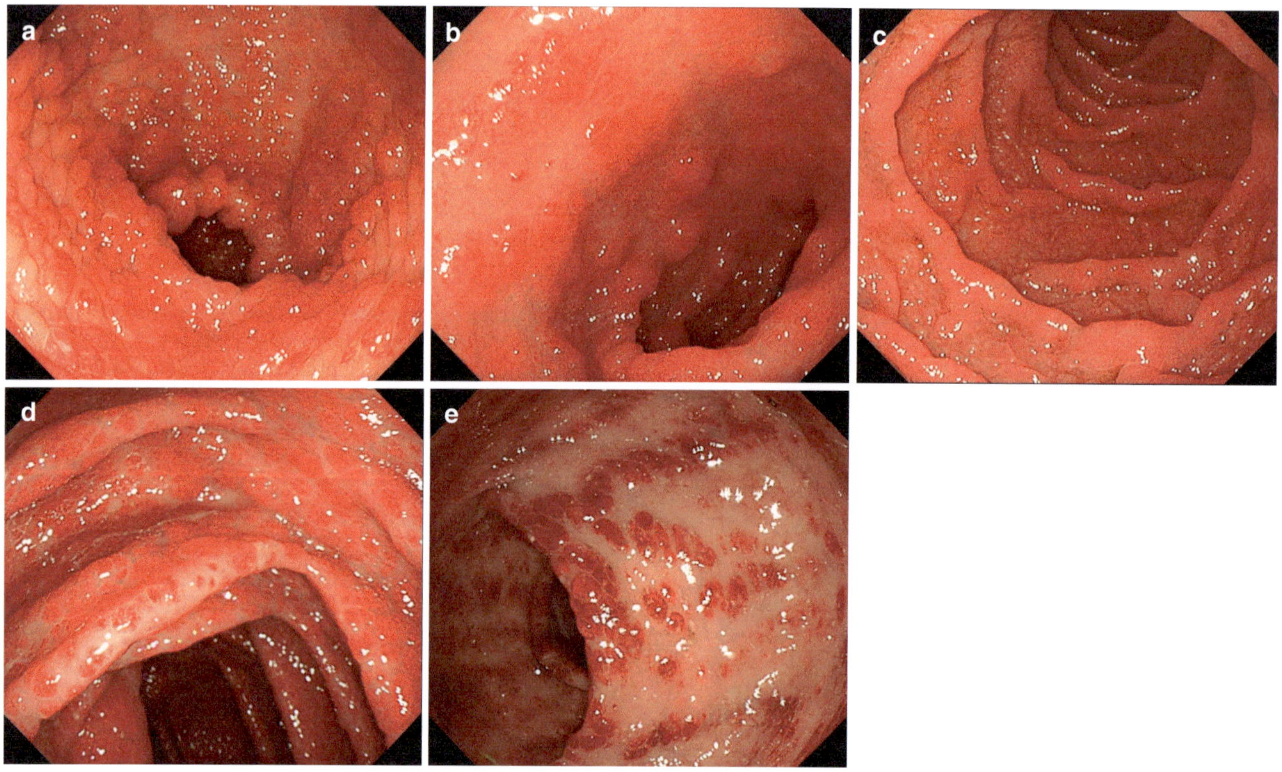

Fig. 25 (**a**) Stomach: Confluent type. Small polyps. (**b**) Duodenal bulb: Sparse type. Small polyps. (**c**) Duodenal second portion: Fold thickening type. (**d**) Transverse colon: Semi-confluent type. Small polyps. (**e**) Rectum: Semi-confluent type. Small polyps

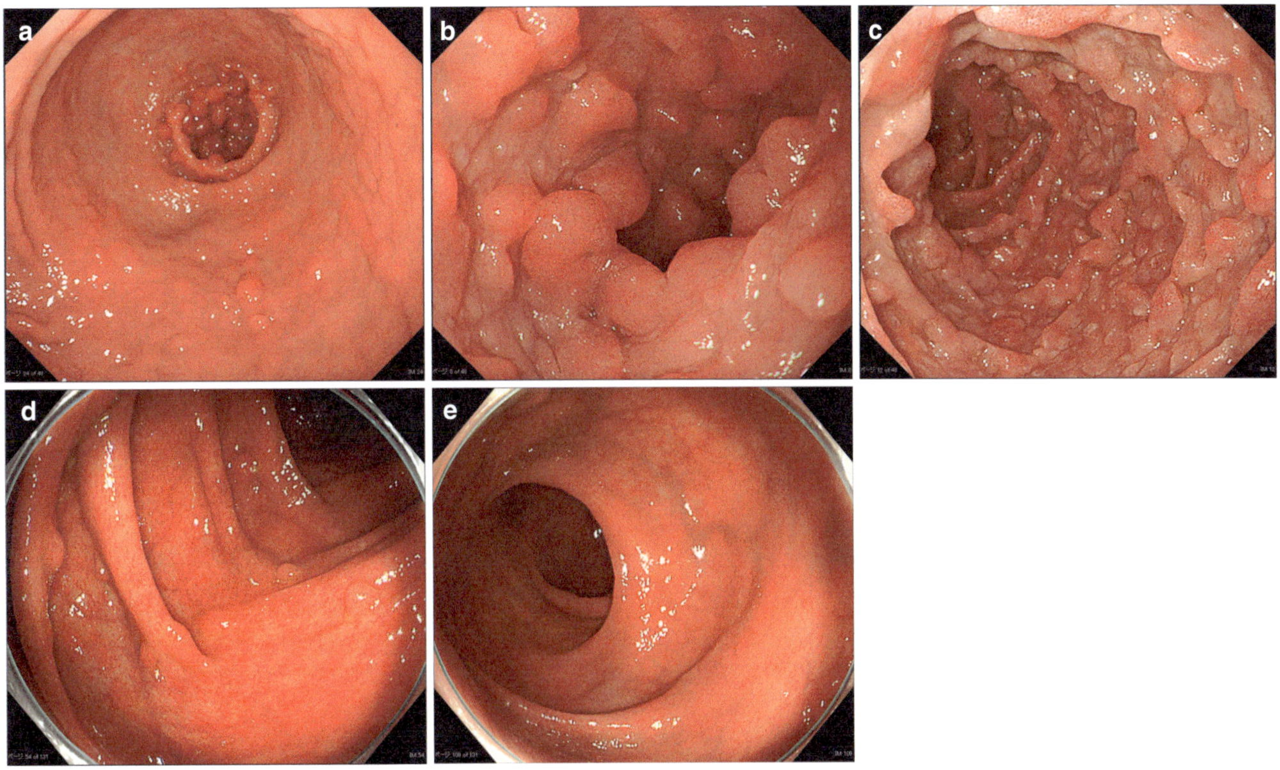

Fig. 26 (**a**) Gastric antrum: Edematous mucosa was present, but the polyps markedly shrunk. (**b**) Duodenal bulb: The polyps became swollen. (**c**) Duodenal second portion: Worsening of fold thickening and newly appeared white villi. (**d**) Transverse colon: Erythematous and edematous mucosa improved with a few residual scattered small polyps. (**e**) Rectum: Polyps almost disappeared with less edematous intervening mucosal

Case 18: A typical case who responded markedly to corticosteroids and had only a few residual polyps.

Provided by Tsukasa Yamakawa and Hiroshi Nakase

[Patient]

A 61-year-old male. CC: Diarrhea.

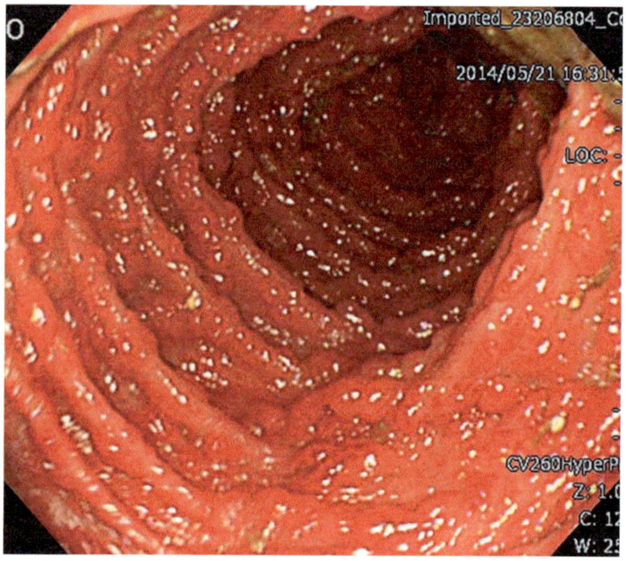

Fig. 27 Colon: Confluent type. Small, erythematous polyps. Edematous intervening mucosa

[Clinical findings]

Alopecia (+), onychodystrophy (+), hyperpigmentation (−), defecation: 5–6 times, mild edema.

[Laboratory findings]

Alb 3.6 mg/dL, CRP <0.10 mg/dL, Hb 15.7 g/dL.

[Endoscopic images 1] (Fig. 27)

[Clinical course]

First attack type.

Initial treatment: PSL 30 mg for 4 weeks.

Clinical response: 4 weeks.

Maintenance dose: PSL 0 mg.

[Endoscopic images 2] (Fig. 28)

EGD and CS during remission 5 years after the diagnosis.

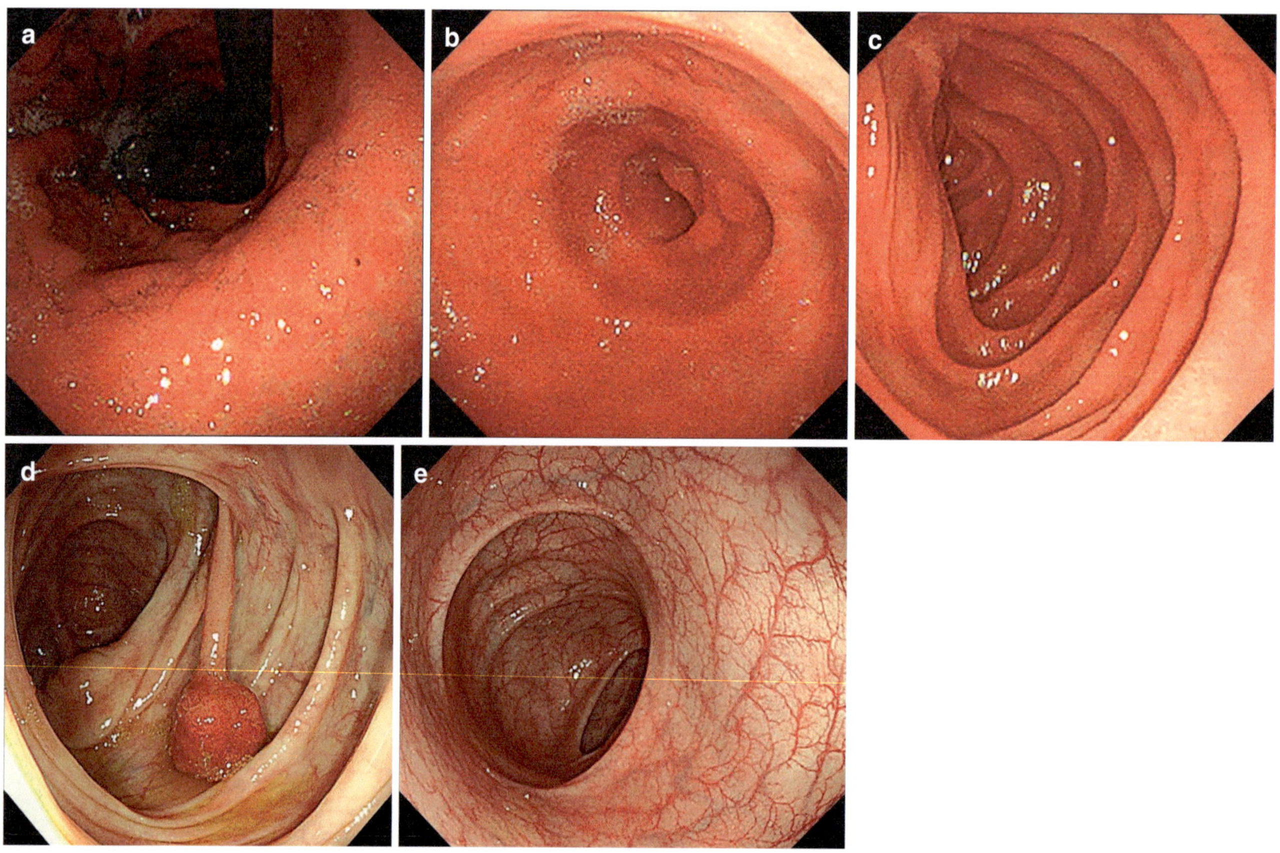

Fig. 28 (**a**), (**b**) Stomach: Erythematous and edematous polyps disappeared. (**c**) Duodenum: Normal findings. (**d**), (**e**) Colon: A large, erythematous stalked polyp. Normalized mucosa

Case 19: A typical case who responded markedly to corticosteroids and had only a few residual polyps

Provided by Tsukasa Yamakawa and Hiroshi Nakase

[Patient]

A 74-year-old man. CC: Dysgeusia, diarrhea.

[Clinical findings]

Alopecia (+), onychodystrophy (+), hyperpigmentation (+), defecation: 15 times/day, mild edema.

[Laboratory findings]

Alb 3.4 mg/dL, CRP 0.79 mg/dL, Hb 12.3 g/dL.

[Endoscopic images 1] (Fig. 29a–j)

Erosive and erythematous intervening mucosa.

[Clinical course]

First attack type.

Initial treatment: PSL 40 mg for 1 week.

Clinical response: 1 week.

Maintenance dose: PSL 0 mg.

[Endoscopic images 2] (Fig. 30a–e)

EGD and CS during remission.

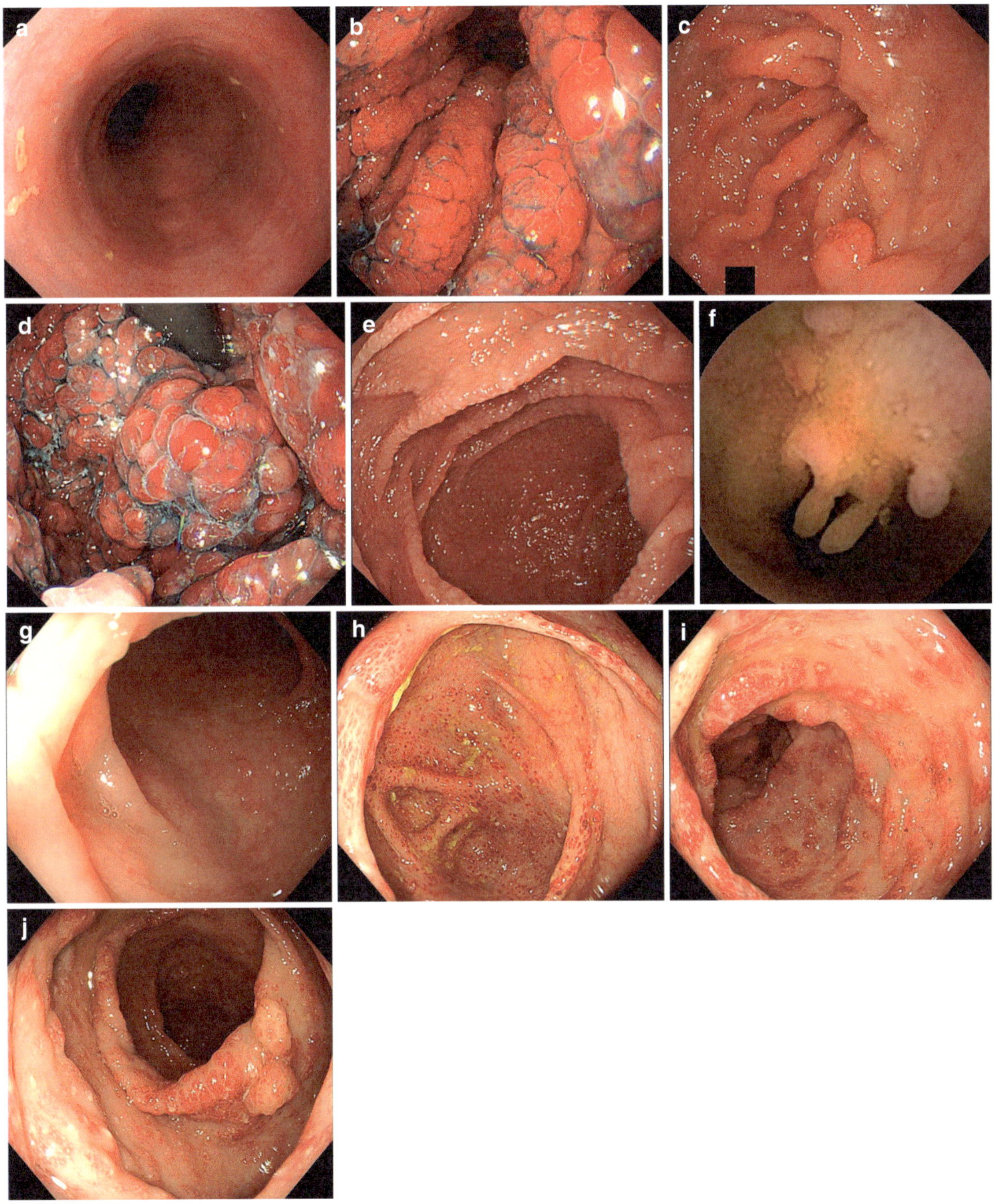

Fig. 29 (**a**) Esophagus: Normal. (**b**), (**c**), (**d**) Stomach: Confluent type. Medium, edematous, and erythematous polyps. Edematous intervening mucosa. Indigocarmine dyeing in (**b**), (**d**). (**e**) Duodenum: Edematous and granular mucosa with no obvious polyps. (**f**) Jejunum (SBCE): Sparse type. Small semipedunculated polyps. (**g**) Terminal ileum: Sparse type. Small polyps. (**h**), (**i**), (**j**) Colon: Semi-confluent type. Medium, erythematous, flat to hemispherical polyps

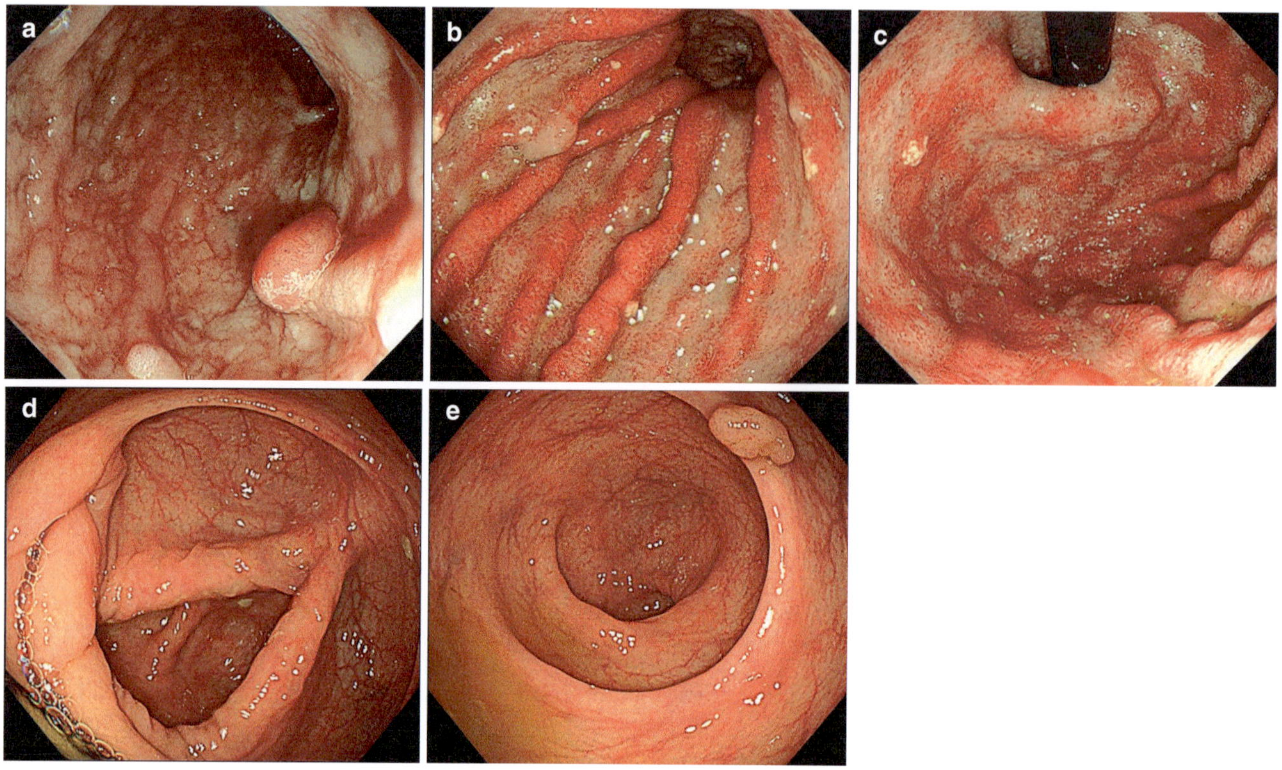

Fig. 30 (**a**), (**b**), (**c**) Stomach (1 year after the diagnosis): Mucosa remained erythematous and edematous, while polyps almost disappeared. (**d**), (**e**) Colon: Only a few polyps remained. Erythematous and erosive mucosa improved

Case 20: A mostly typical case who responded markedly to corticosteroids and had only a few residual polyps

Provided by Makoto Ooi and Yuzo Kodama

[Patient]

A 74-year-old woman. CC: Diarrhea.

[Clinical findings]

Alopecia (−), onychodystrophy (+), hyperpigmentation (+), severe edema.

[Laboratory findings]

Alb 2.3 mg/dL, CRP 0.05 mg/dL, Hb 10.6 g/dL.

[Endoscopic images 1] (Fig. 31a–f)

[Clinical course]

First attack type.

Initial treatment: PSL 40 mg for 4 weeks.

Clinical response: 7 weeks.

Clinical remission: 8 weeks.

Endoscopic response: 2 months.

Endoscopic remission: 11 months.

Maintenance dose: PSL 0 mg.

[Endoscopic images 2] (Fig. 32a–e)

11 months after the diagnosis.

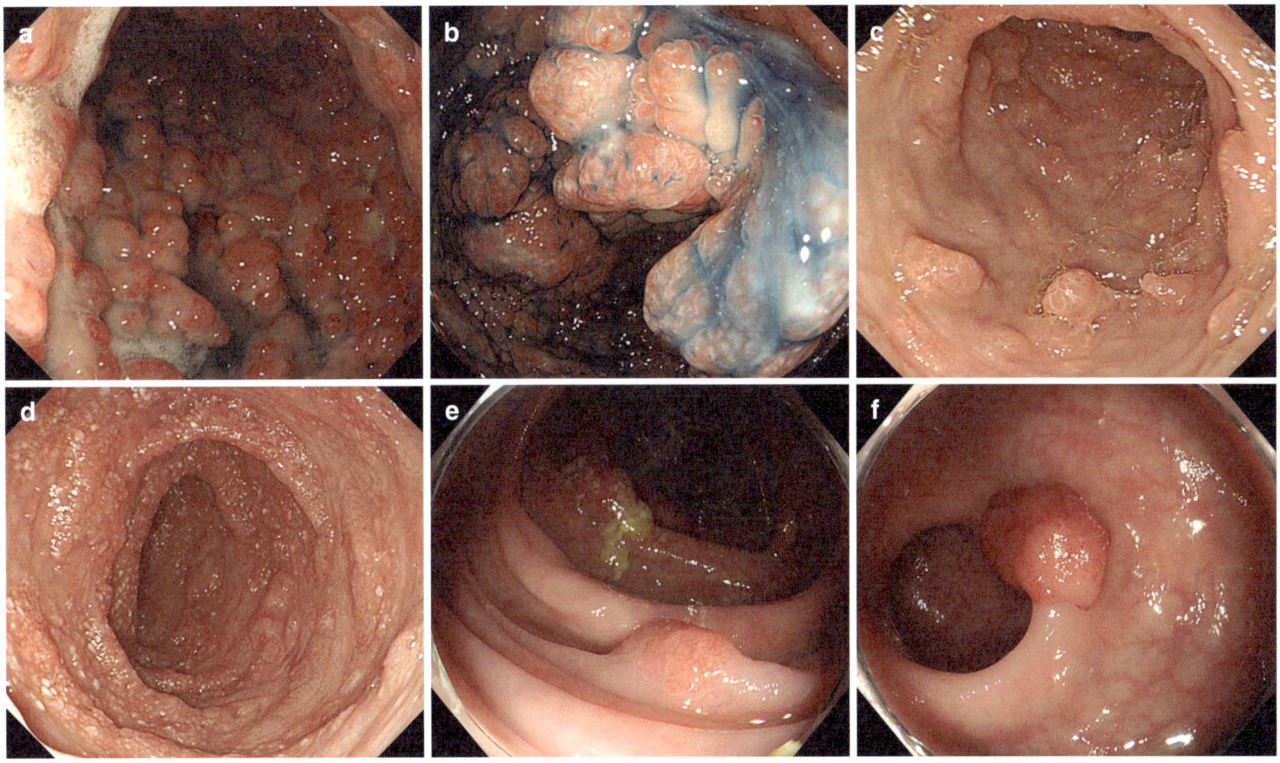

Fig. 31 (**a**), (**b**) Stomach: Confluent type. Medium, edematous, and whitish mucus adhered polyps. Indigocarmine dyeing in (**b**). (**c**), (**d**) Duodenum: Confluent type. Small polyps. (**e**), (**f**) Colon: Sparse type. Medium, erythematous polyps

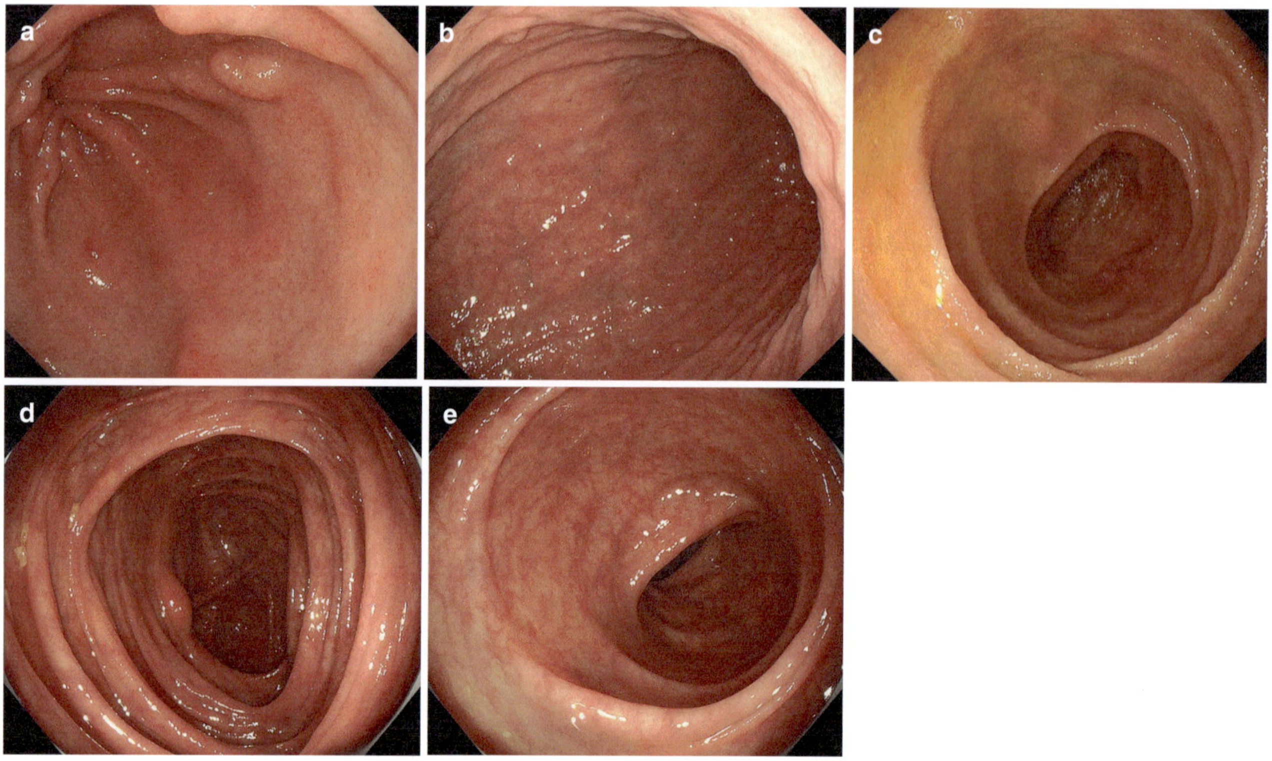

Fig. 32 (**a**), (**b**) Stomach: Polyps almost disappeared. (**c**) Duodenum: Normalized endoscopic findings. (**d**), (**e**) Colon: Normalized endoscopic findings

Case 21: A mostly typical case who responded markedly to corticosteroids and had only a few residual polyps

Provided by Masakazu Nagahori

[Patient]

A 75-year-old man. CC: Diarrhea.

[Clinical findings]

Alopecia (−), onychodystrophy (+), hyperpigmentation (−), dysgeusia (−), defecation: 12 times/day, severe edema.

[Laboratory findings]

Alb 1.3 mg/dL, CRP 0.22 mg/dL, Hb 15.2 g/dL.

[Endoscopic images 1] (Fig. 33a, b)

[Clinical course]

First attack type.

Initial treatment: PSL 40 mg for 2 weeks.

Clinical response: 2 weeks.

Clinical remission: 8 weeks.

Maintenance dose: PSL 0 mg.

[Endoscopic images 2] (Fig. 34)

EGD 6 months after the diagnosis.

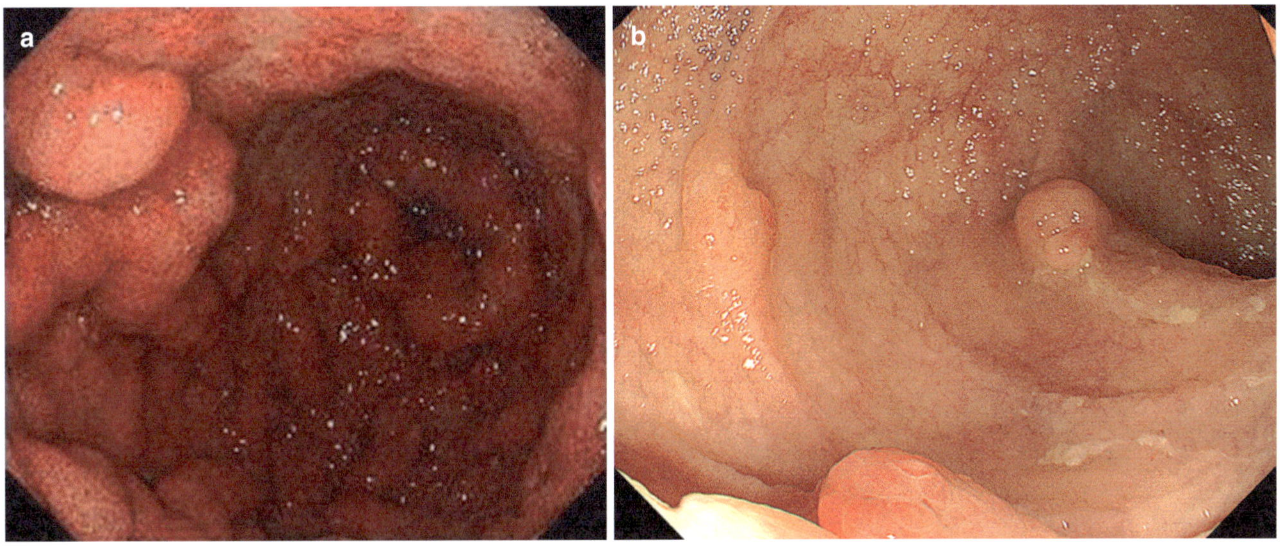

Fig. 33 (**a**) Stomach: Confluent type. Large, edematous, and erythematous polyps. (**b**) Duodenum: Sparse type. Small polyps

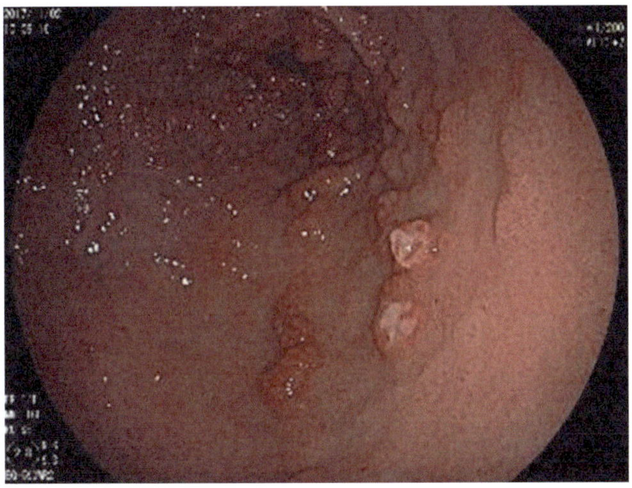

Fig. 34 Gastric antrum: Endoscopic findings improved

Case 22: A mostly typical case who achieved clinical remission with corticosteroids and had gradual endoscopic improvements

Provided by Katsuyoshi Ando and Mikihiro Fujiya

[Patient]

An 81-year-old woman. CC: Dysgeusia, diarrhea, alopecia.

[Clinical findings]

Alopecia (+), onychodystrophy (+), hyperpigmentation (−), dysgeusia (+), defecation 4 times/day.

[Laboratory findings]

Alb 2.8 mg/dL, CRP 0.61 mg/dL, Hb 13.7 g/dL.

[Endoscopic images 1] (Fig. 35a–d)

[Clinical course]

First attack type.

Initial treatment: PSL 30 mg for 7 weeks.

Clinical response: 7 weeks.

Clinical remission: 10 weeks.

Maintenance dose: PSL 0 mg.

[Endoscopic images 2] (Fig. 36a–d)

EGD after treatments.

After 4 weeks of treatments with 20–30 mg of PSL, there was flattening of the polyps and improvement in redness. Reevaluation at 13 weeks showed further flattening of the polyps and improvement in redness.

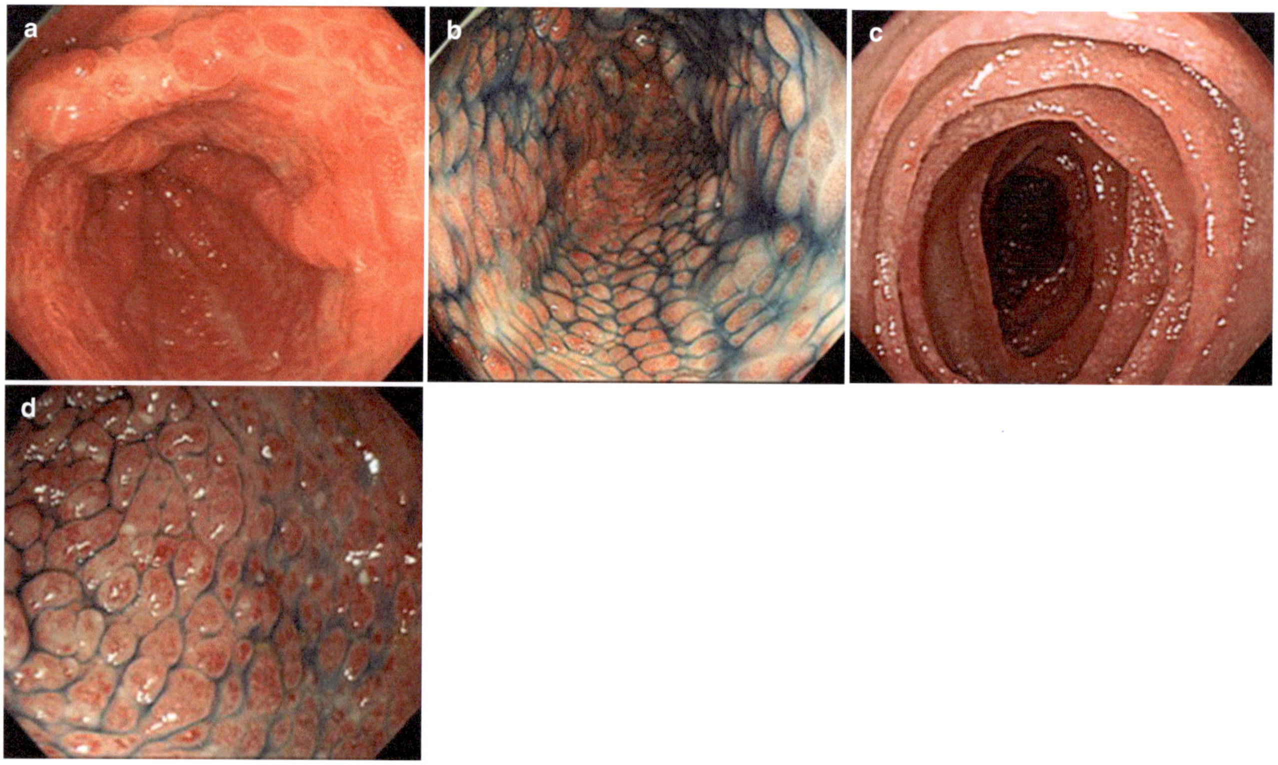

Fig. 35 (**a**) Stomach: Confluent type. Medium, edematous, and erythematous polyp. (**b**) Indigocarmine dyeing of (**a**). (**c**) Jejunum: Fold thickening type with white villi. (**d**) Rectum: Confluent type. Medium, edematous, and erythematous polyps

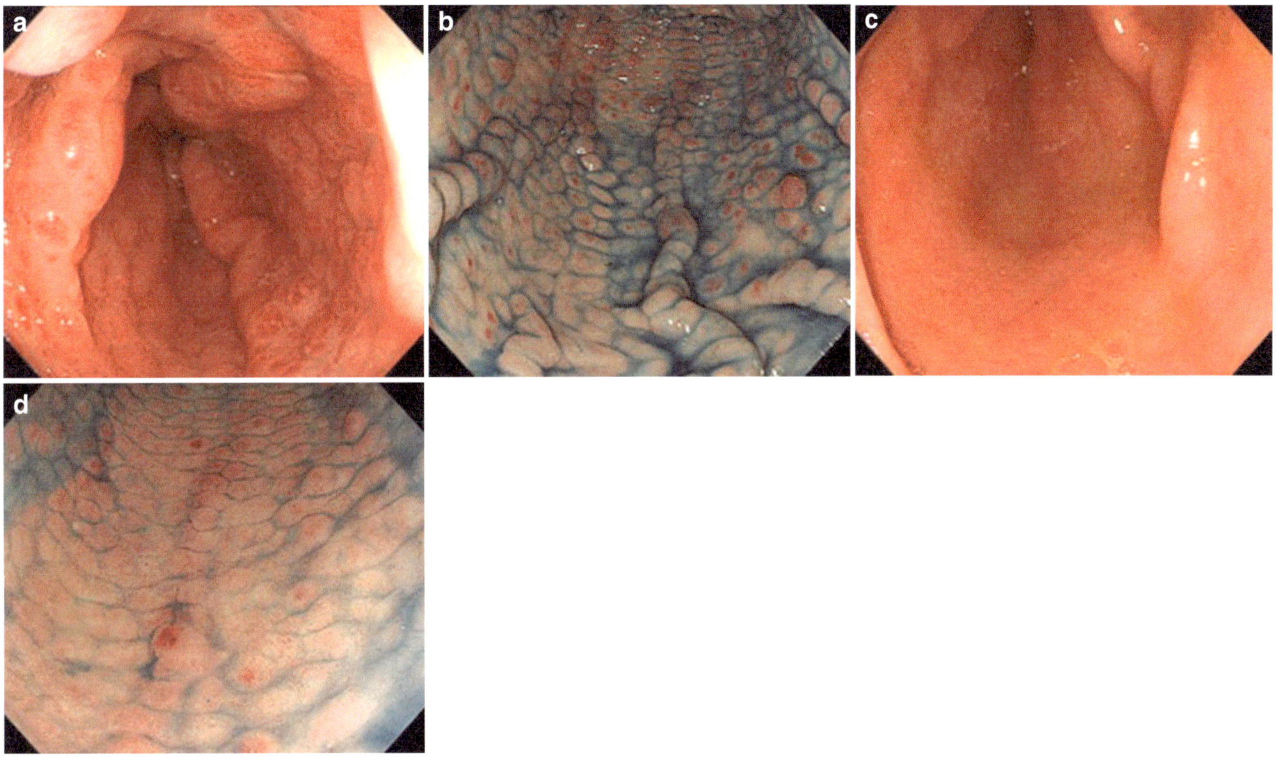

Fig. 36 (**a**) Gastric antrum (4 weeks after treatments). (**b**) Indigocarmine dyeing of (**a**). (**c**) Gastric antrum (13 weeks after treatments). (**d**) Indigocarmine dyeing of (**c**)

Case 23: A typical case who responded markedly to corticosteroids but had some residual polyps

Provided by Ken Sugimoto and Naoto Shirai

[Patient]

A 64-year-old man.

CC: Abdominal pain, diarrhea, melena.

[Clinical findings]

Alopecia (+), onychodystrophy (+), hyperpigmentation (+), dysgeusia (−), defecation: 9 times/day.

[Laboratory findings]

Alb 3.8 mg/dL, CRP 0.27 mg/dL, Hb 17.9 g/dL.

[Endoscopic images 1] (Fig. 37a–c)

[Clinical course]

First attack type.

Initial treatment: PSL 30 mg for 4 weeks.

Clinical response 1 week.

Clinical remission 3 weeks.

Maintenance dose: PSL 5 mg.

[Endoscopic images 2] (Fig. 38a–c)

EGD after treatments.

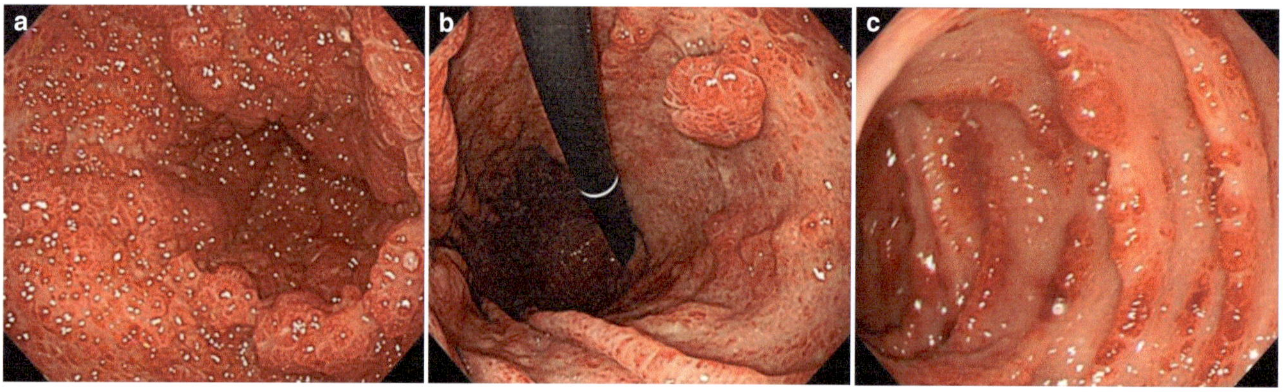

Fig. 37 (**a**), (**b**) Stomach: Confluent type. Medium, edematous, and erythematous polyps. (**c**) Colon: Semi-confluent type. Medium, edematous, and erythematous polyps

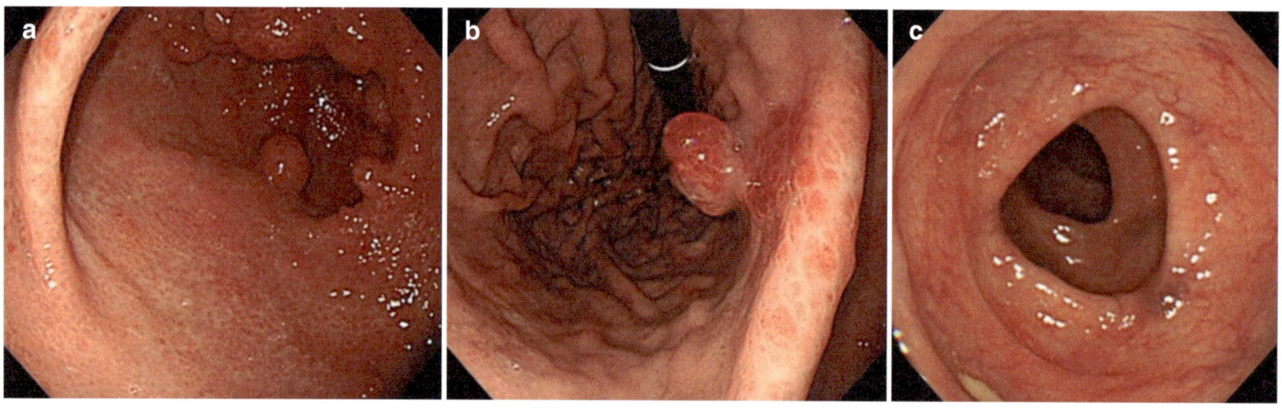

Fig. 38 (**a**), (**b**) Stomach: polyps mostly disappeared and inflammatory findings improved. (**c**) Colon: Polyps disappeared, and inflammatory findings improved

Case-Based Images: Relapse-Remitting Cases/Chronic Continuous Cases

Ryota Hokari, Tadakazu Hisamatsu, and Masaaki Higashiyama

1 Relapse-Remitting Cases

Case 24: A relapse-remitting case who required PSL 2.5 mg for endoscopic remission

Provided by Katsuyuki Fukuda

[Patient]

A 60-year-old woman. CC: Tinnitus, dysgeusia, abdominal pain, diarrhea, facial edema, alopecia, onycholysis.

[Clinical findings]

Alopecia (+), onychodystrophy (+), hyperpigmentation (−), dysgeusia (+), defecation: 3 times/day.

[Laboratory findings]

Alb 3.3 mg/dL, CRP 0.14 mg/dL, Hb 13.8 g/dL.

[Endoscopic images 1] (Fig. 1a, b)

[Clinical course]

Relapse-remitting type.

Initial treatment: PSL 30 mg for 2 weeks.

Clinical response: 1 week.

Maintenance dose: PSL 2.5 mg.

Therapeutic dose at relapse: PSL 40 mg.

[Endoscopic images 2] (Fig. 2a, b)

EGD and CS after treatments.

Endoscopic remission was achieved in both lesions.

R. Hokari (✉) · M. Higashiyama
Department of Internal Medicine, National Defense Medical College, Tokorozawa, Saitama, Japan
e-mail: ryota@ndmc.ac.jp; masaakih@ndmc.ac.jp

T. Hisamatsu
Department of Gastroenterology and Hepatology, Kyorin University School of Medicine, Mitaka, Tokyo, Japan

R. Hokari, T. Hisamatsu (eds.), *Atlas of Cronkhite-Canada Syndrome*, https://doi.org/10.1007/978-981-19-0652-7_7

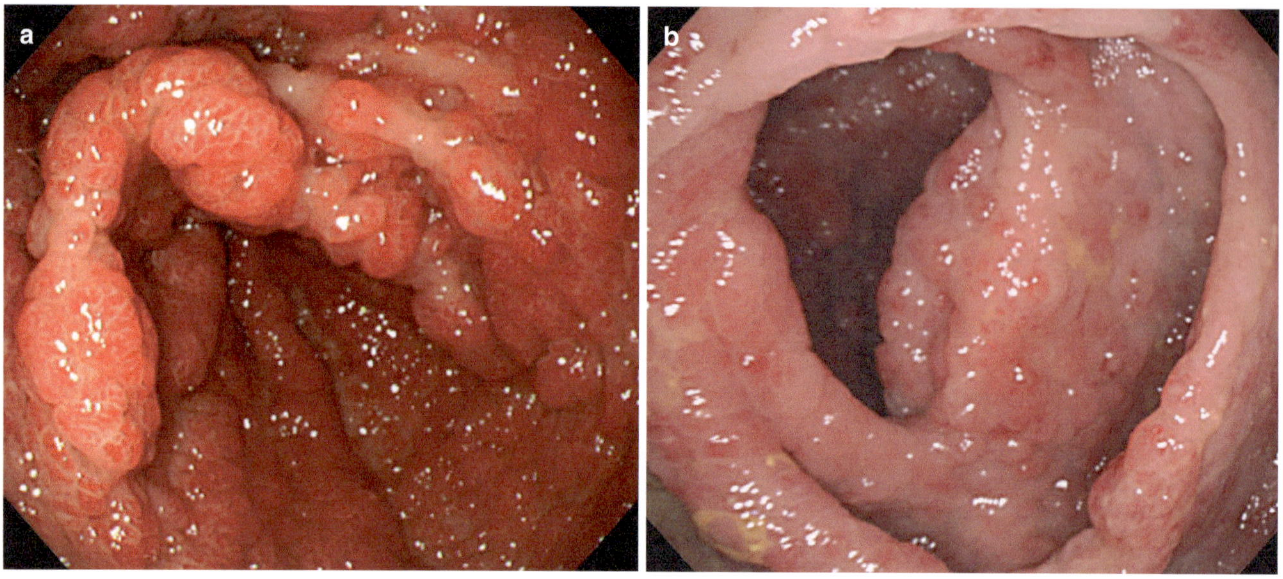

Fig. 1 (**a**) Stomach: Confluent type. Medium, edematous, and erythematous polyps. (**b**) Colon: Confluent type. Medium, edematous, and erythematous polyps

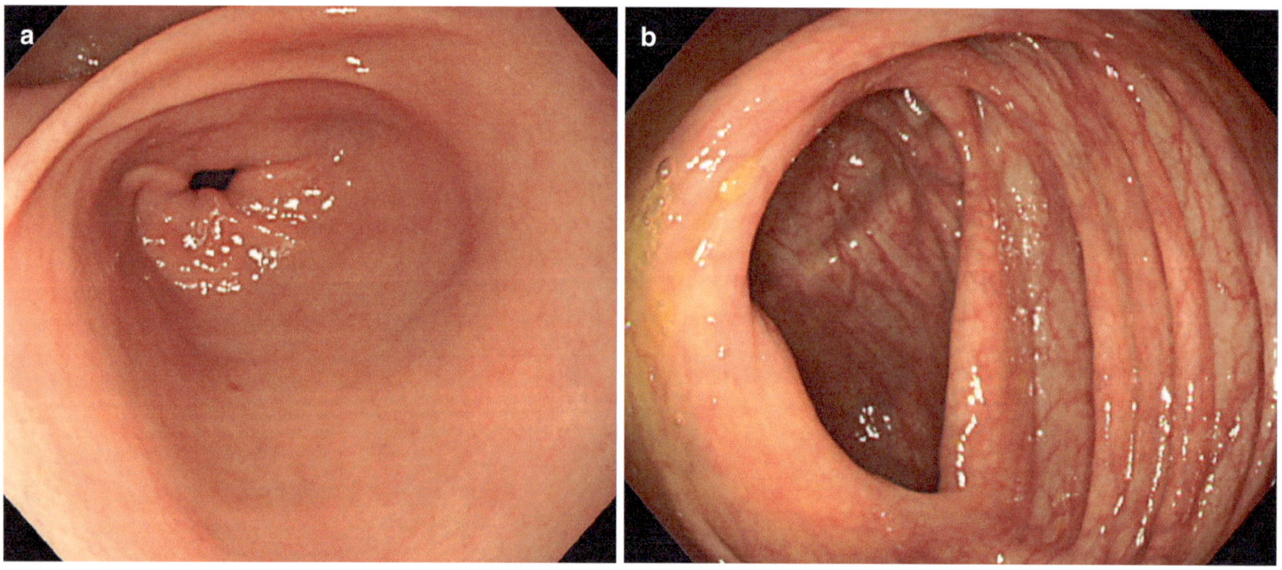

Fig. 2 (**a**) Stomach. (**b**) Colon

Case 25: A case who responded markedly to corticosteroids clinically and endoscopically, but suffered from relapsing when PSL was tapered to 5 mg

Provided by Noriko Kamata

[Patient]

A 77-year-old woman. CC: Diarrhea, melena, alopecia, hyperpigmentation.

[Clinical findings]

Alopecia (+), onychodystrophy (+), hyperpigmentation (+), dysgeusia (+), defecation: 4 times/day.

[Laboratory findings]

Alb 3.0 mg/dL, CRP 2.87 mg/dL, Hb 13.6 g/dL.

[Clinical course]

Relapse-remitting type.

Initial treatment: PSL 40 mg for 2 weeks.

Clinical response: 2 weeks.

Endoscopic response: 2 months.

Endoscopic remission: 6 months.

Therapeutic dose at relapse: PSL 30 mg.

[Endoscopic images 1] (Fig. 3a–g)

[Endoscopic images 2] (Fig. 4a–f)

Symptoms flared up 9 months after the diagnosis when the dosage of PSL was reduced to 5 mg.

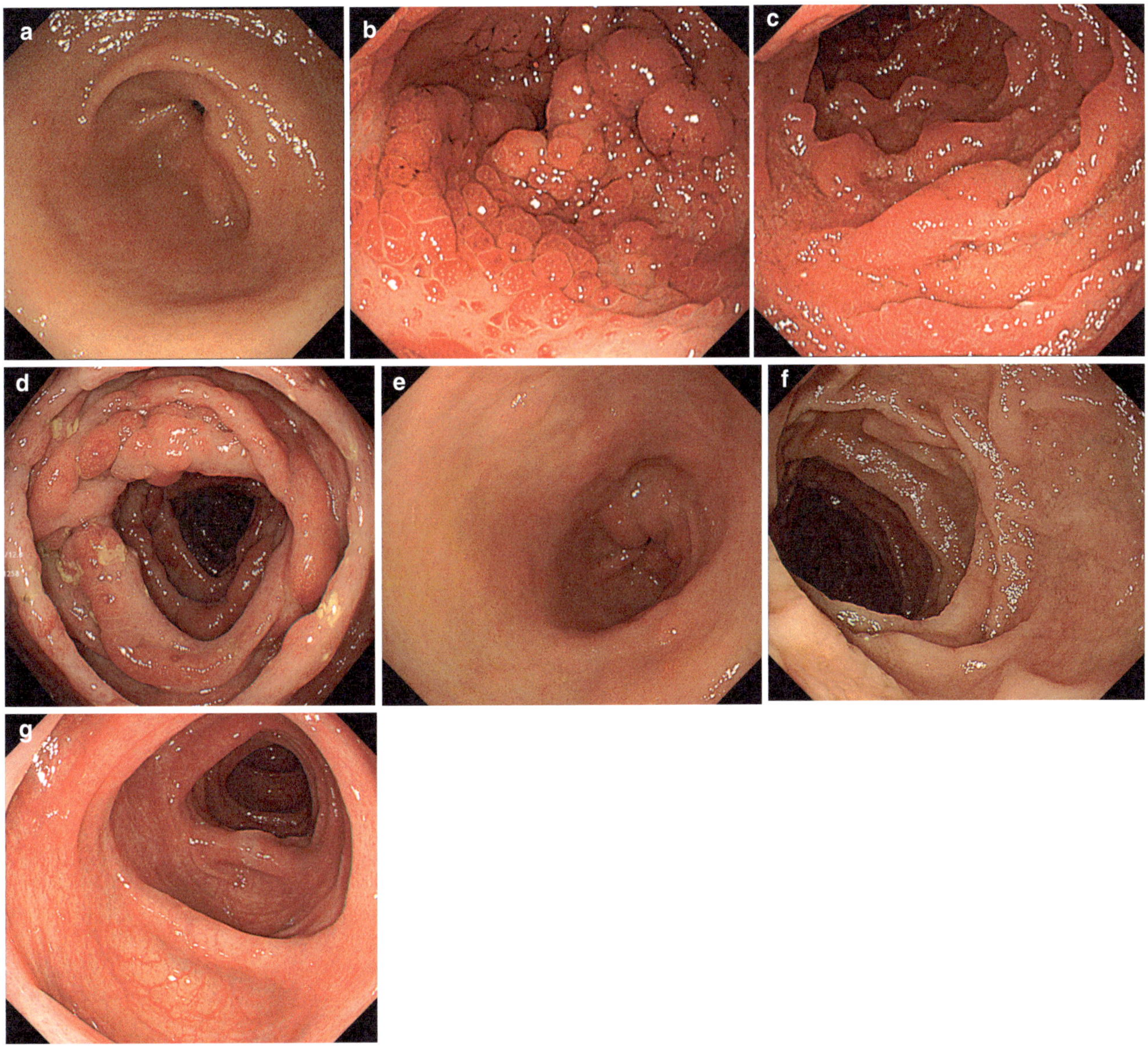

Fig. 3 (**a**), (**b**), (**e**) Gastric antrum. (**c**), (**f**) Duodenum. (**d**), (**g**) Colon. (**a**) Two years prior to the onset of disease at medical checkup. Neither inflammation nor polyps were present. (**b**), (**c**), (**d**) At onset. Stomach: Confluent type. Small to medium-sized polyps. Duodenum: Fold thickening type. Colon: Semi-confluent type. Medium polyps. (**e**), (**f**), (**g**) 6 months after the onset and treatments. Polyps and inflammatory findings disappeared with slightly edematous mucosa

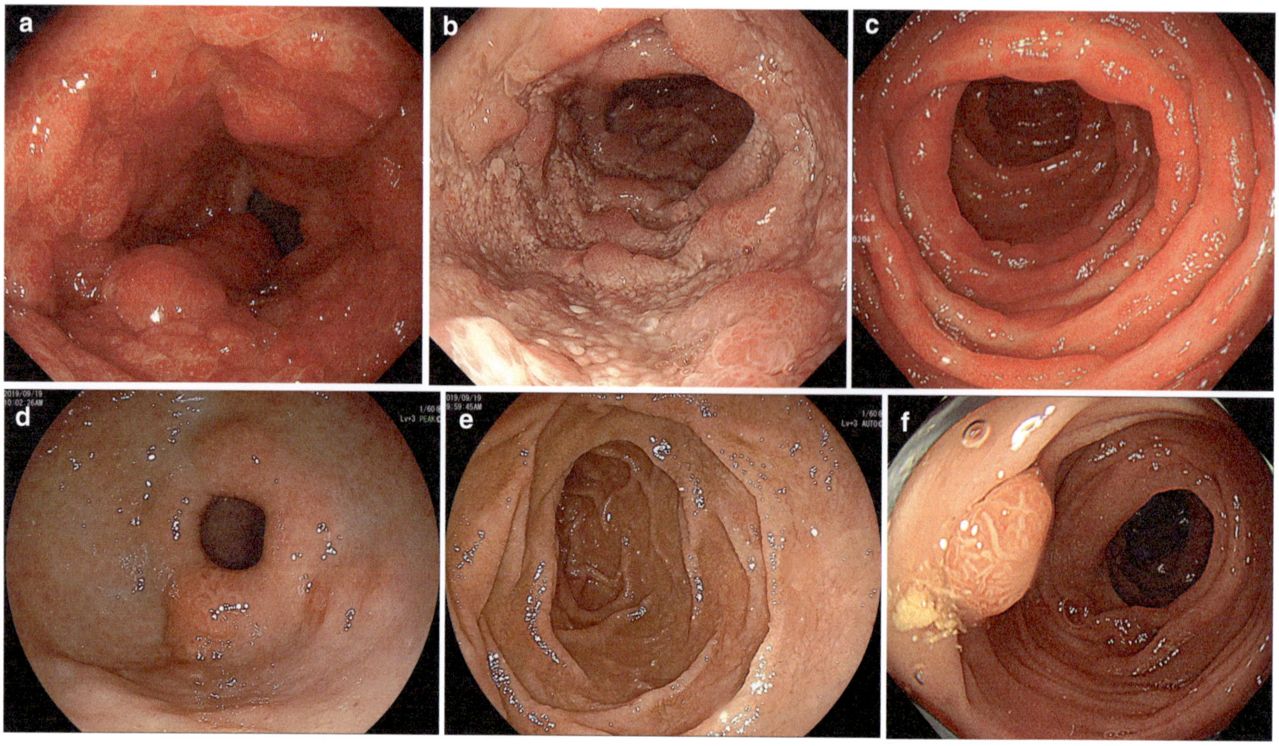

Fig. 4 (**a**), (**d**) Gastric antrum. (**b**), (**e**) Duodenum. (**c**), (**f**). Colon. (**a**), (**b**), (**c**) At relapse. Stomach: Confluent type. Medium polyps. Duodenum: Fold thickening type with white villi. Colon: Semi-confluent type. Small to medium polyps. Relapsing endoscopic finding similar to those of pre-treatments. (**d**), (**e**), (**f**) After reinduction of remission. Polyps disappeared with slightly edematous changes remained

Case 26: A case who achieved endoscopic remission by low-dose corticosteroids, but suffered from relapsing

Provided by Teppei Omori

[Patient]

A 66-year-old male. CC: Dysgeusia, onycholysis, hyperpigmentation of distal portion of extremities and palms, alopecia (head and beard).

[Clinical findings]

Alopecia (+), onychodystrophy (+), hyperpigmentation (+), dysgeusia (+), defecation: 15 times/day, mild edema.

[Laboratory findings]

Alb 3.9 mg/dL, CRP 0.13 mg/dL.

[Clinical course]

Relapse-remitting type.

Initial treatment: PSL 5 mg for 12 weeks.

Clinical response: 12 weeks.

Clinical remission: 24 weeks.

Therapeutic dose at relapse: PSL 3 mg.

Maintenance dose: PSL 0 mg.

[EGD findings] (Fig. 5a–i)

[CS findings] (Fig. 6a–f)

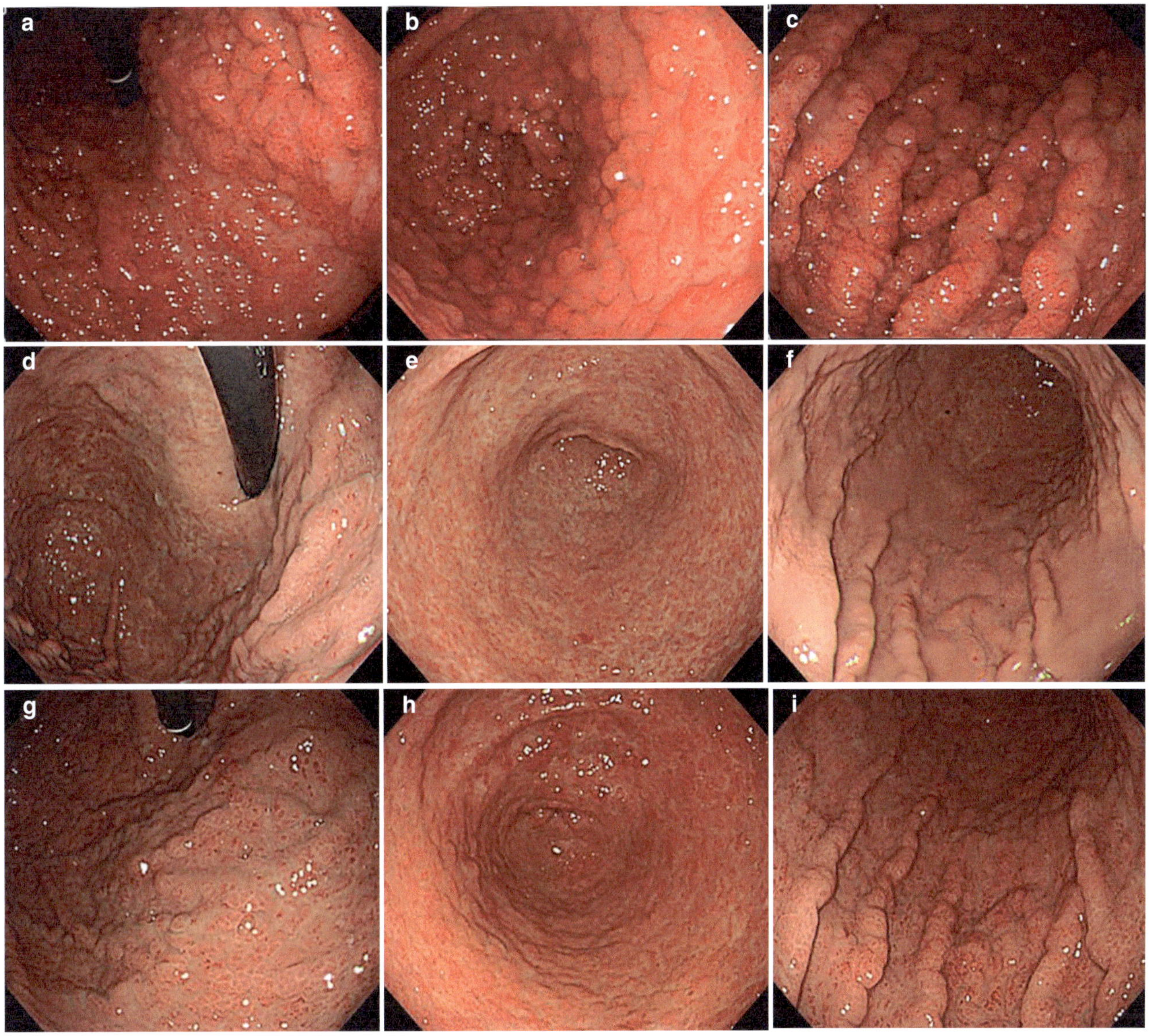

Fig. 5 (**a**), (**b**), (**c**) At the start of treatments. Confluent type. (**d**), (**e**), (**f**) Remission maintained with no PSL (60 months later). (**g**), (**h**), (**i**) At relapse

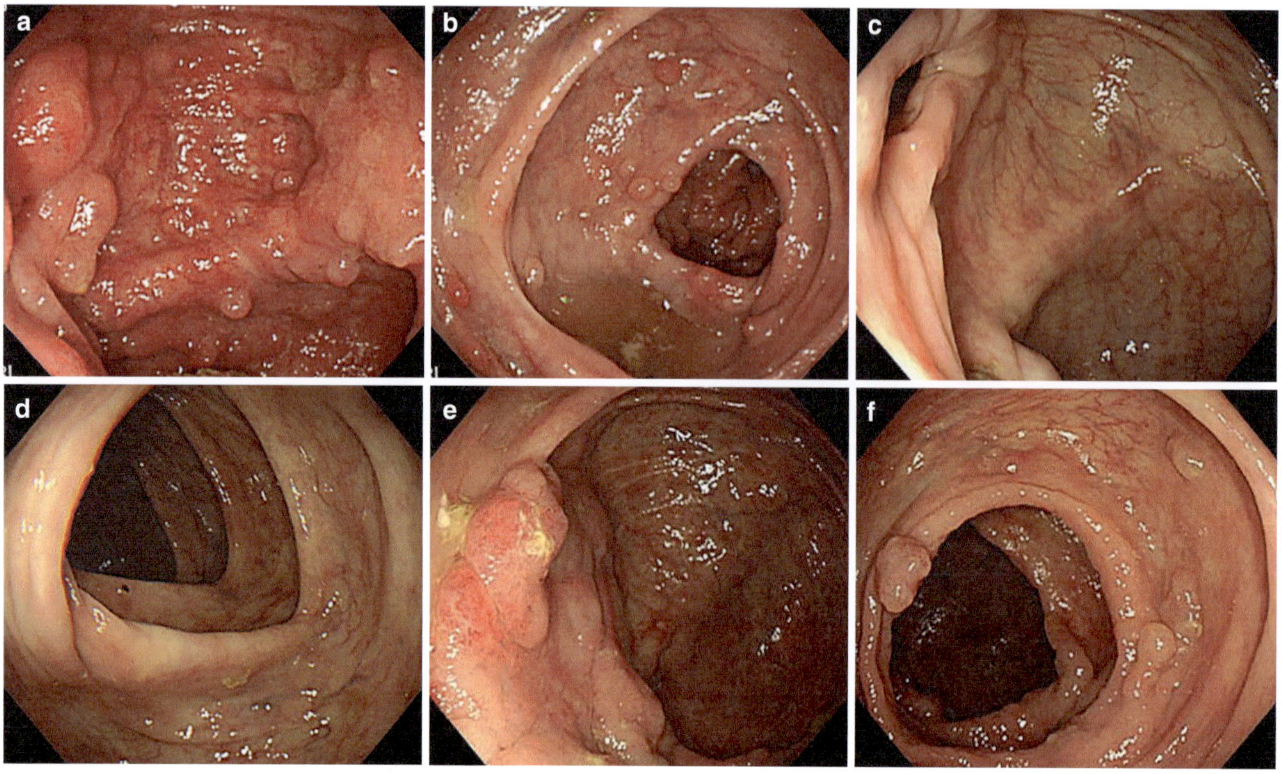

Fig. 6 (**a**), (**b**) At the start of treatments. Semi-confluent type. (**c**), (**d**) Remission maintained with no PSL (60 months later). (**e**), (**f**) At relapse

Case 27: A relapse-remitting case who required PSL 5 mg for maintenance and had a few residual polyps

Provided by Masakazu Nagahori

[Patient]

A 69-year-old man. CC: Dysgeusia, onychodystrophy, diarrhea.

[Clinical findings]

Alopecia (−), onychodystrophy (+), hyperpigmentation (−), dysgeusia (+), defecation: 4 times/day, mild edema.

[Laboratory findings]

Alb 3.3 mg/dL, CRP 1.84 mg/dL, Hb 14.6 g/dL.

[Endoscopic images 1] (Fig. 7a–d)

[Clinical course]

Relapse-remitting type.

Initial treatment: PSL 30 mg for 2 weeks.

Clinical response: 1 week.

Clinical remission: 6 weeks.

Therapeutic dose at relapse: PSL 30 mg.

Maintenance dose: PSL 5 mg.

[Endoscopic images 2] (Fig. 8)

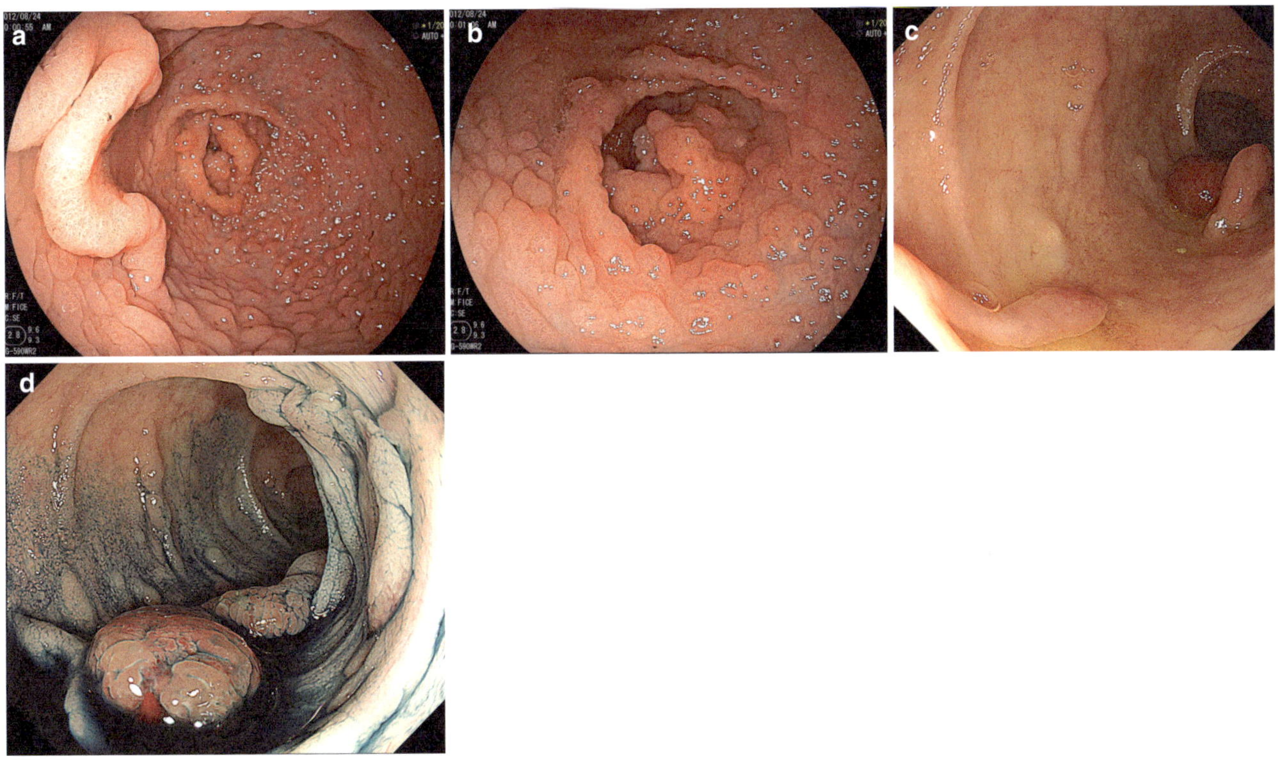

Fig. 7 (**a**), (**b**) Stomach: Confluent type. Small, edematous polyps. (**c**), (**d**) Terminal ileum: Sparse type. Medium polyps. Indigocarmine dyeing in (**d**)

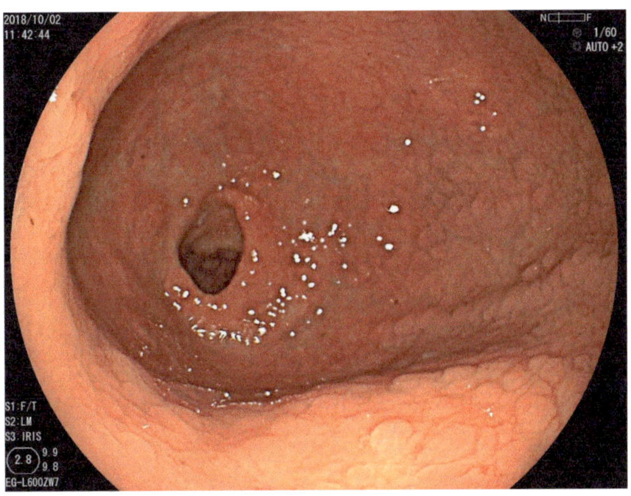

Fig. 8 EGD 6 years after the diagnosis. Although polyps remained, they shrunk

Case 28: A relapse-remitting case who required PSL 2.5 mg for maintenance and had residual endoscopic findings

Provided by Ken Sugimoto

[Patient]

A 73-year-old man. CC: Dysgeusia, diarrhea.

[Clinical findings]

Alopecia (+), onychodystrophy (+), hyperpigmentation (−), dysgeusia (+), defecation: 6 times/day. mild edema.

[Laboratory findings]

Alb 2.9 mg/dL, CRP 1.67 mg/dL, Hb 14.7 g/dL.

[Endoscopic images 1] (Fig. 9a, b)

[Clinical course]

Relapse-remitting type.

Initial treatment: PSL 20 mg for 2 weeks.

Clinical response: 2 weeks.

Clinical remission: 4 weeks.

Maintenance dose: 2.5 mg.

Therapeutic dose at relapse: PSL 20 mg.

[Endoscopic images 2] (Fig. 10a–c)

EGD and CS after treatments.

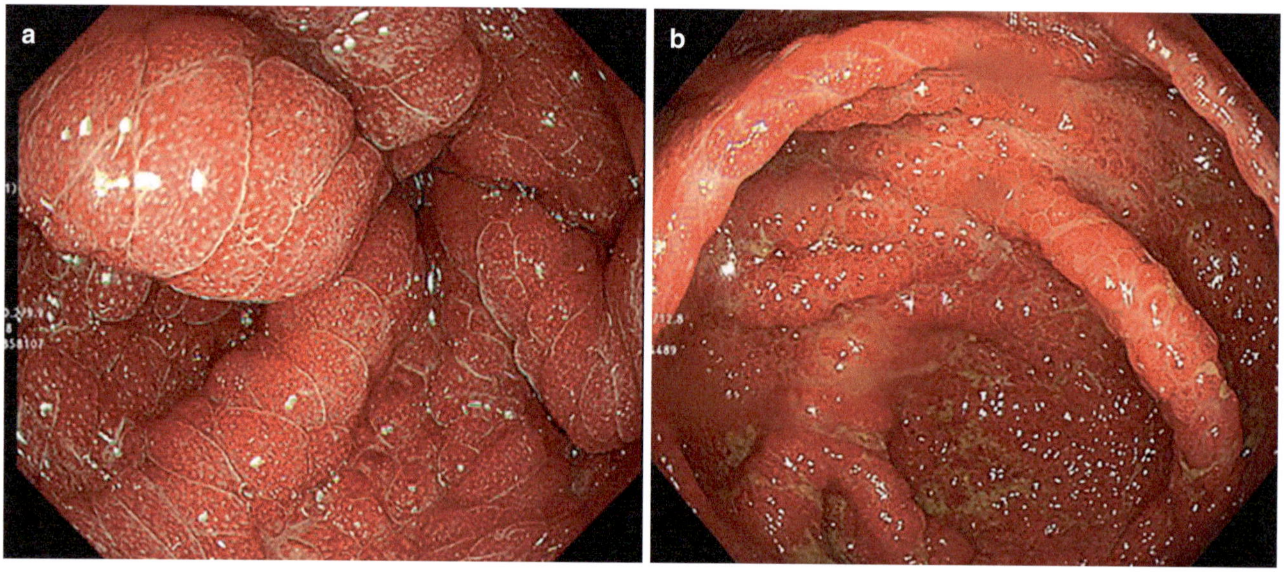

Fig. 9 (**a**) Stomach: Confluent type. Medium, edematous, and erythematous polyps. (**b**) Colon: Confluent type. Small, edematous, and erythematous polyps

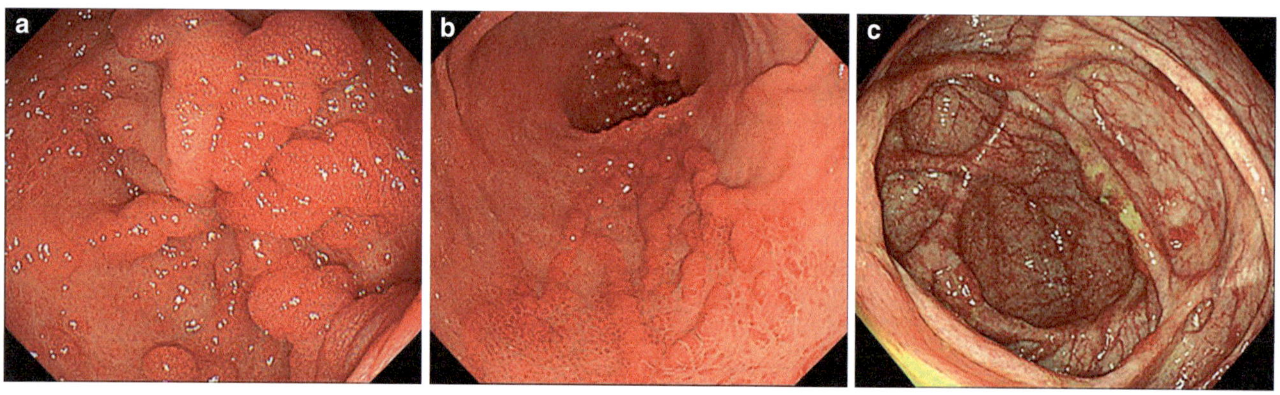

Fig. 10 (**a**), (**b**) Gastric polyps mostly disappeared, but redness and edema of the mucosa remained. (**c**) Colon: Only some erythematous polyps remained

Case 29: A relapse-remitting case who required PSL 2.5 mg for maintenance and increased the dose to 5 mg at relapse

Provided by Naoki Hosoe and Takanori Kanai

[Patient]

A 60-year-old man. CC: Dysgeusia, diarrhea, alopecia, onychodystrophy.

[Clinical findings]

Alopecia (+), onychodystrophy (+), hyperpigmentation (+), dysgeusia (+), mild edema.

[Laboratory findings]

Alb 3.8 mg/dL, CRP 0.05 mg/dL, Hb 15.9 g/dL.

[Endoscopic images] (Fig. 11)

[Clinical course]

Relapse-remitting type

Initial treatment: PSL 30 mg for 4 weeks.

Clinical response: 8 weeks.

Clinical remission: 12 weeks.

Maintenance dose: PSL 2.5 mg.

Therapeutic dose at relapse: PSL 5 mg.

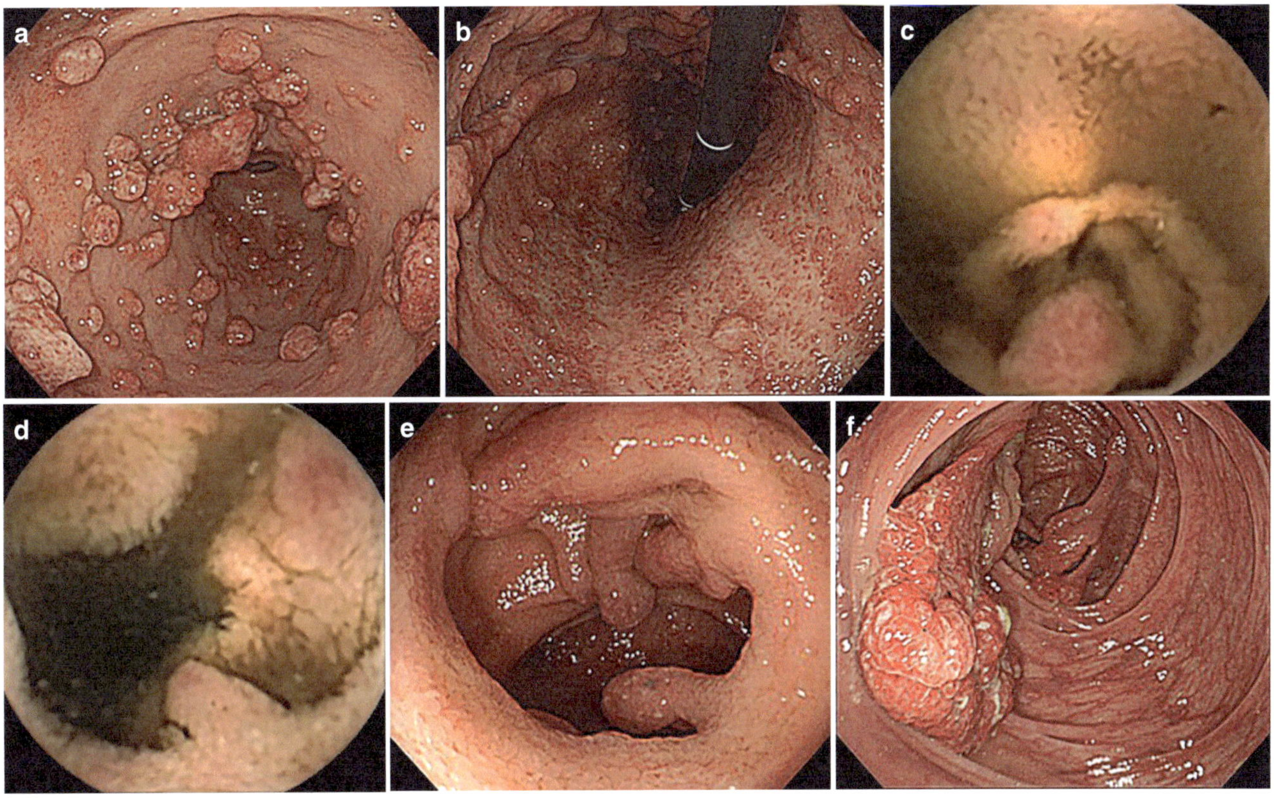

Fig. 11 (**a**), (**b**) Stomach: Semi-confluent type. Large, edematous, and erythematous polyps. (**c**), (**d**) Jejunum and ileum (SBCE): Sparse type. Small polyps. (**e**) Terminal ileum: Semi-confluent type. Small polyps. (**f**) Colon: Prolapsing polyps from the ileum

Case 30: A relapse-remitting case who responded to combination of corticosteroids and tranexamic acid at relapse and achieved steroid-free clinical remission

Provided by Makoto Ooi and Yuzo Kodama

[Patient]

A 65-year-old man. CC: Watery diarrhea, dysgeusia, onychodystrophy.

[Clinical findings]

Alopecia (−), onychodystrophy (+), hyperpigmentation (+), dysgeusia (+).

[Laboratory findings]

Alb 2.6 mg/dL, CRP 3.29 mg/dL, Hb 7.7 g/dL.

[Endoscopic images 1]

No image before treatments because he was diagnosed at another hospital

[Clinical course]

Relapse-remitting type.

Initial treatment: PSL 20 mg.

Therapeutic does at relapse: PSL 40 mg with tranexamic acid 750 mg.

Endoscopic remission: 41 months.

Maintenance dose: PSL 0 mg.

[Endoscopic images 2] (Fig. 12)

EGD and CS after treatments.

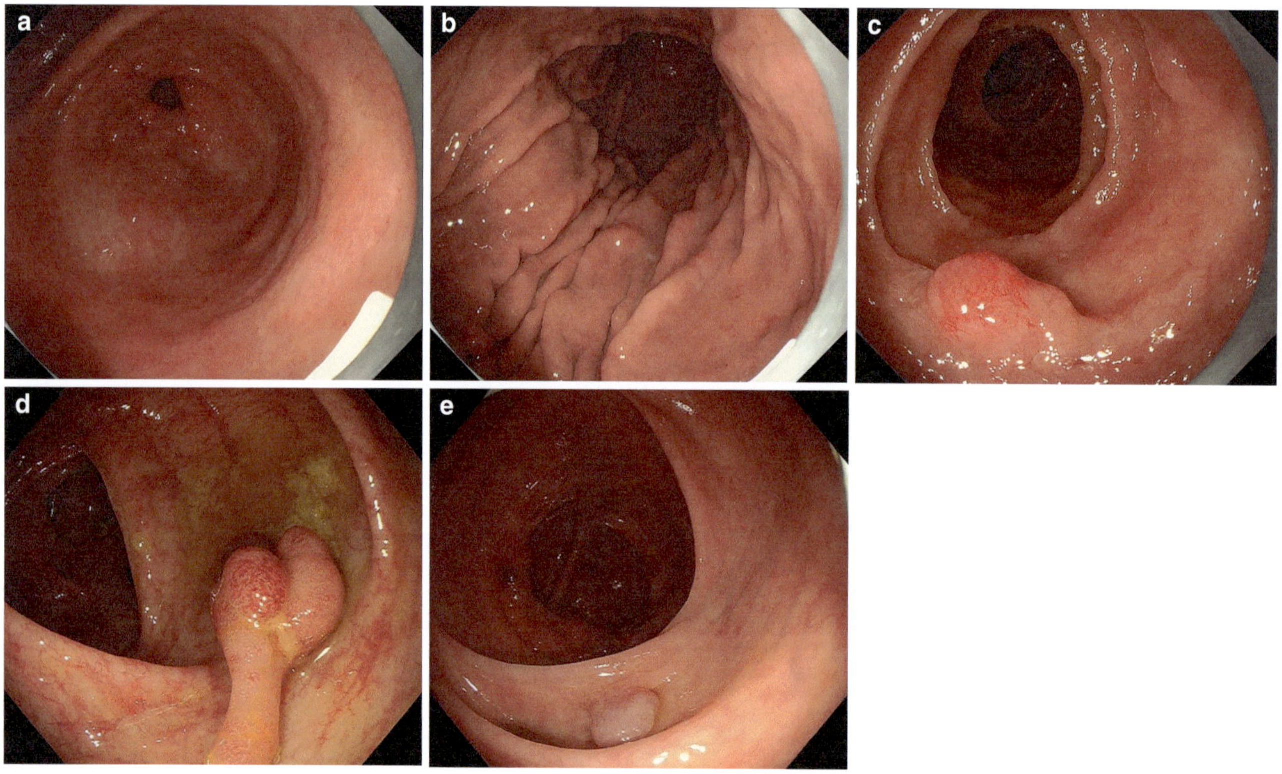

Fig. 12 (**a**), (**b**) Gastric polyps almost completely disappeared. (**c**) Duodenum: Single medium-sized polyp. (**d**), (**e**) Colon: Sparse type. Medium polyps

Case 31: A relapse-remitting case who was diagnosed at age 33 and suffered from relapsing after 20 years' stable disease

Provided by Noriko Kamata

[Patient]

A 53-year-old female. She had been diagnosed as Cronkhite–Canada syndrome 20 years ago and had been stable but developed following symptoms again. CC: General malaise, diarrhea, dysgeusia, alopecia (hair, eyebrows, eyelashes), diarrhea, and edema of the lower legs.

[Clinical findings]

Alopecia (+), onychodystrophy (+), hyperpigmentation (−), dysgeusia (+), defecation: 3 times/day.

[Laboratory findings]

Alb 2.2 mg/dL, CRP 0.79 mg/dL, Hb 12.5 g/dL.

[Endoscopic images 1] (Fig. 13a–d)

[Clinical course]

Relapse-remitting type.

Initial treatment: PSL 30 mg for 2 weeks.

Clinical response: 2 weeks.

Endoscopic response: 2 months.

Endoscopic remission: 3 months.

Therapeutic dose at relapse: PSL 60 mg.

Maintenance dose: PSL 0 mg.

[Endoscopic images 2] (Fig. 14a–d)

EGD and CS 10 months after the diagnosis.

Inflammation improved and polyps almost disappeared in the stomach and colon.

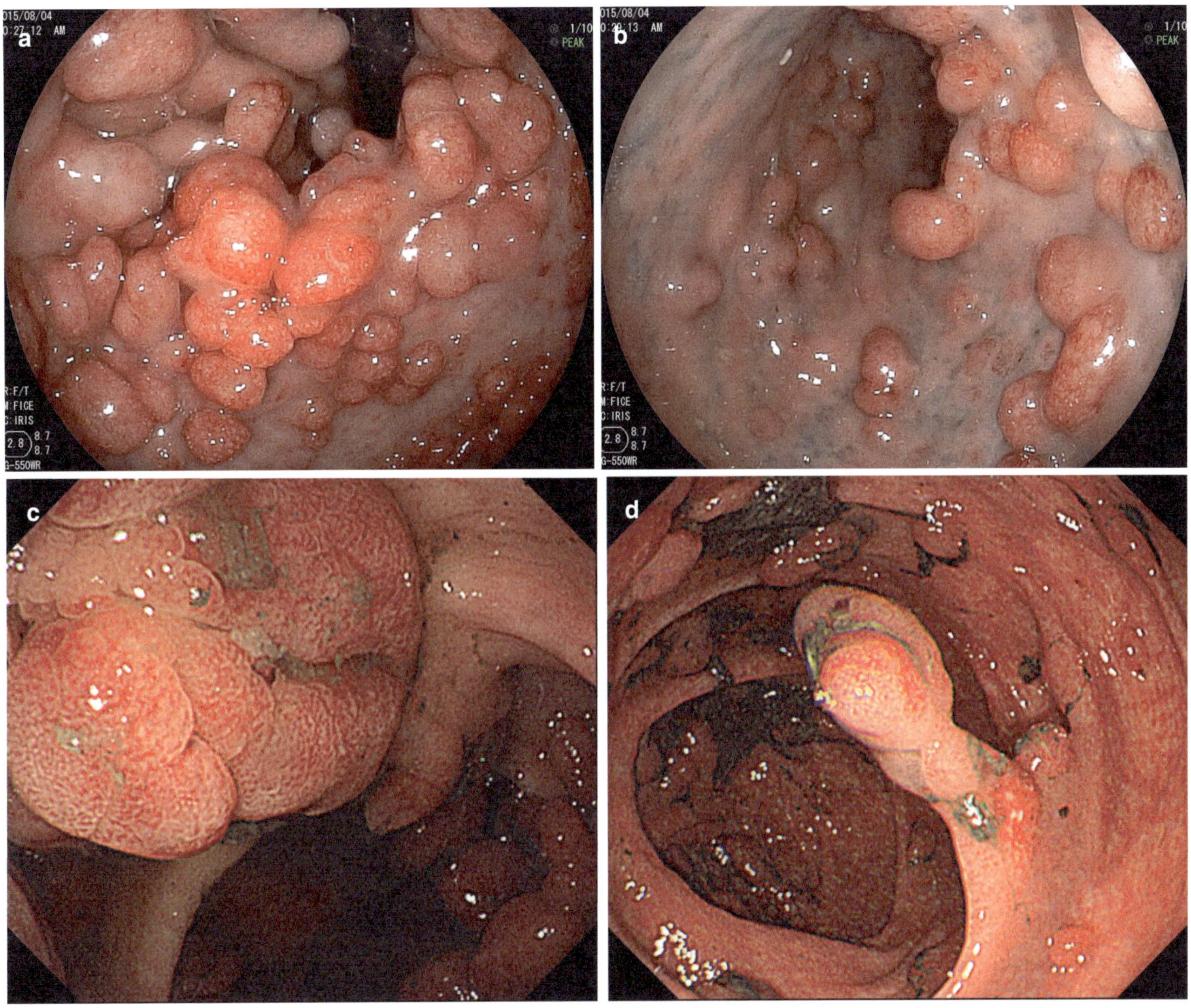

Fig. 13 (**a**), (**b**) Stomach: Confluent type. Medium, edematous, erythematous, and hemorrhagic polyps. (**c**), (**d**) Colon: Sparse type. Medium, edematous, and erythematous polyps

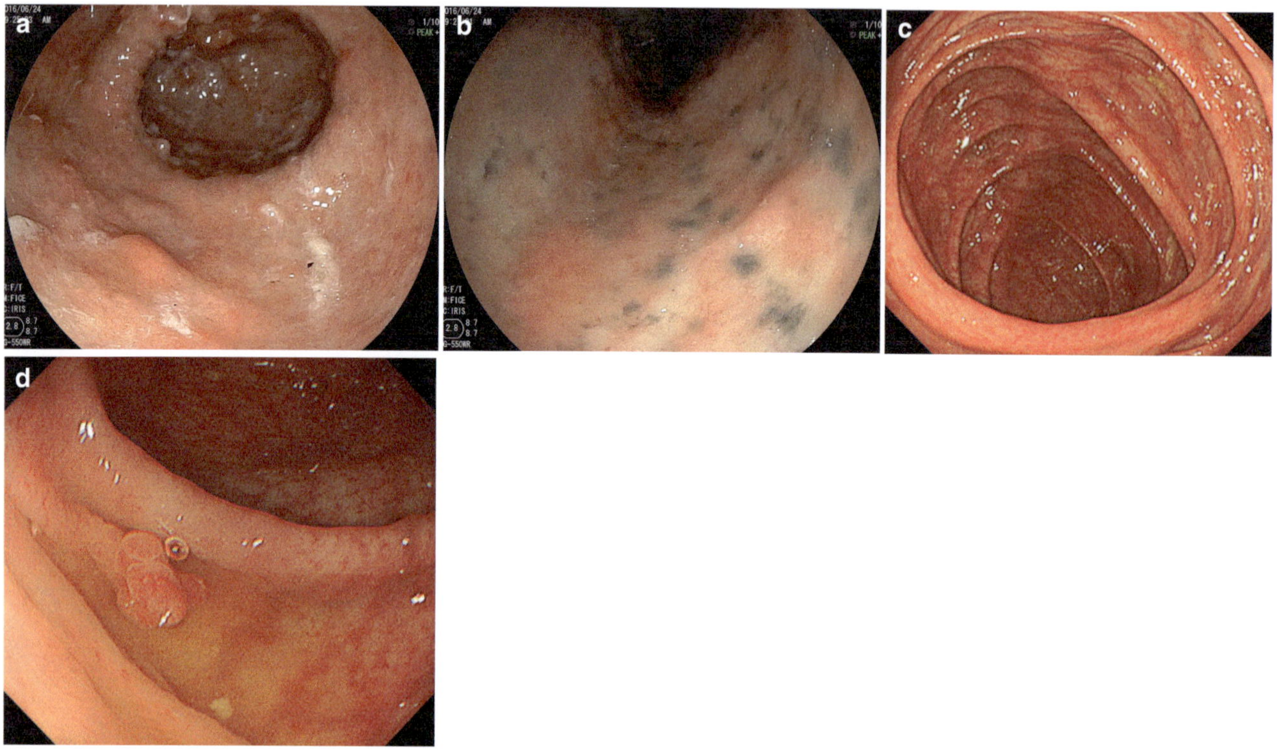

Fig. 14 (**a**), (**b**) Stomach. (**c**), (**d**) Colon

Case 32: A relapse-remitting case who achieved reinduction of remission with a small amount of PSL at relapse and maintained steroid-free remission

Provided by Teppei Omori

[Patient]

A 53-year-old man. CC: Diarrhea, dysgeusia, onycholysis, weakness, edema of lower limbs.

[Clinical findings]

Alopecia (−), onychodystrophy (+), hyperpigmentation (−), dysgeusia (+), mild edema.

[Laboratory findings]

Alb 1.4 mg/dL, CRP negative, Hb 16.9 g/dL.

[Endoscopic images] (Fig. 15)

[Clinical course]

Relapse-remitting type.

Initial treatment: PSL 40 mg for 3 weeks.

Clinical response: 3 weeks.

Clinical remission: 8 weeks.

Therapeutic dose at relapse: PSL 5 mg.

Maintenance dose: PSL 0 mg.

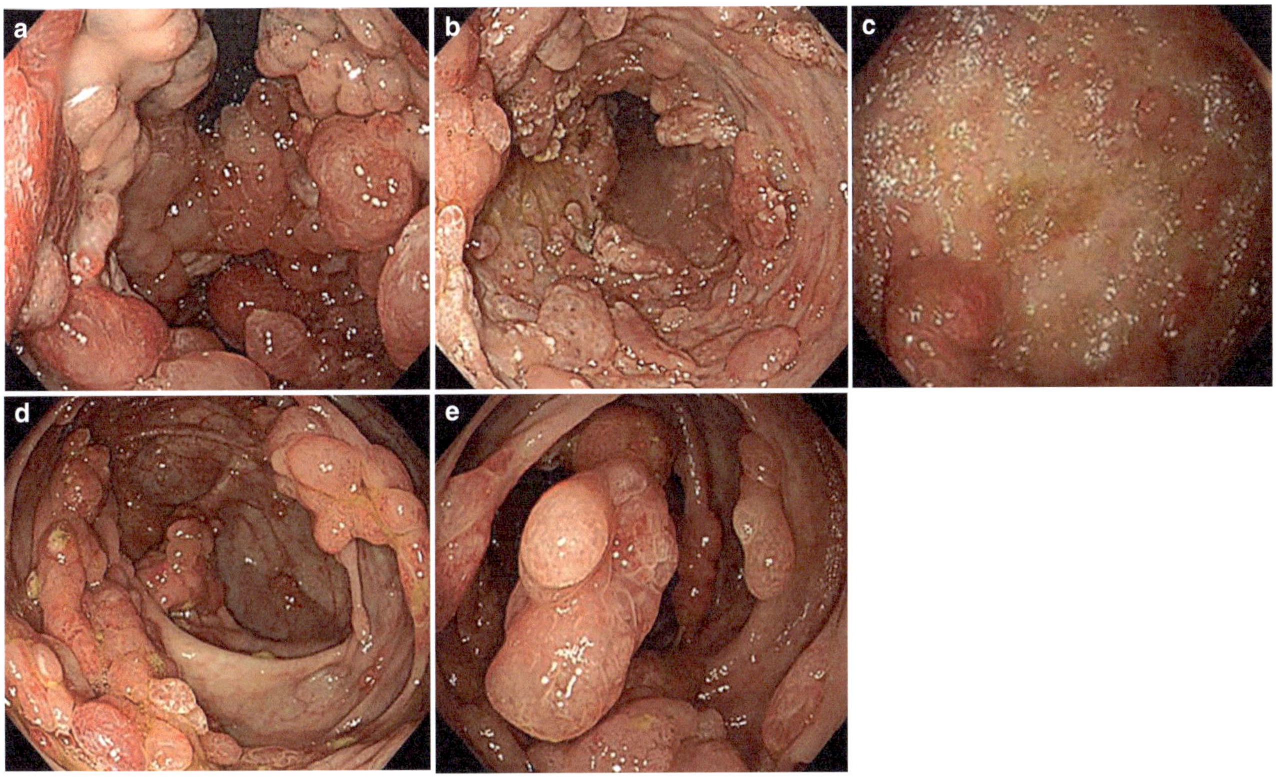

Fig. 15 (**a**) Stomach: Confluent type. Medium, edematous, and erythematous polyps. (**b**) Duodenum: Semi-confluent type. Medium polyps with white villi. Edematous intervening mucosa. (**c**) Ileum: Sparse type. Small polyps. (**d**), (**e**) Colon: Sparse type. Large, edematous polyps

Case 33: A relapse-remitting case who achieved reinduction of remission with a small amount of PSL at relapse and maintained steroid-free remission

Provided by Teppei Omori

[Patient]

A 53-year-old man. CC: Diarrhea, dysgeusia, onycholysis, weakness, edema of lower limbs.

[Clinical findings]

Alopecia (−), onychodystrophy (+), hyperpigmentation (−), dysgeusia (+), mild edema.

[Laboratory findings]

Alb 1.6 mg/dL, CRP 0.13 mg/dL, Hb 10.0 g/dL.

[Clinical course]

Initial treatment: PSL 40 mg for 3 weeks.

Clinical response: 3 weeks.

Clinical remission: 8 weeks.

Therapeutic dose at relapse: PSL 5 mg.

Maintenance dose: 0 mg.

[Endoscopic images] (Fig. 16)

(a) ~ (d): Before treatments.

(e) ~ (h): After treatments.

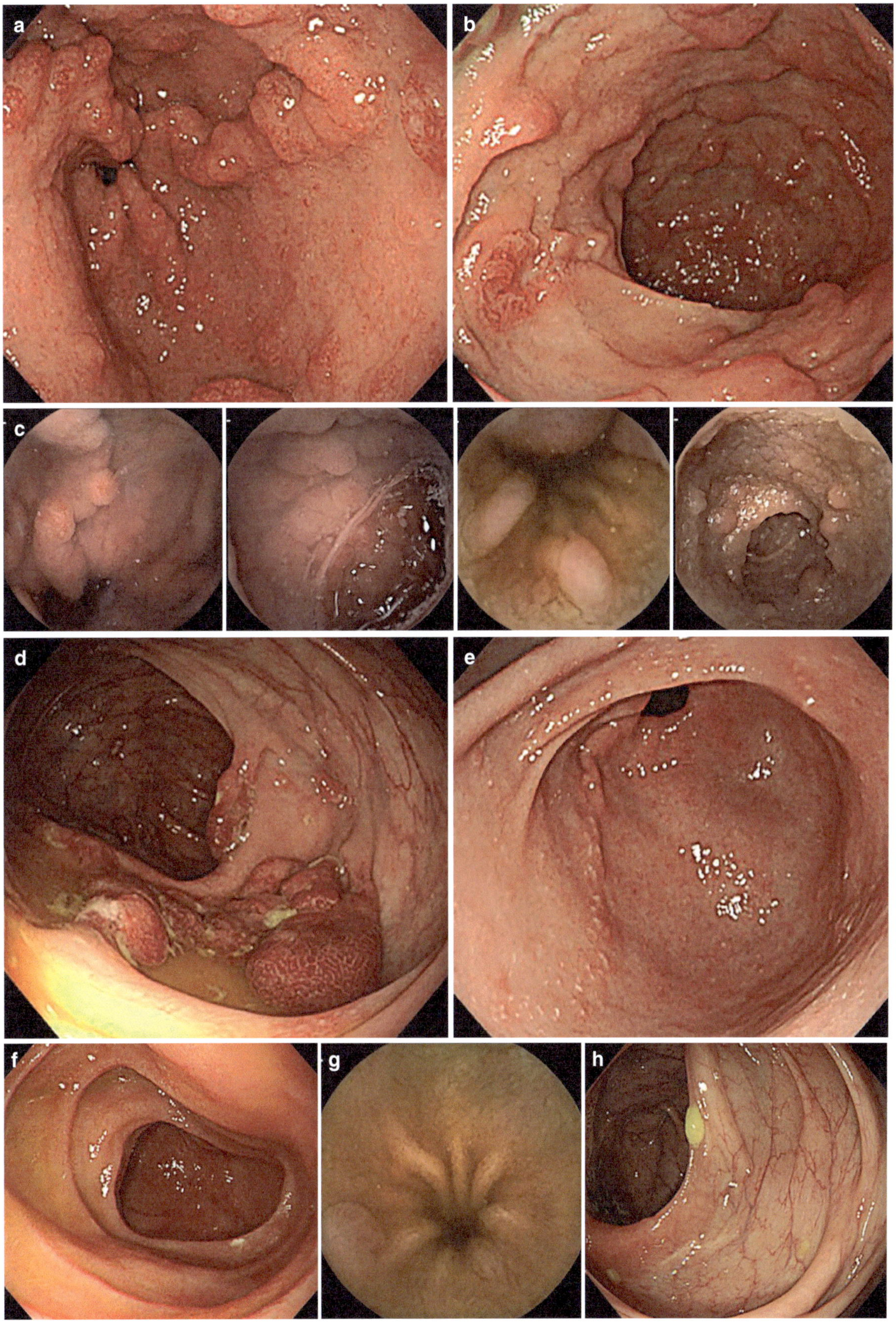

Fig. 16 (**a**) Stomach: Semi-confluent type. Medium, edematous, and erythematous polyps. (**b**) Duodenum: Semi-confluent type. Small polyps. (**c**, 4 images) Small intestine (SBCE): Semi-confluent type. Small polyps. (**d**) Colon: Sparse type. Large, edematous polyps. Polyps diminished and inflammatory findings improved in the stomach (**e**), duodenum (**f**), small intestine (**g**) and colon (**h**) after treatments

Case 34: A relapse-remitting case who did not respond to PSL 30 mg but responded when increased to 60 mg

Povided by Katsuyoshi Matsuoka and Yasuo Suzuki

[Patient]

An 83-year-old man. CC: Diarrhea, alopecia, dysgeusia.

[Clinical findings]

Alopecia (+), onychodystrophy (−), hyperpigmentation (−), dysgeusia (+), defecation: 6 times/day.

[Laboratory findings]

Alb 3.6 mg/dL, CRP 0.93 mg/dL, Hb 16.1 g/dL.

[Endoscopic images 1] (Fig. 17a–c)

[Clinical course]

Relapse-remitting type.

Oral intake of PSL 30 mg was ineffective.

Symptoms improved after intravenous administration of PSL 60 mg.

Clinical response: 1 week.

Clinical remission: 4 weeks.

Therapeutic dose at relapse: PSL 30mg.

Maintenance dose: PSL 2.5 mg.

[Endoscopic images 2] (Fig. 18a, b)

EGD and CS during remission.

Endoscopic findings improved but did not achieve remission.

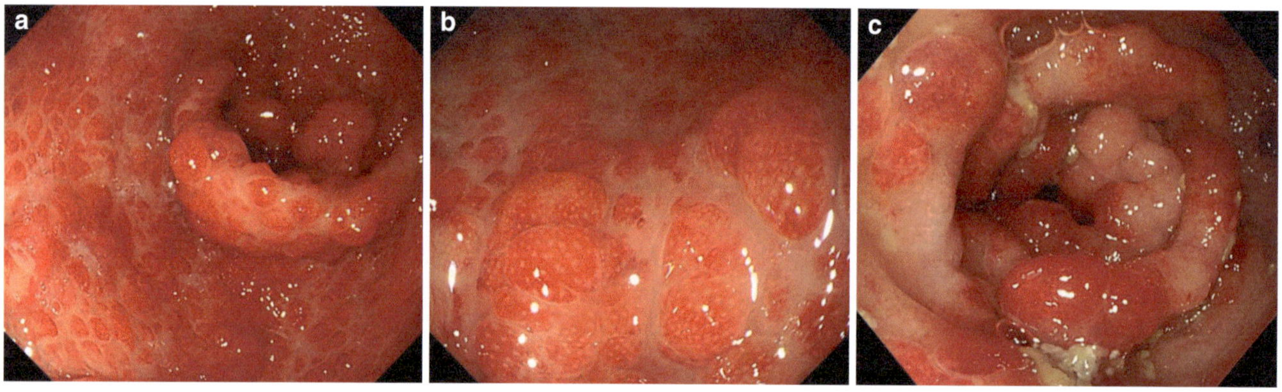

Fig. 17 (**a**), (**b**) Stomach: Confluent type. Small, erythematous polyps. (**c**) Colon: Confluent type. Medium, edematous, and erythematous polyps

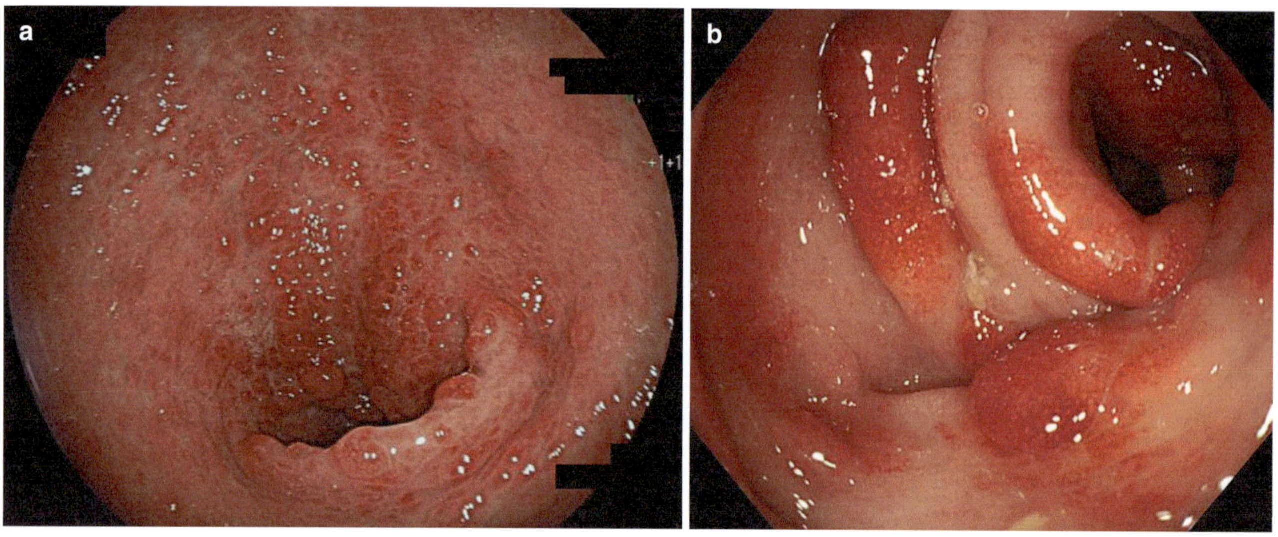

Fig. 18 (**a**) Stomach (1 year after the diagnosis). (**b**) Colon (3 years after the diagnosis)

Case 35: A relapse-remitting case who required PSL 4 mg for maintenance and increased the dose to 20 mg at relapse

Provided by Miwa Sada and Kiyonori Kobayashi

[Patient]

A 52-year-old woman. CC: Diarrhea, weight loss, hyperpigmentation of extremities.

[Clinical findings]

Alopecia (+), onychodystrophy (+), hyperpigmentation (+), dysgeusia (+), defecation: 10 times/day, mild edema.

[Laboratory findings]

Alb 4.1 mg/dL, CRP 0.01 mg/dL, Hb 11.8 g/dL.

[Endoscopic images] (Fig. 19)

[Clinical course]

Relapse-remitting type.

Initial treatment: PSL 50 mg for 1 week.

Clinical response: 3 weeks.

Clinical remission: 5 weeks.

Maintenance dose: PSL 4 mg.

Therapeutic dose at relapse: PSL 20 mg.

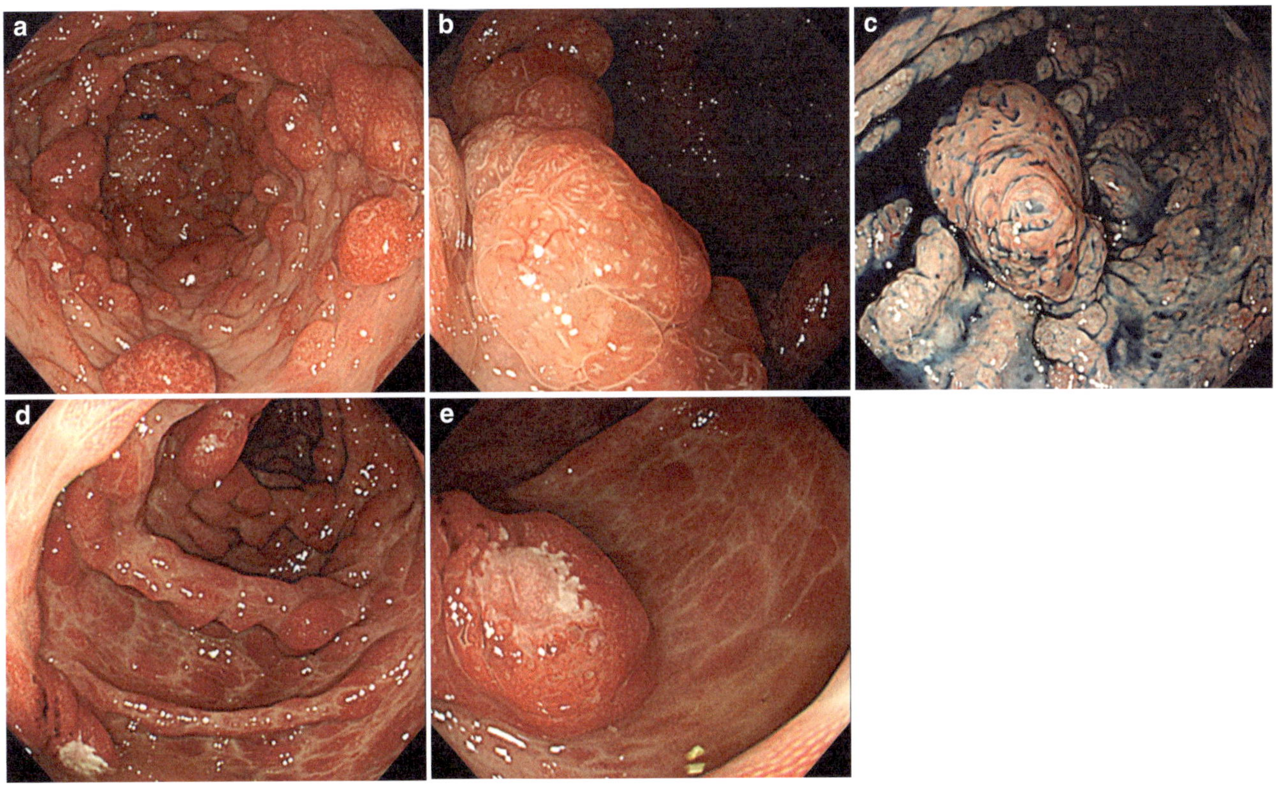

Fig. 19 (**a**), (**b**), (**c**) Stomach: Confluent type. Large, edematous, and erythematous polyps. Indigocarmine dyeing in (**c**). (**d**), (**e**) Colon: Confluent type. Large, edematous, erosive, and whitish mucus adhered polyps

Case 36: A relapse-remitting case who achieved reinduction of remission by PSL 2 mg at relapse

Provided by Mari Hayashida

[Patient]

A 68-year-old man.CC: Abnormal findings by barium contrast X-ray and hypoproteinemia in medical checkup.

[Clinical findings]

Alopecia (+), onychodystrophy (+), hyperpigmentation (−), dysgeusia (+), defecation: 3 times/day, mild edema.

[Laboratory findings]

Alb 2.1 mg/dL, CRP 0.2 mg/dL, Hb 13.3 g/dL.

Fecal alpha1-antitrypsin clearance: 215 mL/day

[Endoscopic images] (Fig. 20)

[Clinical course]

Relapse-remitting type.

Initial treatment: PSL 40 mg for 2 weeks.

Clinical response: 3 weeks.

Clinical remission: 36 weeks.

Maintenance dose: PSL 0 mg.

Therapeutic dose at relapse: PSL 2 mg.

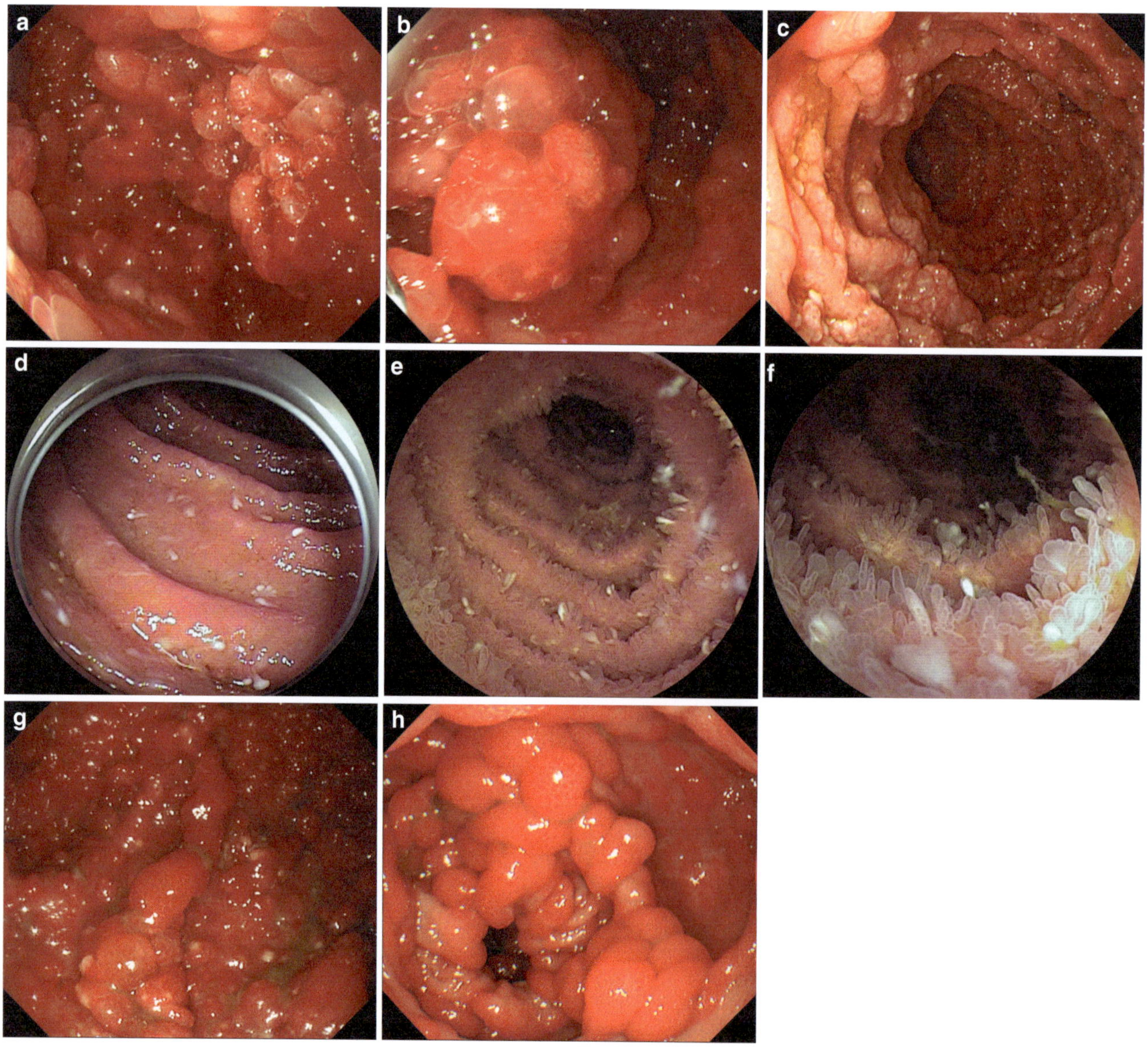

Fig. 20 (**a**), (**b**) Stomach: Confluent type. Medium, edematous, erythematous, and hemorrhagic polyps. Edematous intervening mucosa. (**c**) Duodenum: Fold thickening type with small polyps and white villi. (**d**), (**e**), (**f**) Jejunum: Fold thickening type with small polyps. Scattered polypoid lesions with elongated villi containing whitish material inside. (**g**), (**h**) Colon: Confluent type. Small, edematous, erythematous, and whitish mucus adhered polyps

Case 37: A relapse-remitting case who required PSL 6 mg for maintenance and increased the dose to 8 mg at relapse

Provided by Mari Hayashida

[Patient]

A 73-year-old male. CC: Diarrhea, hypoproteinemia, and leg edema appeared during follow-up for multiple colorectal polyps.

[Clinical findings]

Alopecia (+), onychodystrophy (+), hyperpigmentation (+), dysgeusia (+), defecation: 10 times/day, severe edema.

[Laboratory findings]

Alb 1.6 mg/dL, CRP 0.3 mg/dL, Hb 12.5 g/dL.

[Endoscopic images 1] (Fig. 21)

[Clinical course]

Relapse-remitting type.

Initial treatment: PSL 30 mg for 3 weeks.

Clinical response: 1 week.

Clinical remission: 3 weeks.

Maintenance dose: PSL 6 mg.

Therapeutic does at relapse: PSL 8 mg.

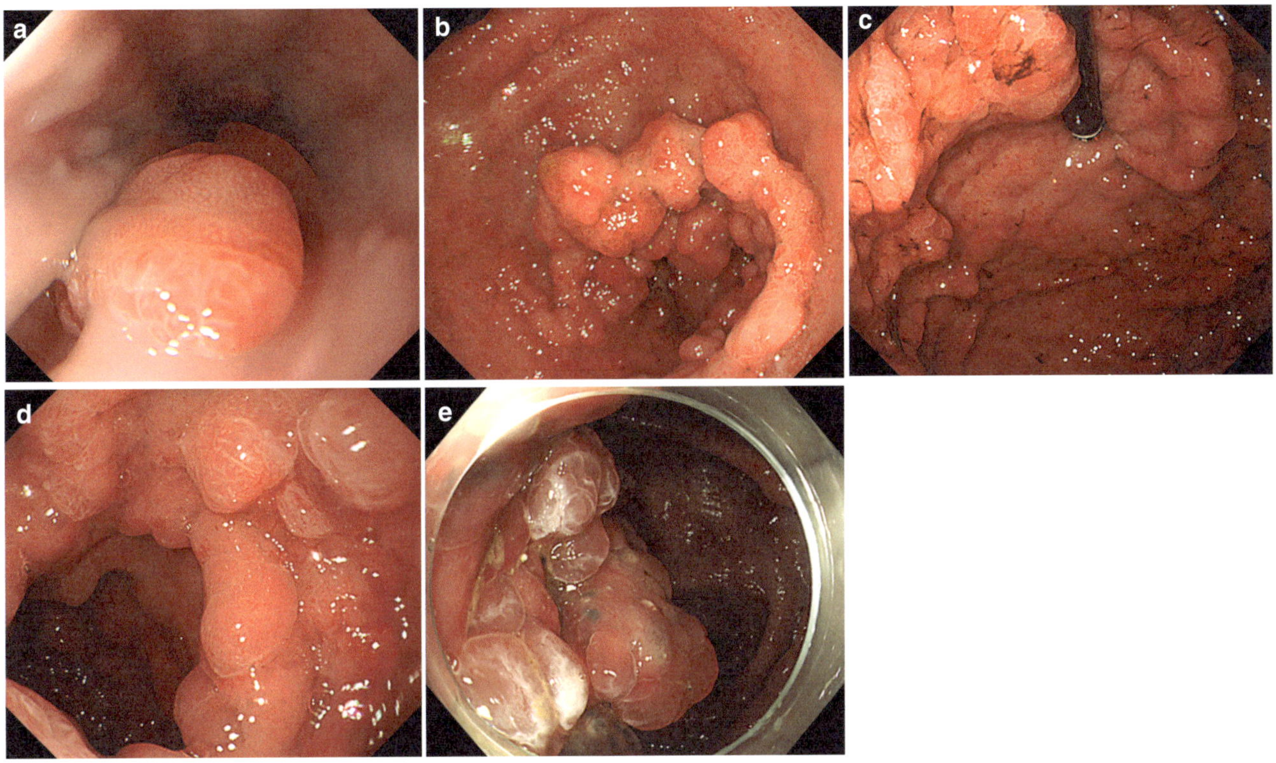

Fig. 21 (**a**) Esophagus: Sparse type. Medium, edematous, and erythematous polyps. (**b**), (**c**) Stomach: Confluent type. Large, edematous, erythematous, and hemorrhagic polyps. (**d**) Duodenum: Confluent type. Small polyps. (**e**) Colon: Confluent type. Large, edematous, erythematous, erosive, and white mucus adhered polyps

Case 38: A case who required PSL 2.5 mg for maintenance and increased the dose to 30 mg at relapse

Provided by Takehiro Torisu and Junji Umeno

[Patient]

A 69-year-old male. CC: Dysgeusia, diarrhea

[Clinical findings]

Alopecia (+), onychodystrophy (+), hyperpigmentation (−), defecation: 5 times/day.

[Laboratory findings]

Alb 3.6 mg/dL, CRP 1.24 mg/dL, Hb 12.9 g/dL.

[Endoscopic images] (Fig. 22)

[Clinical course]

Relapse-remitting type.

Initial treatment: PSL 60 mg for 2 weeks.

Clinical response: 8 weeks.

Clinical remission: 12 weeks.

Maintenance dose: PSL 2.5 mg.

Therapeutic dose at relapse: PSL 30 mg.

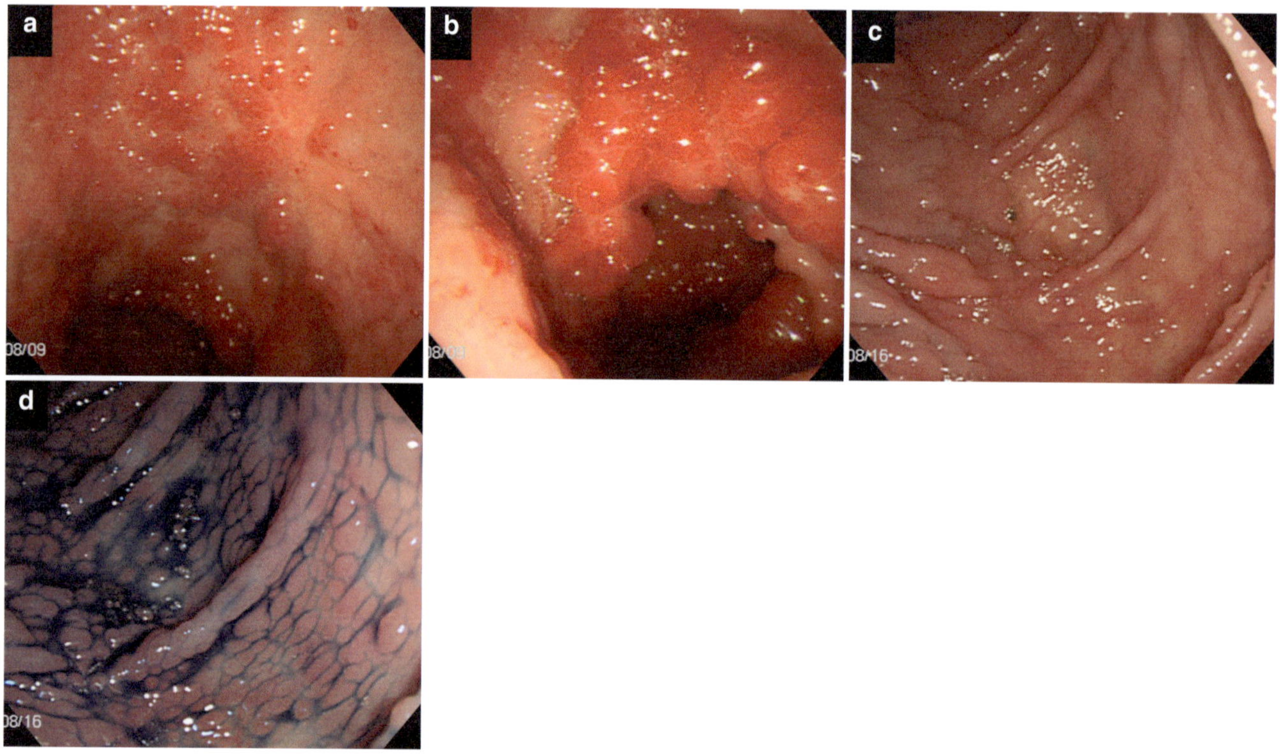

Fig. 22 (**a**), (**b**) Stomach: Semi-confluent type. Medium, erythematous, edematous, and hemorrhagic polyps. (**c**) Colon: Confluent type. Edematous and erythematous polyps. (**d**) Indigocarmine dyeing of (**c**)

Case 39: A relapse-remitting case who maintained steroid-free remission

Provided by Noriko Kamata

[Patient]

A 65-year-old male. CC: Dysgeusia, alopecia (hair, eyebrows, eyelashes, beard), diarrhea, leg edema.

[Clinical findings]

Alopecia (+), onychodystrophy (+), hyperpigmentation (−), dysgeusia (+), defecation: 4 times/day.

[Laboratory findings]

Alb 3.0 mg/dL, CRP 0.12 mg/dL, Hb 11.6 g/dL.

[Cutaneous manifestations] (Fig. 23)

[Clinical course]

Relapse-remitting type.

Initial treatment: PSL 30 mg for 2 weeks.

Clinical response: 2 weeks.

Endoscopic response: 2 months.

Endoscopic remission: 3 months.

Maintenance dose: PSL 0 mg.

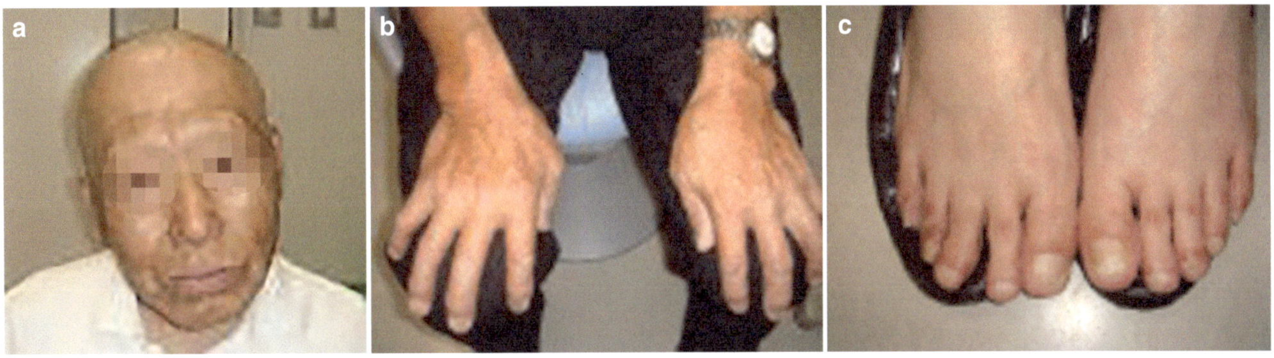

Fig. 23 (**a**) Head: Loss of hair from the face (eyebrows, eyelashes, beard) and head. (**b**) Hands: Onychodystrophy. (**c**) Feet: Onychodystrophy

2 Chronic Continuous Cases

Case 40: A chronic continuous case who responded slowly to corticosteroids

Provided by Masaru Nakano

[Patient]

A 63-year-old male. CC: Dysgeusia, diarrhea, weight loss, dyschromatosis (pigmentation and depigmentation), onychodystrophy, alopecia, bloody stool.

[Clinical findings]

Alopecia (+), onychodystrophy (+), hyperpigmentation (+), dysgeusia (+), defecation: 10 times/day.

[Laboratory findings]

Alb 3.5 mg/dL, CRP 0.03 mg/dL, Hb 14.4 g/dL.

[Photographs of cutaneous findings] (Fig. 24a–d)

Pigmentation of the fingers and toes peripherally from the distal interphalangeal (DIP) joint.

[Endoscopic images] (Fig. 25a–h)

[Clinical course]

Chronic continuous type.

Initial treatment: PSL 30 mg for 6 weeks.

Clinical response: 8 weeks.

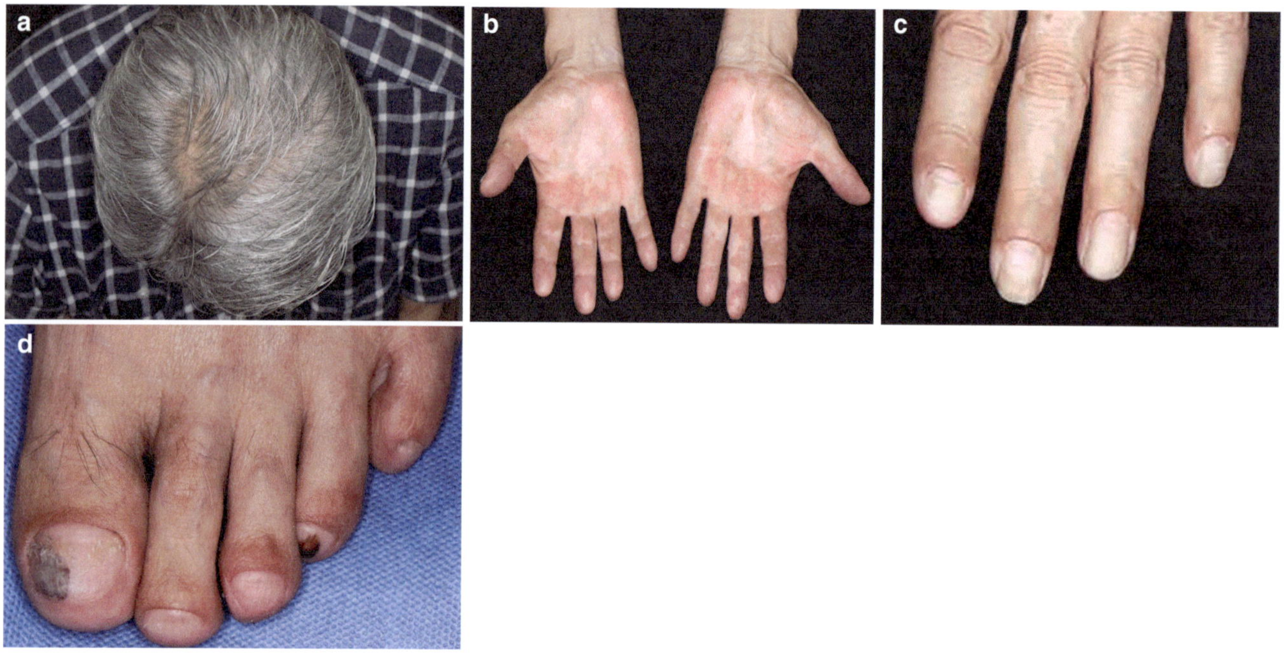

Fig. 24 (**a**) Head: Mild alopecia. (**b**) Hands: Hyperpigmentation of the palms. (**c**) Fingers: Onychodystrophy. (**d**) Toes: Onychodystrophy

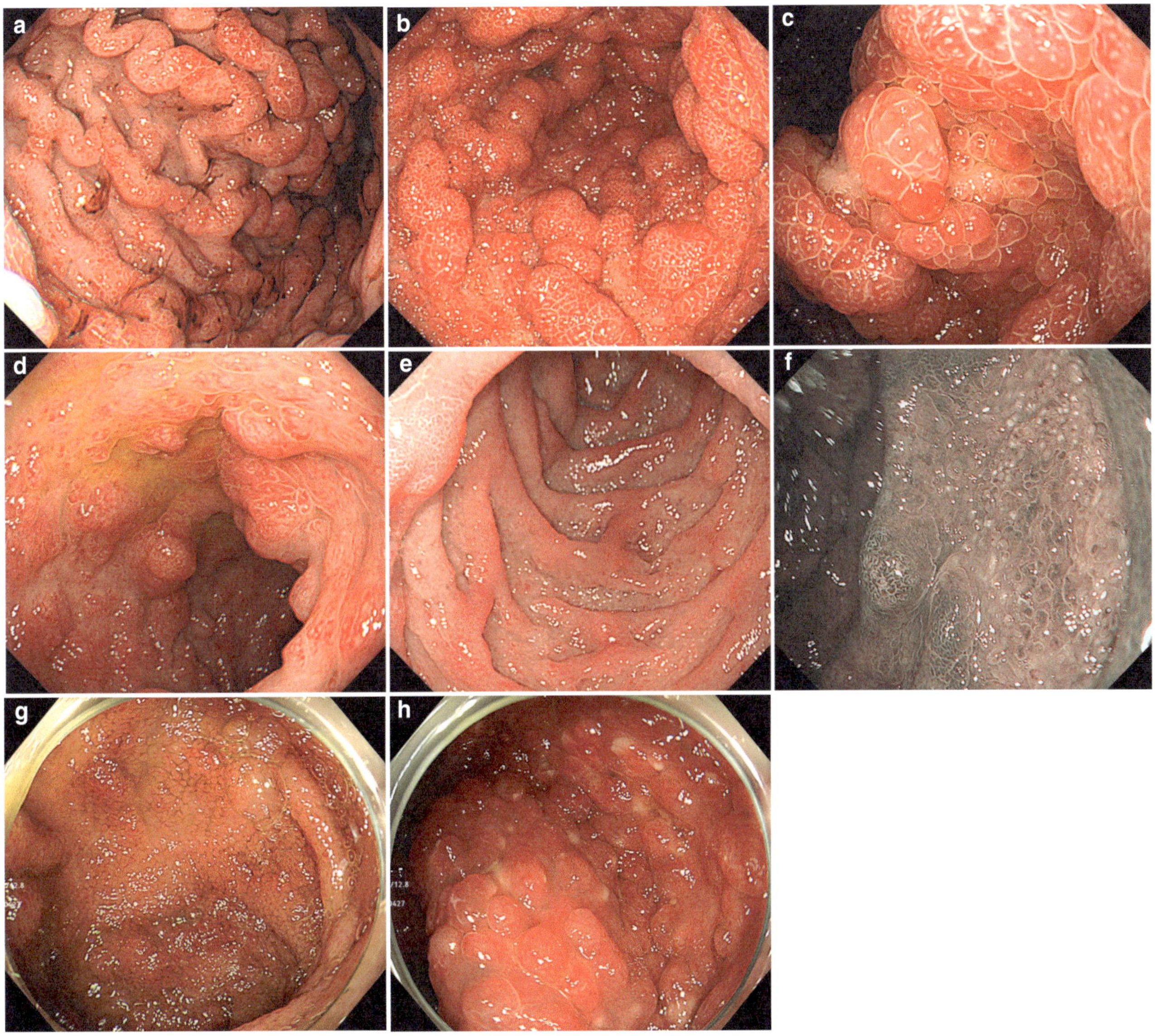

Fig. 25 (**a**), (**b**), (**c**) Stomach: Confluent type. Medium, edematous, and erythematous polyps. Red cavir like appearance. Yamada type I to III (sessile to semi-pedunculated) polyps were confluent in the gastric antrum. Erythematous and edematous intervening mucosa. (**d**), (**e**), (**f**) Duodenum: Fold thickening type with medium polyps. NBI observation in (**f**). (**g**) Ileum: Fold thickening type. (**h**) Colon: Confluent type. Medium, edematous, erythematous, and whitish mucus adhered polyps

Case-Based Images: Steroid-Resistant/ Refractory/Intolerant Cases

Ryota Hokari, Tadakazu Hisamatsu, and Masaaki Higashiyama

Case 41: A case who died of sepsis because of resistance to initial treatment with PSL 30 mg and following corticosteroid pulse therapy

Provided by Mikihiro Fujiya and Katsuyoshi Ando

[Patient]

A 59-year-old male. CC: Dysgeusia, diarrhea, skin rash, leg edema.

[Clinical findings]

Alopecia (+), onychodystrophy (+), hyperpigmentation (+), dysgeusia (+), defecation: more than 10 times/day, severe edema.

[Laboratory findings]

Alb 1.5 mg/dL, CRP 8.47 mg/dL, Hb 11.6 g/dL.

[Endoscopic images 1] (Fig. 1a–h)

[Clinical course]

Chronic continuous type (steroid-resistant).

Initial treatment: PSL 30 mg for 6 weeks.

No response to PSL, resulting in worsening of generalized edema including pleural effusion and ascites, and sepsis. He died 6 months after the onset of illness due to sepsis caused by marked hypoproteinemia and infection with extended-spectrum β-lactamase-producing bacteria.

[Endoscopic images 2] (Fig. 2a–d)

EGD for evaluation after two courses of PSL 30 mg and steroid pulse therapy.

Polyps in all lesions remained unchanged or showed a slight progression.

R. Hokari (✉) · M. Higashiyama
Department of Internal Medicine, National Defense Medical College, Tokorozawa, Saitama, Japan
e-mail: ryota@ndmc.ac.jp; masaakih@ndmc.ac.jp

T. Hisamatsu
Department of Gastroenterology and Hepatology, Kyorin University School of Medicine, Mitaka, Tokyo, Japan

R. Hokari, T. Hisamatsu (eds.), *Atlas of Cronkhite-Canada Syndrome*, https://doi.org/10.1007/978-981-19-0652-7_8

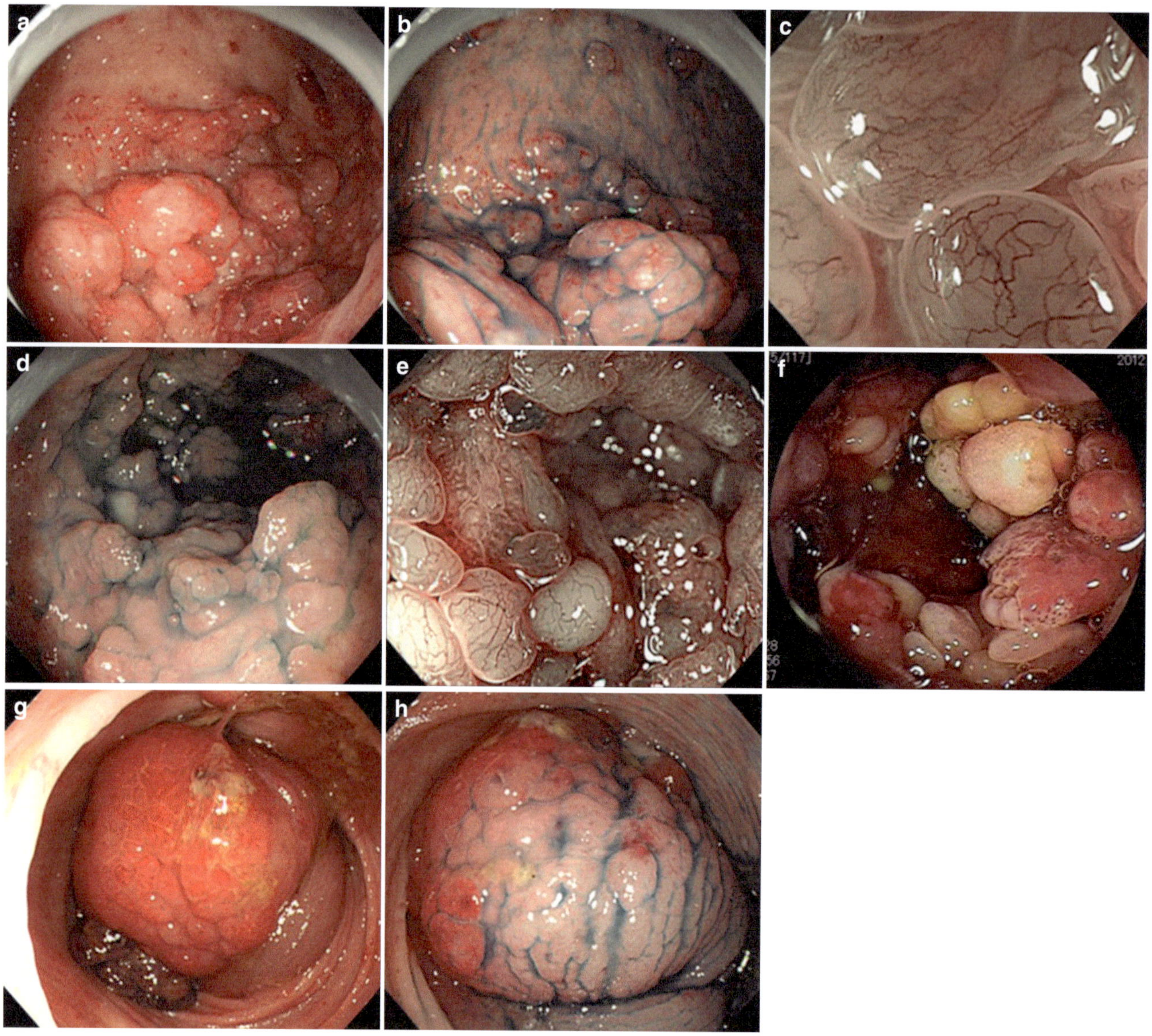

Fig. 1 (**a**), (**b**) Gastric body: Confluent type. Small to large, edematous, and erythematous polyps. (**c**) Gastric body (magnified NBI observation): Obscuration of glandular duct orifices and proliferation, dilation, extension, and tortuosity of superficial vessels without caliber irregularity. (**d**) Duodenum: Confluent type. Small to medium, edematous, and erythematous polyps. (**e**) Duodenum (magnified NBI observation): Proliferation, dilation, and tortuosity of superficial vessels without caliber irregularity. (**f**) Jejunum: Confluent type. Edematous, erythematous, and whitish mucus adhered lobulated polyps. (**g**), (**h**) Colon: Sparse type. Large, edematous, and erythematous protuberant mass occupying the lumen of ascending colon. Indigocarmine dyeing in (**b**), (**d**), (**h**)

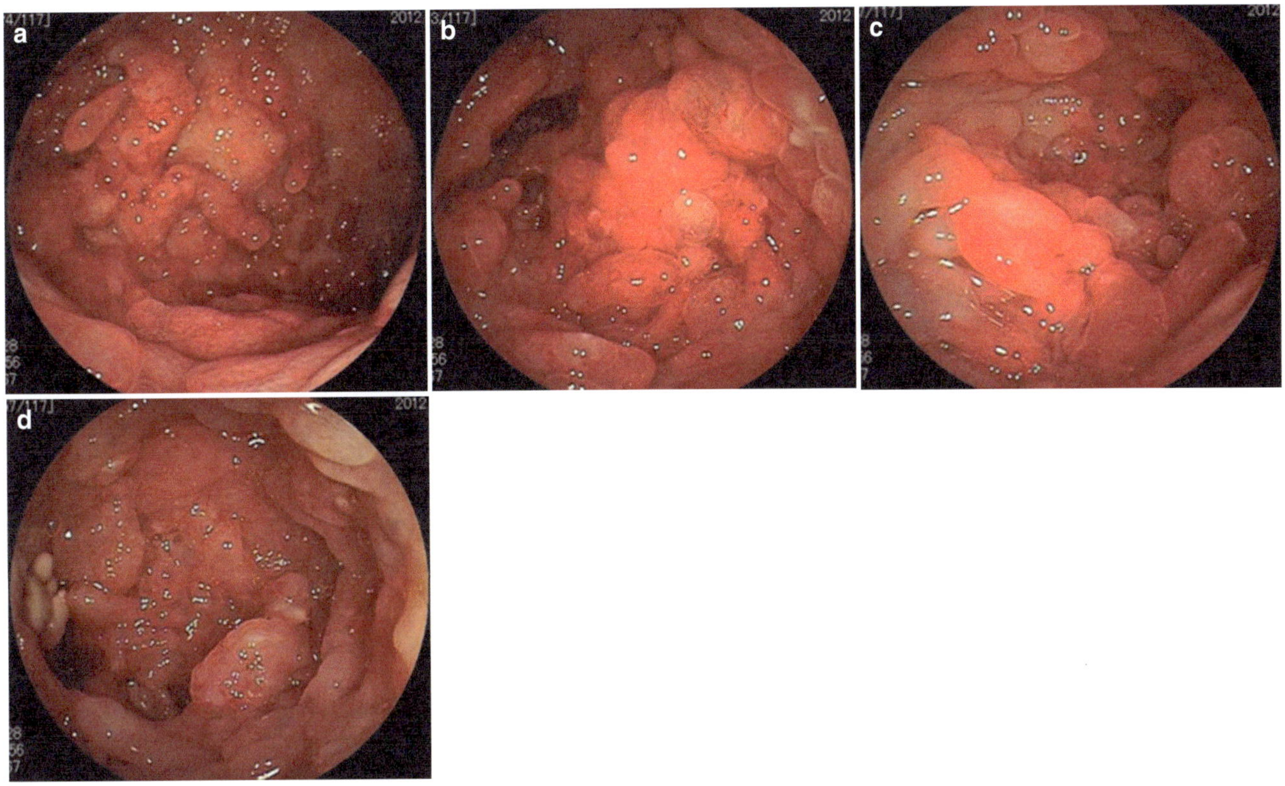

Fig. 2 (**a**) Gastric body. (**b**) Gastric antrum. (**c**) Duodenal bulb. (**d**) Second portion of the duodenum

Case 42: A relapsing case during tapering of PSL, who was induced to remission by corticosteroid pulse therapy and achieved steroid-free remission by combination of azathioprine

Provided by Shuji Kanmura

[Patient]

A 70-year-old male. CC: Diarrhea.

[Clinical findings]

Alopecia (+), onychodystrophy (+), hyperpigmentation (+), dysgeusia (+), defecation: 6 times/day, moderate edema, weight loss: −6 kg/2 months.

[Laboratory findings]

Alb 2.9 mg/dL, CRP 0.96 mg/dL, Hb 15.0 g/dL.

[Endoscopic images 1] (Fig. 3a–g)

[Clinical course]

Relapse-remitting type.

Initial treatment: PSL 30 mg for 2 weeks.

Clinical response: 2 weeks.

Clinical remission: 2 weeks.

Clinical and endoscopic relapse and hypoalbuminemia symptoms were observed at PSL 15 mg/day.

After steroid pulse therapy, combination therapy of PSL 30 mg/day and azathioprine (25 mg/day) started. The dose of PSL was reduced gradually and successfully terminated.

[Endoscopic images 2] (Fig. 4a–f)

Endoscopic findings 2 years after azathioprine use.

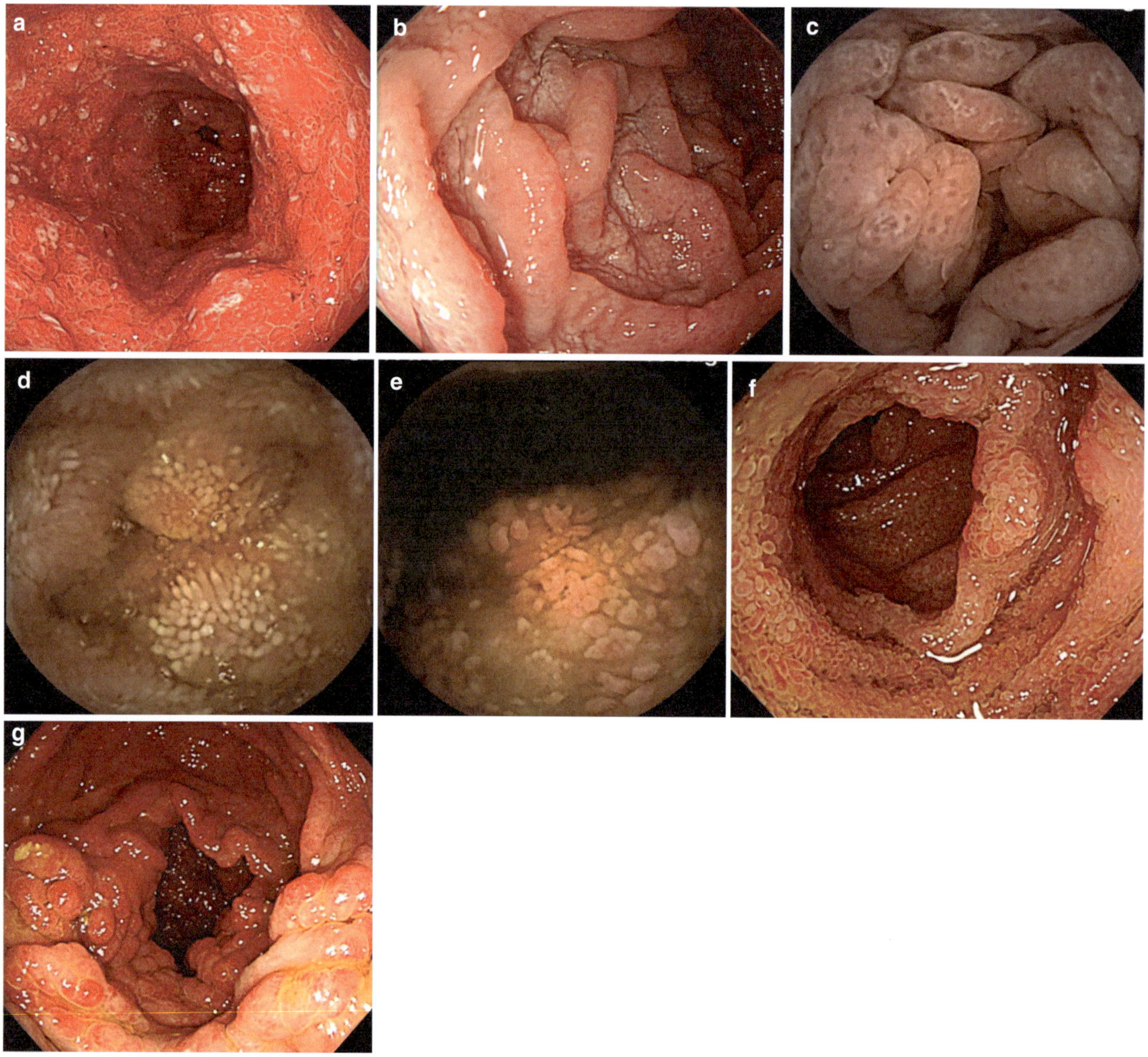

Fig. 3 (**a**) Stomach: Thickening type with edematous, erythematous, erosive, and white mucus adhered polyps. (**b**) Duodenum: Fold thickening type. (**c**) Jejunum (SBCE): Fold thickening type. Edematous polyps containing scattered dark red spots. (**d**) Ileum (SBCE): Fold thickening type. Edematous mucosa with white villi. (**e**) Ileum (SBCE): Unequal-sized villi with some defluxion. (**f**) Terminal ileum: Small polyps and unequal-sized erythematous villi. (**g**) Colon: Semi-confluent type. Medium, edematous, erythematous, and hemorrhagic polyps

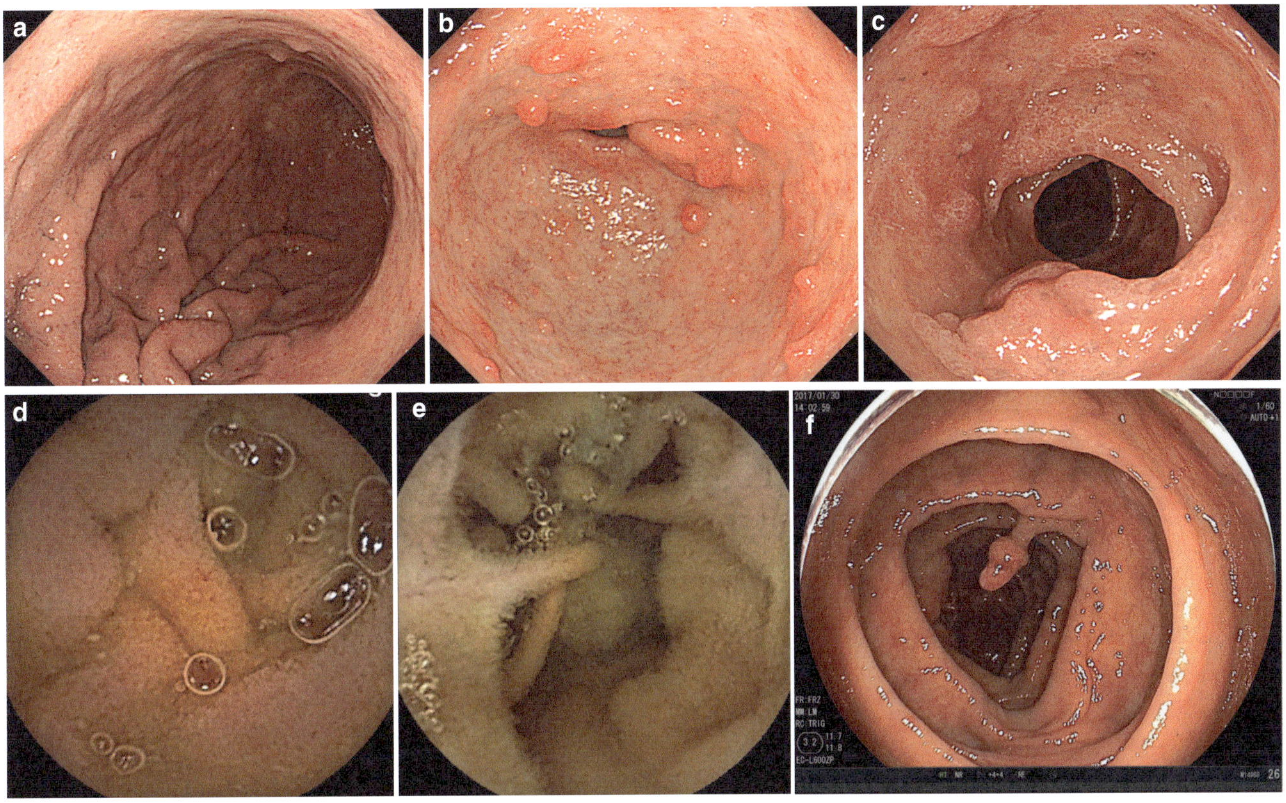

Fig. 4 (**a**), (**b**) Stomach: Although a few polyps were present in the gastric antrum, the number extremely decreased and the mucosal edema improved. (**c**) Duodenum edema was improved. (**d**) Jejunum mucosal lesions disappeared with slightly edematous mucosa remained. (**e**) Ileum: Some polyps with post-inflammatory appearance remained. (**f**) Colon: Polyps almost disappeared. Ip polyp detected in ascending colon was resected endoscopically and diagnosed as adenoma pathologically

Case 43: A case who did not respond to PSL 30 mg and achieved remission with IFX

Provided by Fumikazu Koyama

[Patient]

A 48-year-old woman. CC: Alopecia, diarrhea.

[Clinical findings]

Alopecia (+), onychodystrophy (+), hyperpigmentation (−), dysgeusia (+), defecation: 5 times/day, severe edema.

[Laboratory findings] (Fig. 5)

Alb 1.6 mg/dL, CRP 0.16 mg/dL, Hb 12.3 g/dL.

[Cutaneous findings] (Fig. 6a–d)

[Endoscopic images 1] (Fig. 7a–k)

[Clinical course]

First attack type.

No response to initial treatment with PSL 30 mg for 3 weeks.

Remission was achieved with IFX 200 mg.

[Endoscopic images 2] (Fig. 8a–e)

4 years after the diagnosis.

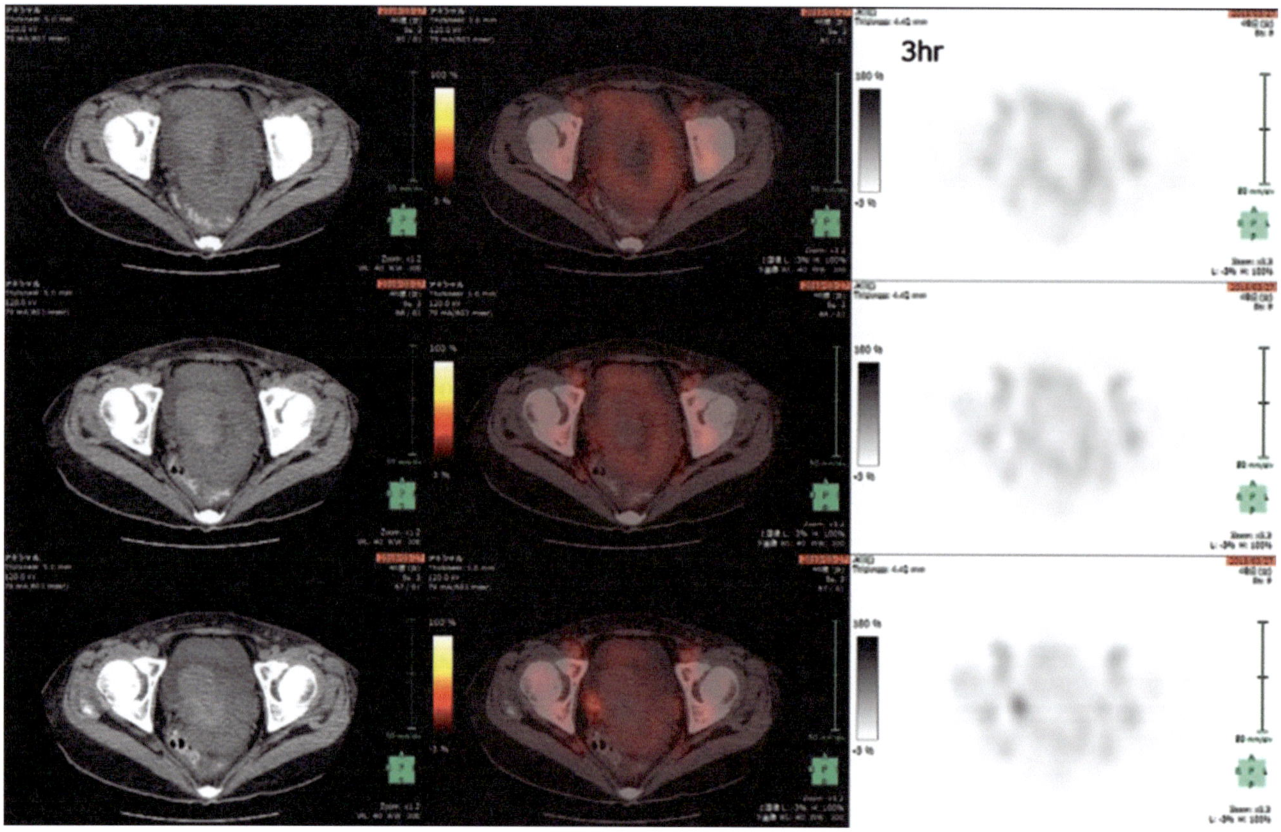

Fig. 5 99Tc-human serum albumin scintigraphy: Abnormal leakage from ileum in the pelvis

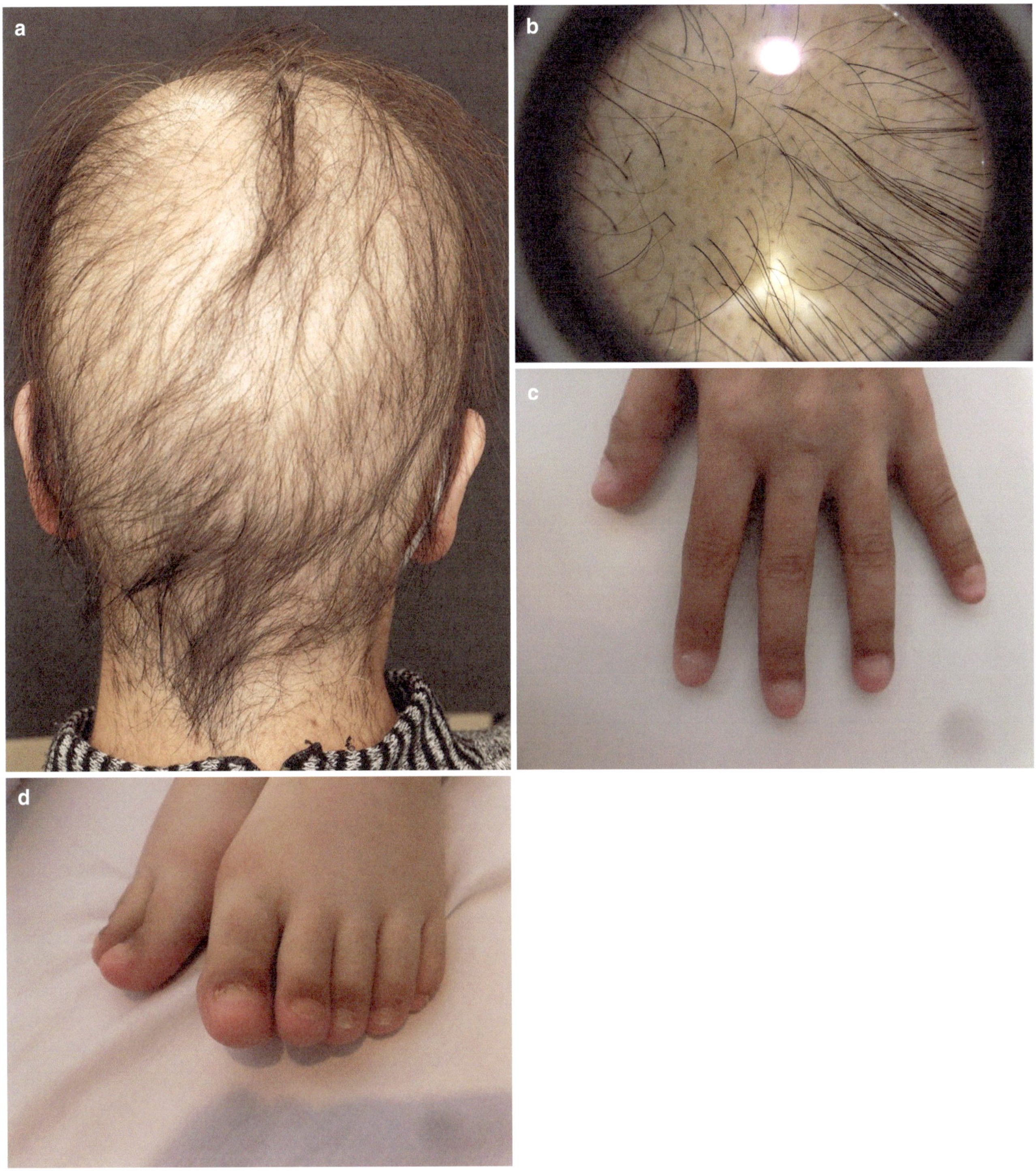

Fig. 6 (**a**) Scalp alopecia. (**b**) Scalp dermoscopy image. (**c**), (**d**) Onychodystrophy of fingernail and toenail. Hyperpigmentation was also observed on the fingers and toes

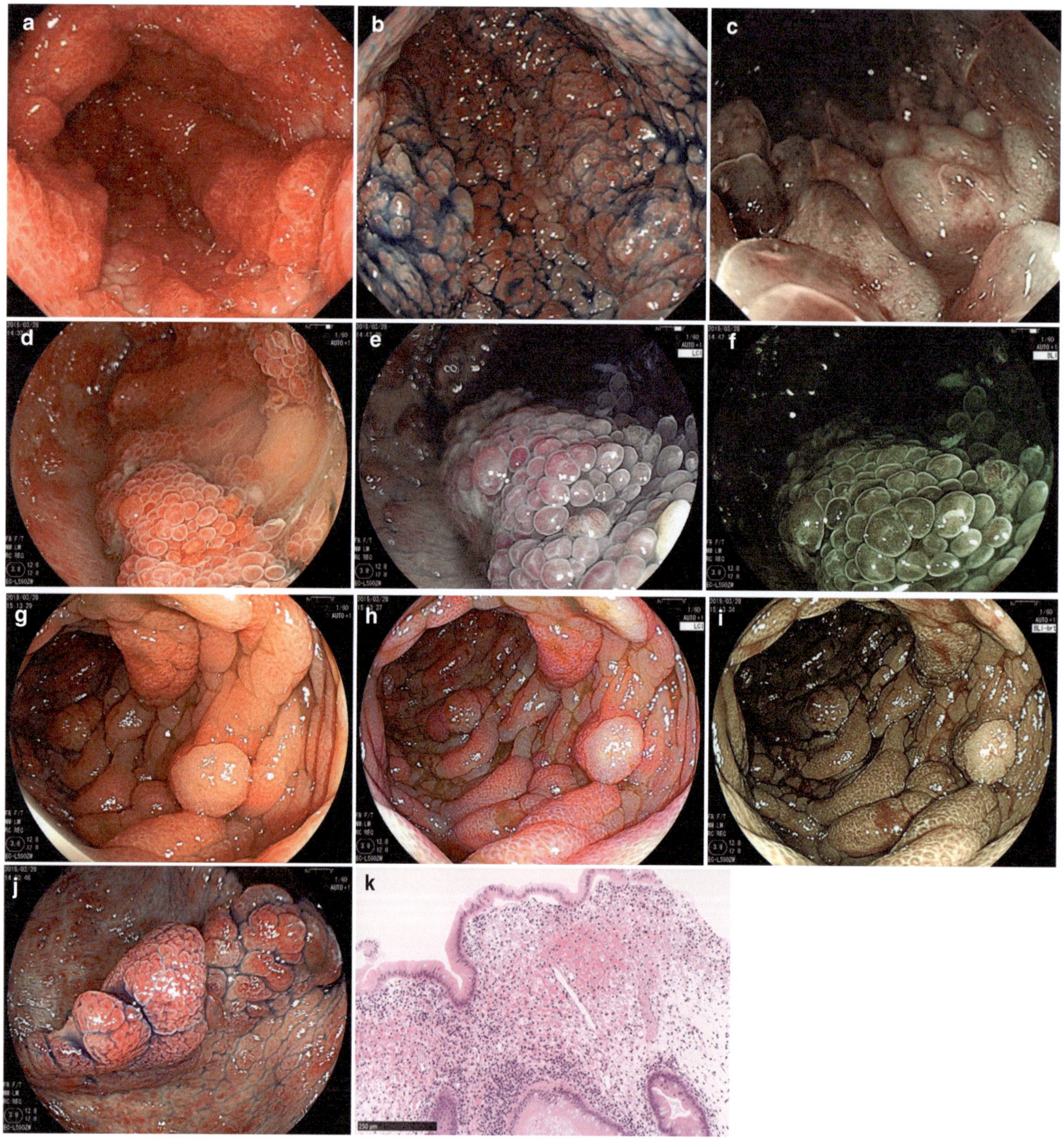

Fig. 7 (**a**) Stomach: Confluent type. Large, edematous polyps. (**b**) Indigocarmine dyeing of (**a**). (**c**) Magnified NBI observation of (**a**). (**d**) Ileum: Confluent type. Large polyps. (**e**) Magnified LCI observation of (**d**). (**f**) Magnified BLI observation of (**d**). (**g**) Colon: Confluent type. Medium, erythematous polyps. (**h**) LCI observation of (**g**). (**i**) BLI observation of (**g**). (**j**) An elevated lesion of the cecum was endoscopically resected. (**k**) Histological examination of (**j**) by HE staining

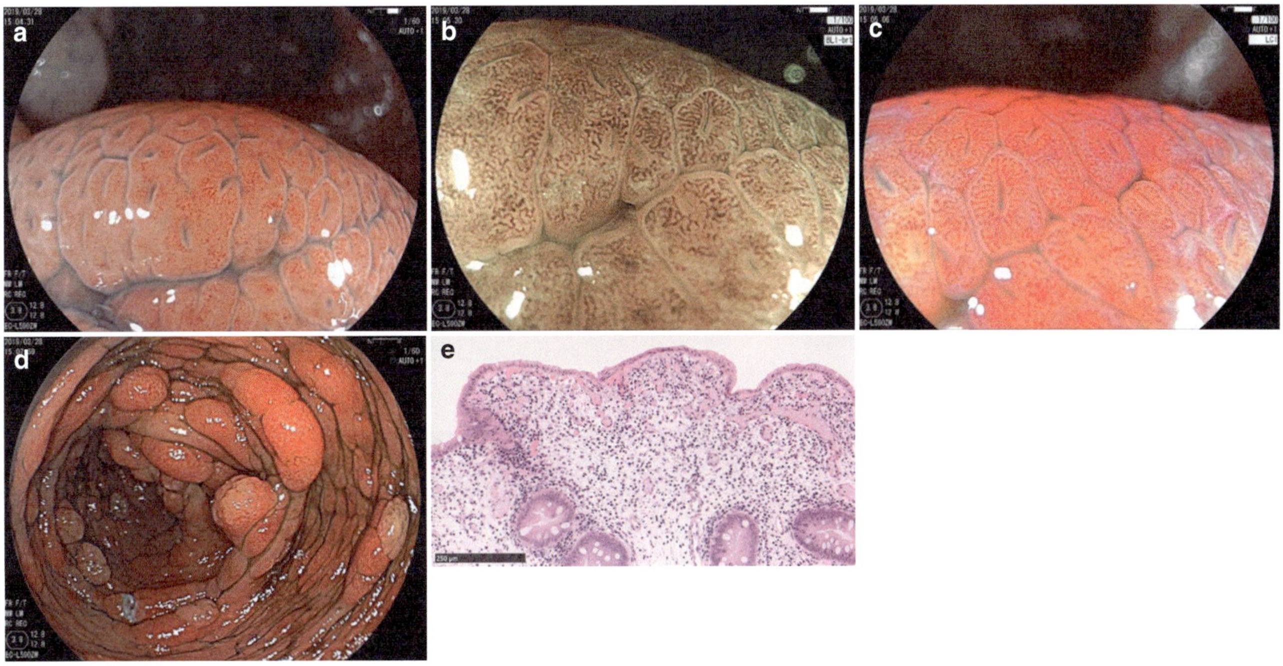

Fig. 8 (**a**) Magnified observation with indigocarmine dyeing. (**b**) Magnified BLI observation of (**a**). (**c**) Magnified LCI observation of (**a**). (**d**) Observation with indigocarmine dyeing. Residual elevated mucosa with marked erythema in descending colon. (**e**) Pathological image of (**d**): Marked vasodilation was observed in the interstitium

Case 44: A case who failed to achieve remission regardless of responding to PSL 40 mg but improved with additional cyclosporine

Provided by Masanao Nakamura and Mitsuhiro Fujishiro

[Patient]

A 70-year-old male. CC: Numbness in the hands and feet, onychodystrophy, dysgeusia, diarrhea.

[Clinical findings]

Alopecia (+), onychodystrophy (+), hyperpigmentation (+), dysgeusia (+), defecation: 6 times/day, mild edema.

[Laboratory findings]

Alb 3.3 mg/dL, CRP 0.49 mg/dL, Hb 15.6 g/dL.

Fecal alpha1-antitrypsin clearance: 54 mL/day

[Endoscopic images 1] (Fig. 9a, b)

[Clinical course]

Chronic continuous type (steroid-resistant).

Initial treatment: PSL 40 mg for 2 weeks.

Clinical response: 2 weeks.

Clinical remission: Not achieved. Additional cyclosporine (target trough: 400 ng/mL) improved clinical response further.

[Endoscopic images 2] (Fig. 10a, b)

2 months after cyclosporine administration

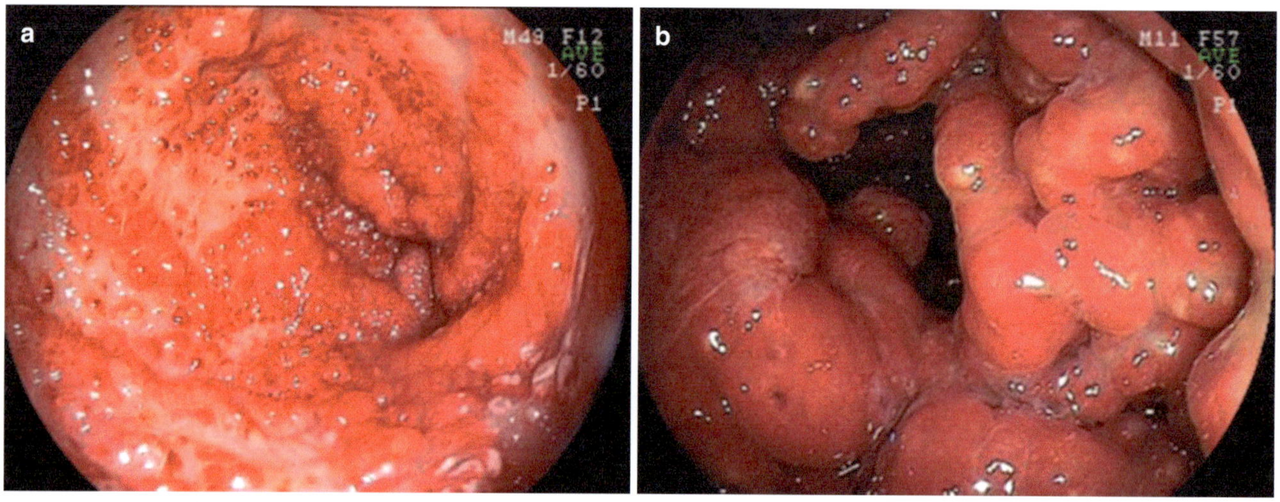

Fig. 9 (**a**) Stomach: Confluent type. Medium, edematous, and erythematous polyps. (**b**) Colon: Confluent type. Large, edematous polyps

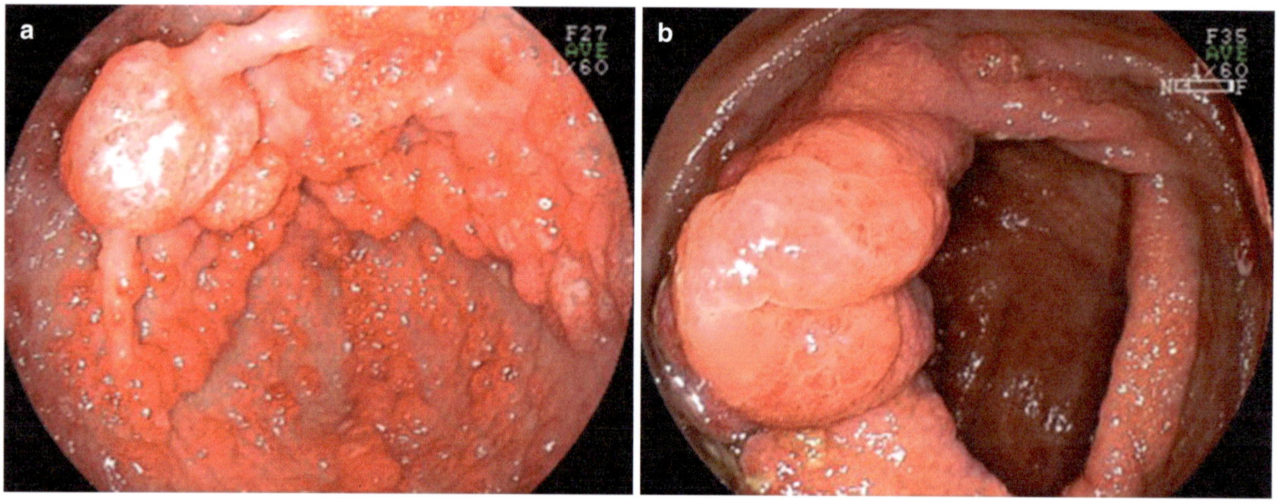

Fig. 10 (**a**) Stomach: Mucosal edema was mildly improved, but the polyps remained unchanged. (**b**) Colon: Polyps remained, but mucosal edema was markedly improved

Case 45: A chronic continuous case who did not respond to steroid and received additional treatment with azathioprine

Provided by Naoki Ohmiya

[Patient]

A 62-year-old woman. CC: Abnormal findings pointed out by barium X-ray radiography of the stomach in medical checkup, positive for occult blood in stool.

[Clinical findings]

Alopecia (+), Onychodystrophy (+), hyperpigmentation (−), dysgeusia (+), defecation: 2 times/day, mild edema.

[Laboratory findings]

Alb 3.0 mg/dL, CRP 1.29 mg/dL, Hb 14.0 g/dL.

[Endoscopic images] (Fig. 11)

[Clinical course]

Chronic continuous type.

Initial treatment: PSL 20 mg for 2 weeks. There was no sufficient improvement by PSL, and 50 mg of azathioprine was added.

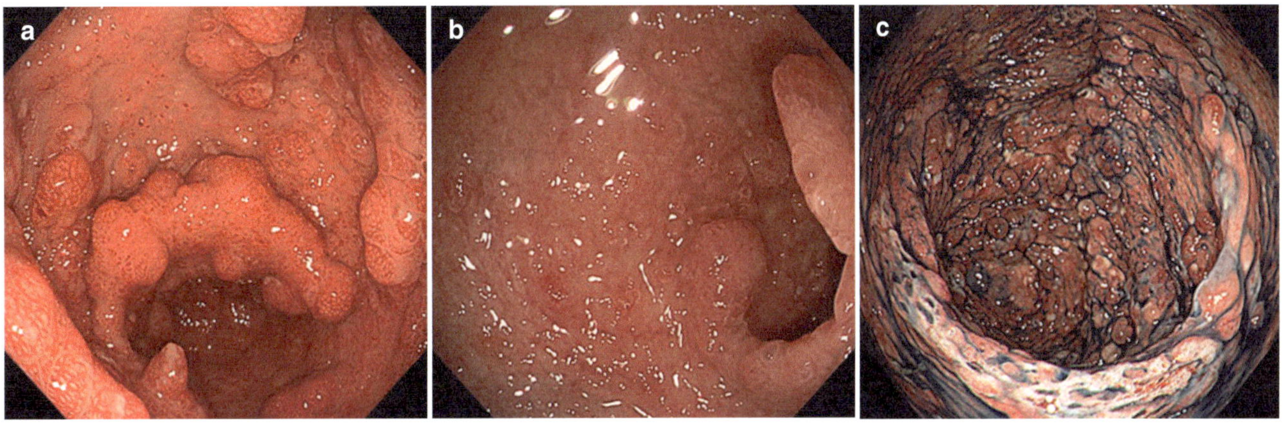

Fig. 11 (**a**) Stomach: Semi-confluent type. Large, edematous, erythematous, and whitish mucus adhered polyps. (**b**) Duodenum: Semi-confluent type. Small polyps. (**c**) Ascending colon (Indigocarmine dyeing): Semi-confluent type. Medium, erythematous, and whitish mucus adhered polyps

Case 46: A chronic continuous case who achieved endoscopic remission with corticosteroids and azathioprine, but developed gastric cancer

Provided by Makoto Ooi and Yuzo Kodama

[Patient]

A 55-year-old woman. CC: Dysgeusia, anorexia, nailfold abnormality, alopecia universalis, diarrhea, weight loss.

[Clinical findings]

Alopecia (+), onychodystrophy (+), hyperpigmentation (+), defecation: 10 times/day, mild edema.

[Laboratory findings]

Alb 2.5 mg/dL, CRP 2.85 mg/dL, Hb 13.1 g/dL.

[Endoscopic images 1] (Fig. 12a–f)

[Clinical course]

Chronic continuous type.

Initial treatment: PSL 40 mg for 1 week with 25 mg of azathioprine.

Endoscopic response: 3 months.

Endoscopic remission: 34 months.

Therapeutic dose at relapse: PSL 30 mg.

Maintenance dose: PSL 10 mg.

[Endoscopic images 2] (Fig. 13a–f)

EGD and CS after induction of remission.

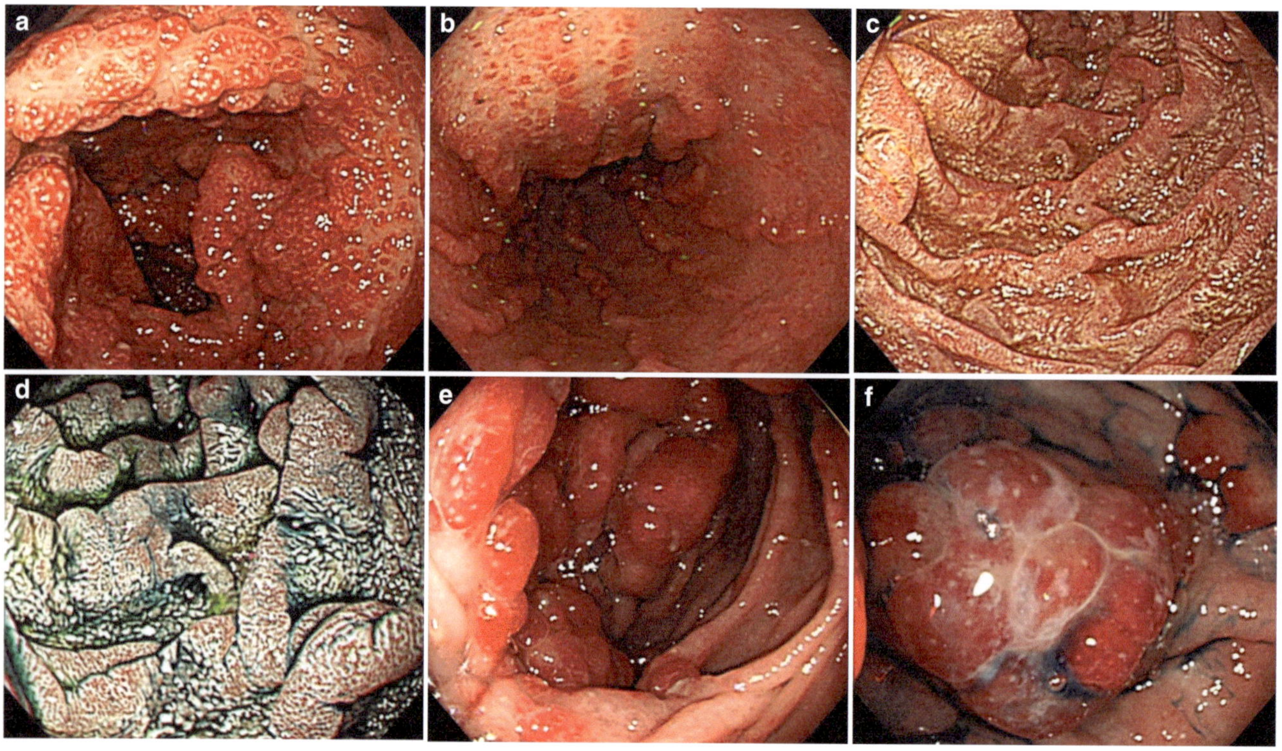

Fig. 12 (**a**), (**b**) Stomach: Confluent type. Medium, erythematous polyps. (**c**) Duodenum: Fold thickening type with white villi. (**d**) Indigocarmine dyeing of (**c**). (**e**), (**f**) Colon: Sparse type. Medium, erythematous and whitish mucus adhered polyps

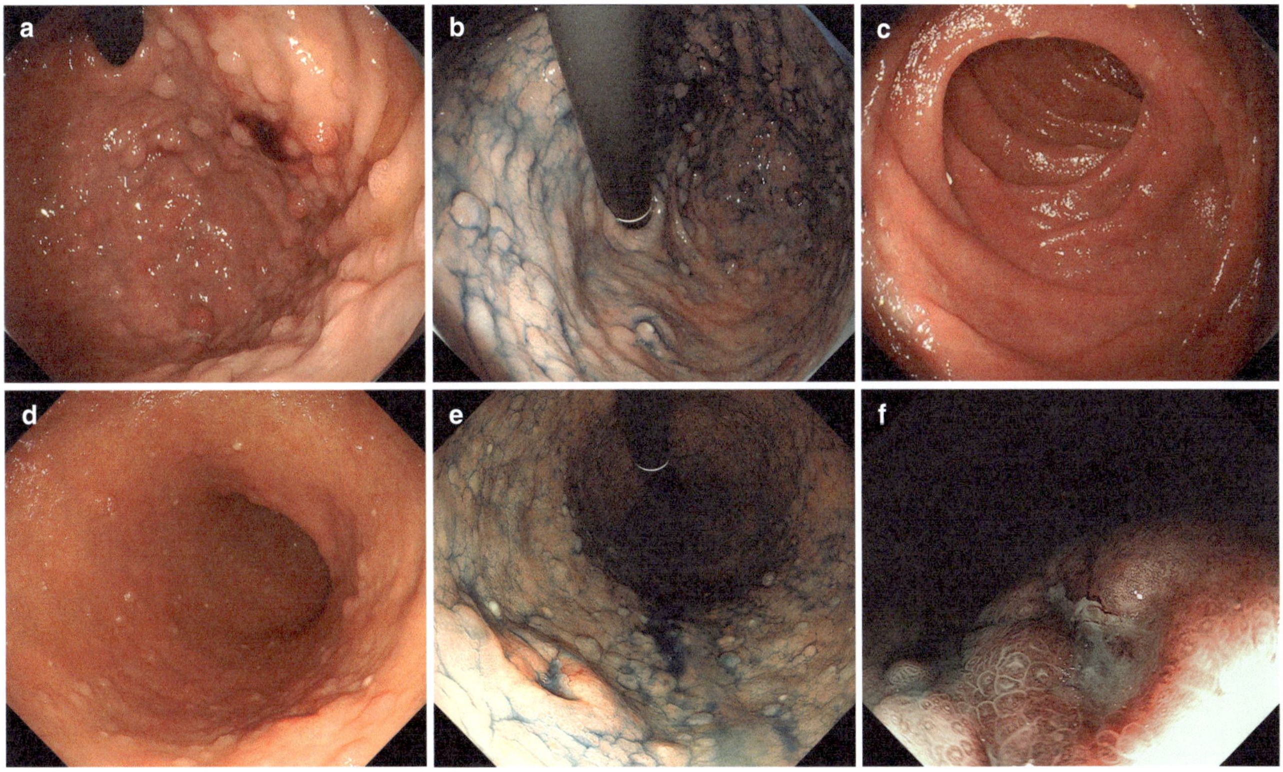

Fig. 13 (**a**) Stomach: Polyps decreased and became less erythematous. (**b**) Indigocarmine dyeing of (**a**). (**c**) Duodenum: Fold thickening improved. (**d**) Carcinoma at the posterior wall of the mid-gastric body was surgically resected. (**e**) Indigocarmine dyeing of (**d**). (**f**) Magnified NBI observation of (**d**)

Case 47: A chronic continuous case who responded to corticosteroids and azathioprine, but required a maintenance dose of PSL 15 mg

Provided by Makoto Ooi and Yuzo Kodama

[Patient]

A 68-year-old male. CC: Dysgeusia, diarrhea, hyperpigmentation, onychodystrophy, alopecia.

[Clinical findings]

Alopecia (+), onychodystrophy (+), hyperpigmentation (+).

[Laboratory findings]

Alb 3.1 mg/dL, CRP 0.99 mg/dL, Hb 11.1 g/dL.

[Endoscopic images 1] (Fig. 14a–e)

[Clinical course]

Chronic continuous type.

Initial treatment: PSL 40 mg for 5 weeks with 50 mg of azathioprine.

Endoscopic response: 49 months.

Endoscopic remission: 90 months.

Maintenance dose: PSL 15 mg.

[Endoscopic images 2] (Fig. 15a–e)

EGD and CS during remission.

Only a few polyps remained and became less erythematous and erosive.

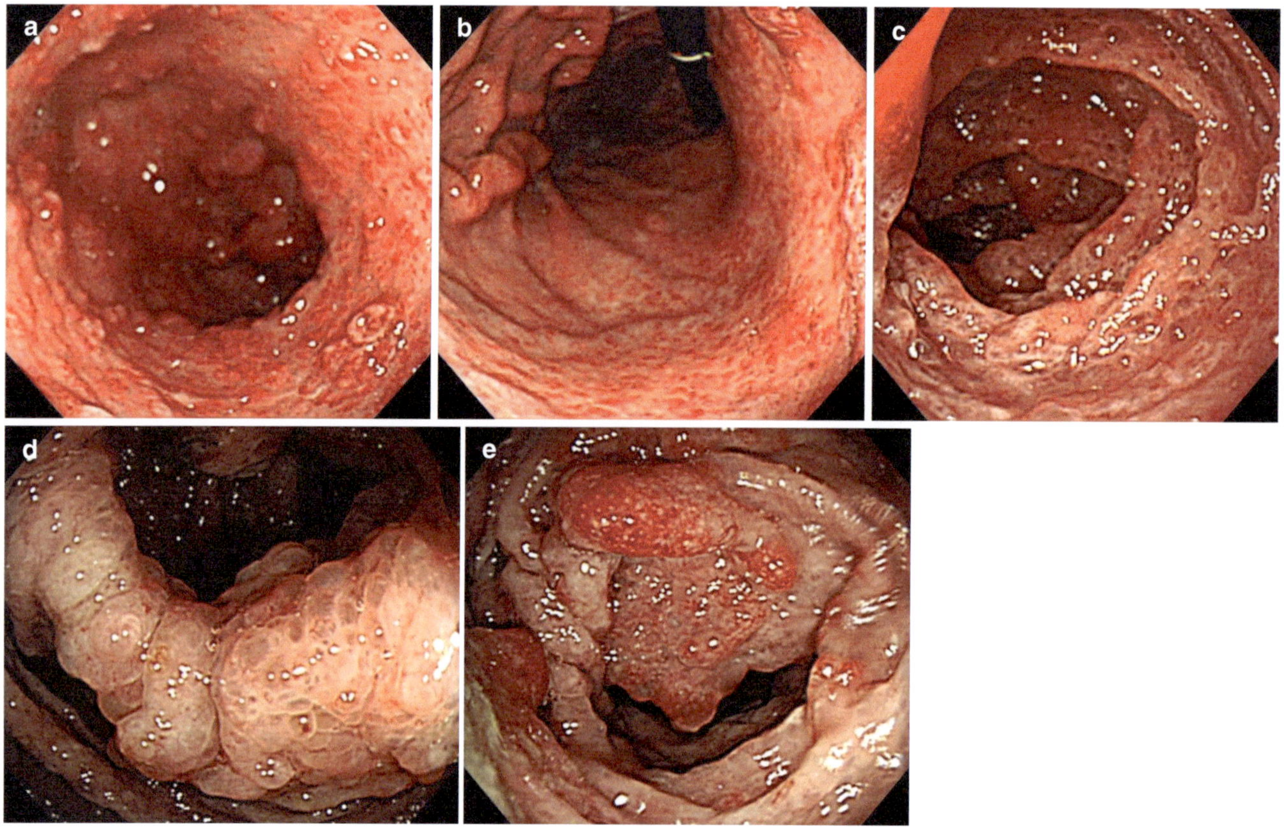

Fig. 14 (**a**), (**b**) Stomach: Confluent type. Small, erythematous polyps. (**c**) Duodenum: Confluent type. Small polyps with white villi. (**d**), (**e**) Colon: Confluent type. Medium, edematous, and erythematous polyps

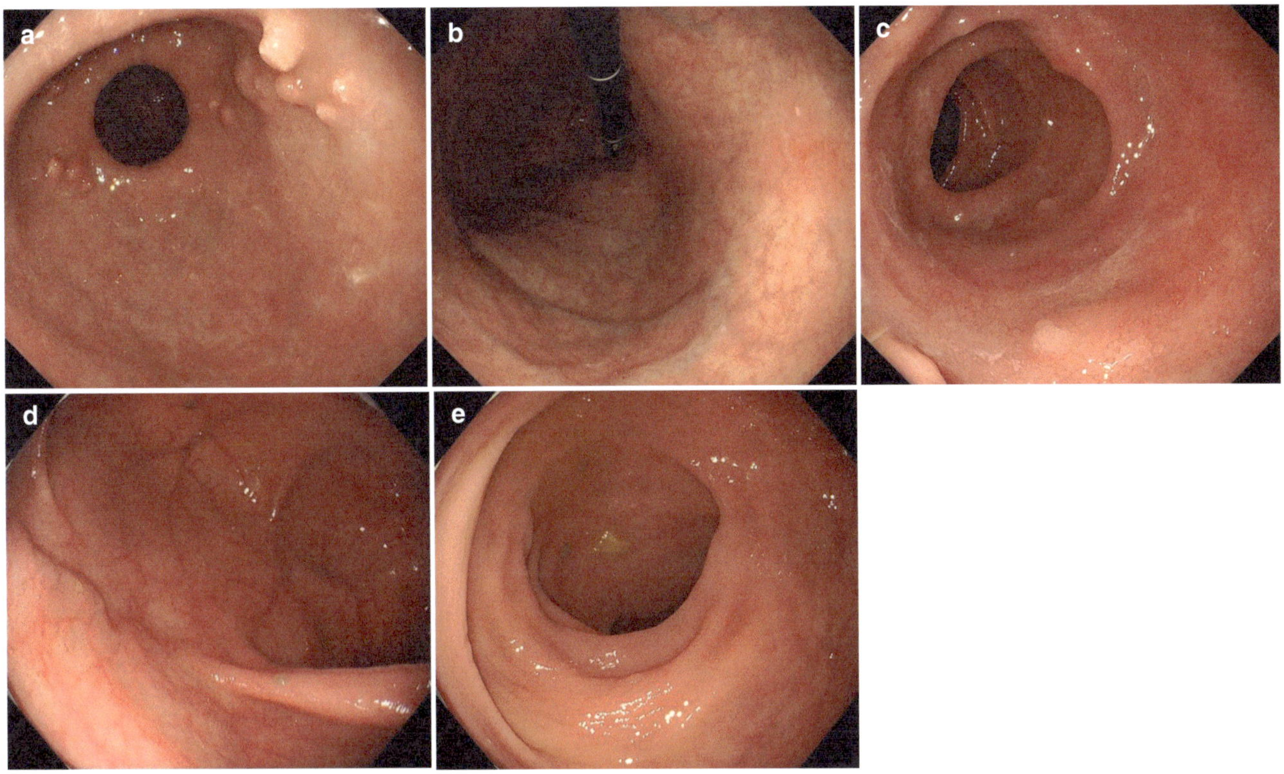

Fig. 15 (**a**), (**b**) Stomach. (**c**) Duodenum. (**d**), (**e**) Colon

Case 48: A case who responded to corticosteroids and azathioprine, but had residual polyps and required a maintenance dose of PSL 7.5 mg

Provided by Masanao Nakamura and Mitsuhiro Fujishiro

[Patient]

A 64-year-old woman. CC: Dysgeusia, anorexia, alopecia.

[Clinical findings]

Alopecia (+), onychodystrophy (+), hyperpigmentation (+), dysgeusia (+), defecation: 5 times/day, mild edema.

[Laboratory findings]

Alb 3.2 mg/dL, CRP 0.06 mg/dL, Hb 11.5 g/dL.

[Endoscopic images 1] (Fig. 16a–f)

[Clinical course]

First attack type (steroid resistant).

Initial treatment with 20 mg of PSL for 4 weeks and 50 mg of azathioprine was added to reduce the PSL.

Maintenance dose: PSL 7.5 mg.

[Endoscopic images 2] (Fig. 17a–g)

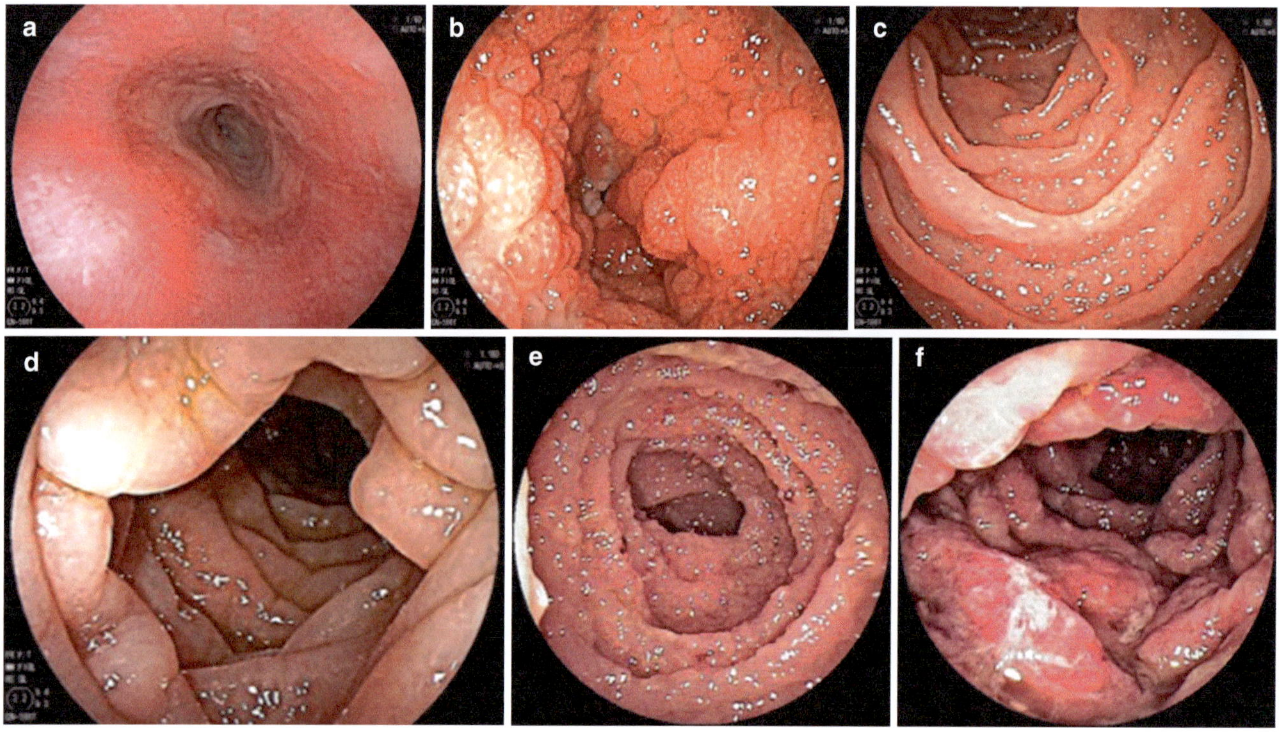

Fig. 16 (**a**) Esophagus: Sparse type. Small, flat to sub-pedunculated polyps. (**b**) Stomach: Confluent type. Medium, edematous, and erythematous polyps. (**c**) Duodenum: Fold thickening type. (**d**) Jejunum: Fold thickening type. (**e**) Ileum: Fold thickening type with small polyps. (**f**) Colon: Thickening type

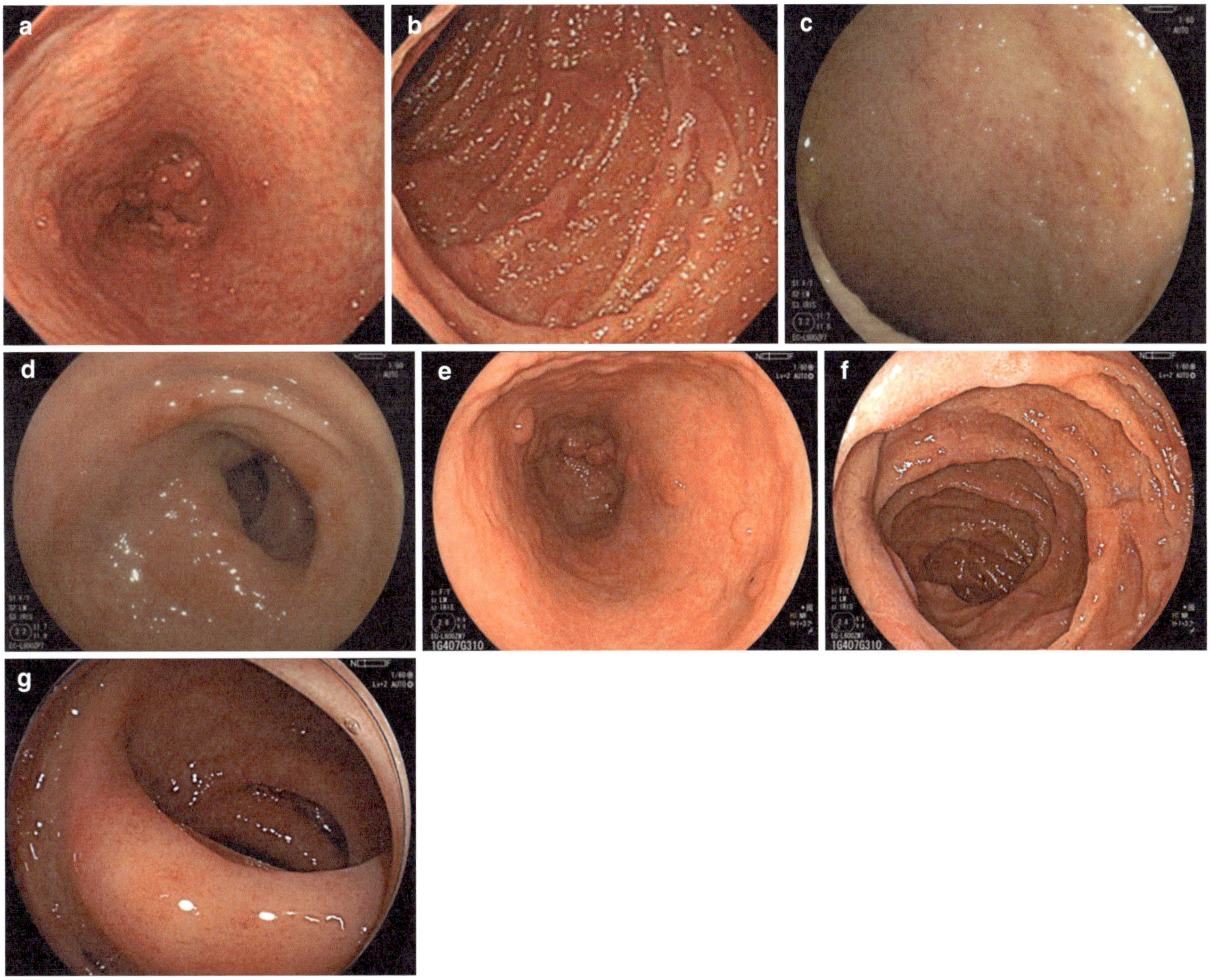

Fig. 17 (**a**), (**b**), (**c**), (**d**) EGD and CS 12 months later, maintained by PSL 10 mg. (**e**), (**f**), (**g**) EGD and CS 5 years later, maintained by PSL 7.5 mg. (**a**), (**e**) Gastric antrum: Red cavir-like polyps diminished, and edema improved. Hemispherical polyps 5–10 mm in diameter remained. (**b**), (**f**) Second portion of duodenum: Fold thickening remained. (**c**) Ileum: Fold thickening remained. (**d**), (**g**) Sigmoid colon: Polyps disappeared

Case 49: A case who responded to corticosteroids and 6-mercaptopurine, but was complicated with colorectal cancer

Provided by Kan Uchiyama

[Patient]

A 52-year-old woman. CC: Anorexia, diarrhea, bloody stool, weight loss.

[Clinical findings]

Alopecia (+), onychodystrophy (+), hyperpigmentation (+), dysgeusia (−), defecation: 10 times/day.

[Laboratory findings]

Alb 1.8 mg/dL, CRP 0.10 mg/dL, Hb 13.0 g/dL.

99Tc-human serum albumin scintigraphy: Abnormal leakage from the cecum.

[Endoscopic images 1] (Fig. 18a–g)

[Clinical course]

Relapse-remitting type.

Initial treatment: PSL 60 mg for 2 weeks with 6-mercaptopurine.

Clinical response: 8 weeks.

Maintenance dose: PSL 0 mg.

[Endoscopic images 2] (Fig. 19a–h)

CS after treatments.

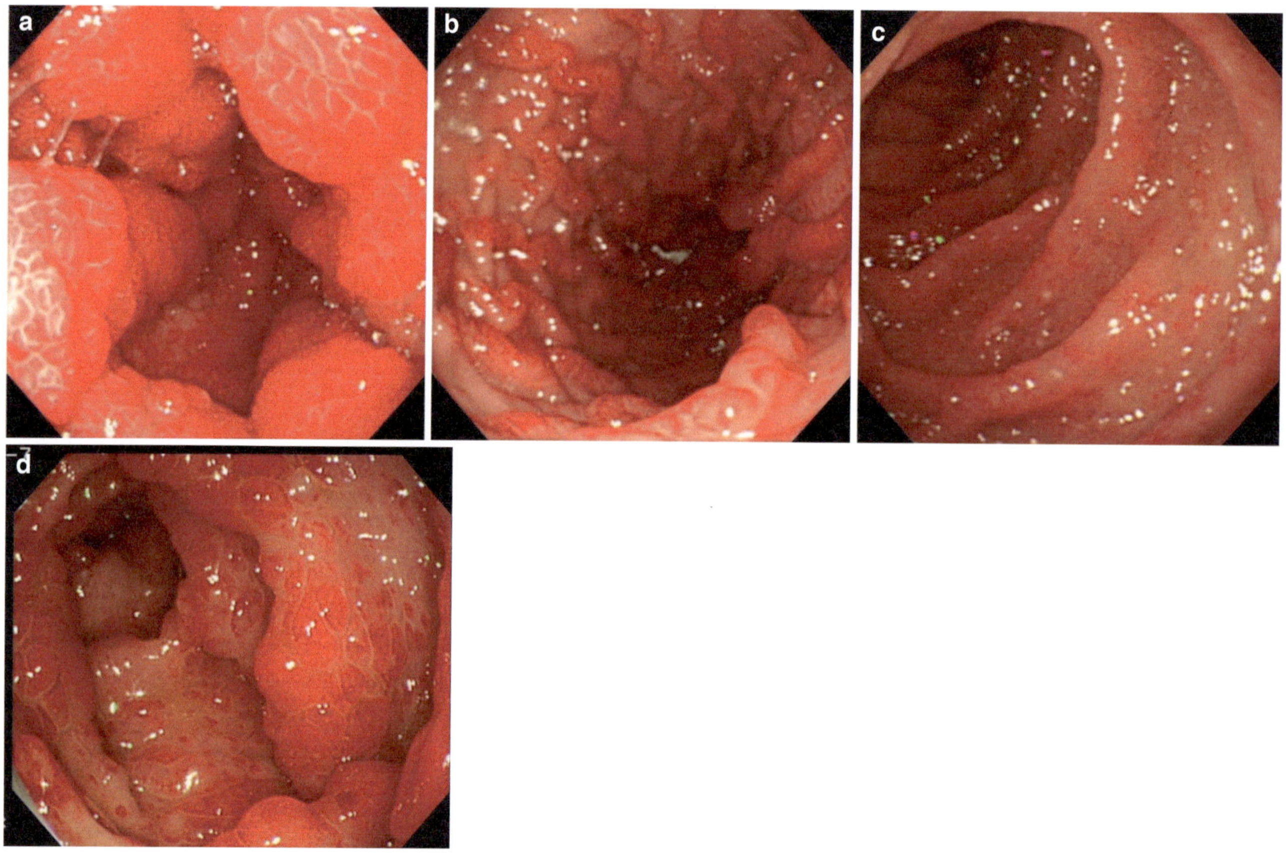

Fig. 18 (**a**), (**b**) Stomach: Confluent type. Medium, edematous, and erosive polyps. (**c**) Duodenum: Fold thickening type. (**d**) Cecum: Confluent type. Small polyps. (**e**) 99Tc-human serum albumin scintigraphy (24 h later): Abnormal leakage from the cecum. (**f**) Transverse colon: A colonic polyp in the transverse colon at the diagnosis. (**g**) The colonic polyp of (**f**) was resected 2 months after the initial treatment. Pathological findings: Polyps consisted of cystically dilated atypical glands, some of which showed cancer cell net of highly differentiated adenocarcinoma and was diagnosed as adenocarcinoma in situ

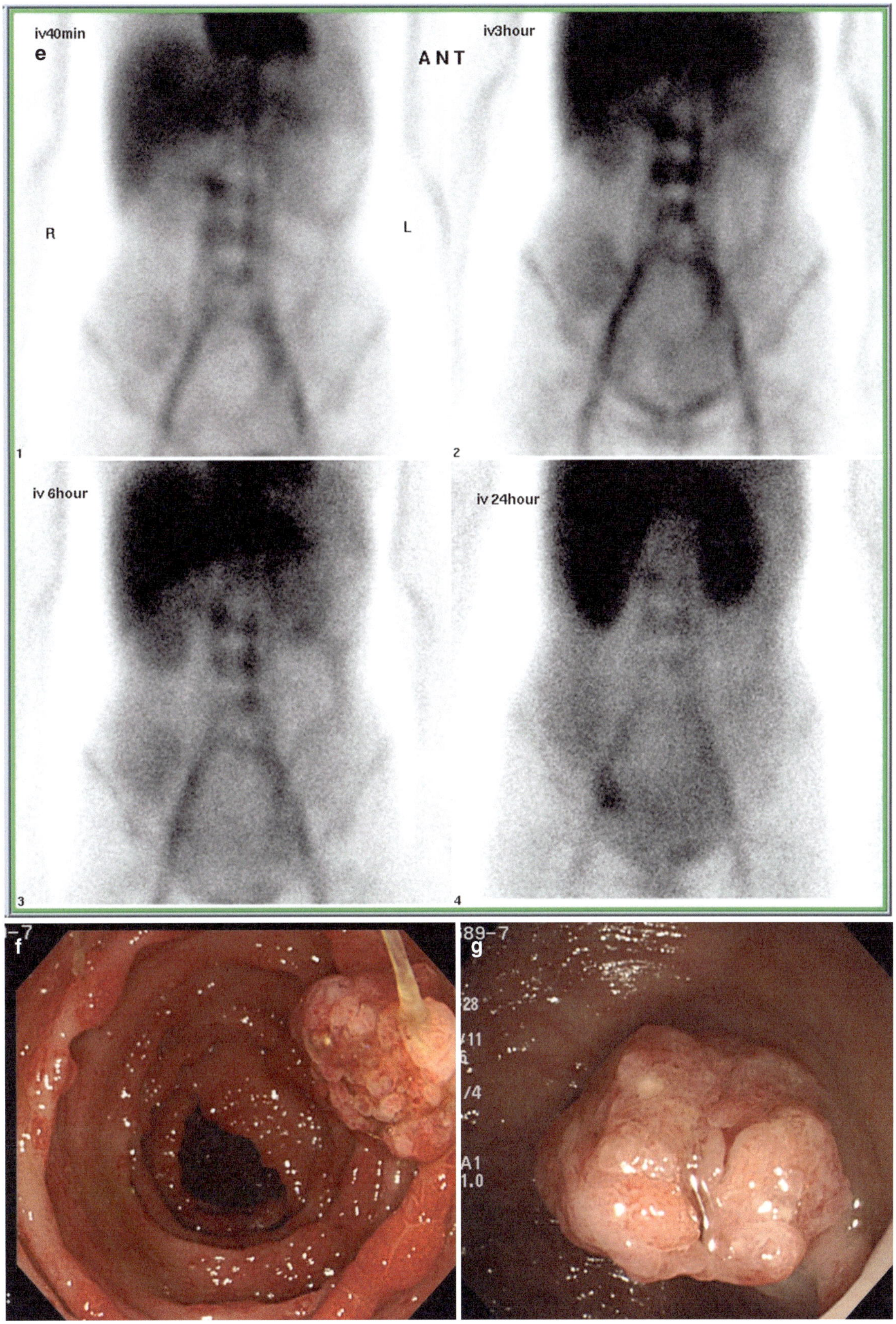

Fig. 18 (continued)

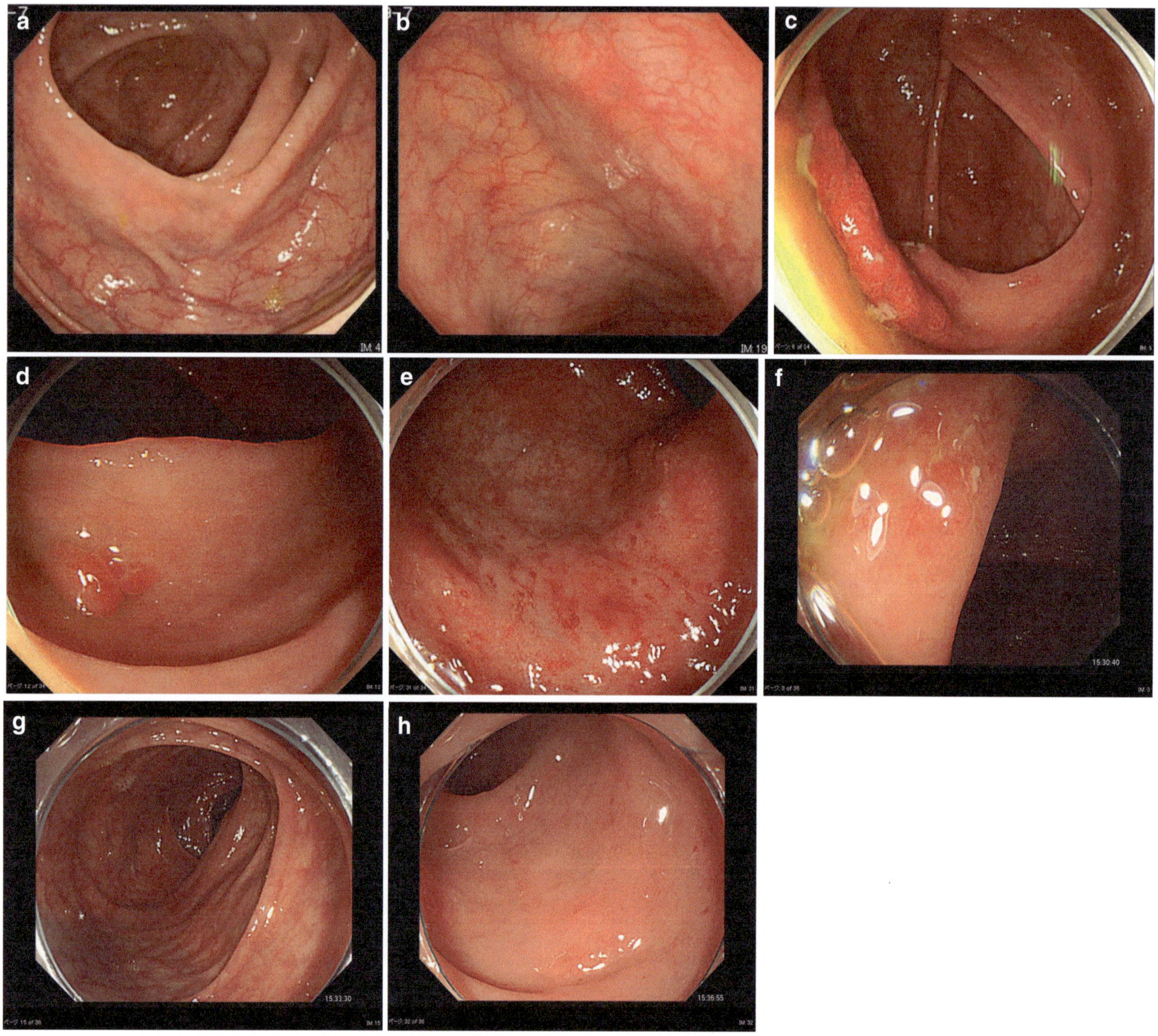

Fig. 19 (**a**), (**b**) 1 year after treatments. Endoscopic findings improved. (**c**), (**d**), (**e**) 5 years after treatments at relapse. Serum albumin decreased to 2.6 mg/dL, but no apparent subjective symptoms appeared. Short-term PSL was temporarily administered. (**f**), (**g**), (**h**) 7 years after treatments. Although polyps disappeared, erythematous, edematous, and microerosive mucosa remained in some places

Case 50: A chronic continuous case who could not keep taking steroid due to steroid psychosis and diabetes mellitus

Provided by Kingo Hirasawa and Reiko Kunisaki

[Patient]

A 54-year-old male. CC: Dysgeusia, anorexia, weight loss.

[Clinical findings]

Alopecia (−), onychodystrophy (+), hyperpigmentation (−), dysgeusia (+), defecation: 2 times/day, mild edema.

[Laboratory findings]

Alb 1.8 mg/dL, CRP 1.96 mg/dL, Hb 15.1 g/dL.

[Endoscopic images 1] (Fig. 20a–n)

[Clinical course]

Chronic continuous type.

Initial treatment: PSL 30 mg for 4 weeks. PSL treatment was terminated due to adverse effects including diabetes mellitus and steroid psychosis.

[Endoscopic images 2] (Fig. 21a–f)

CS 1 year after the treatment.

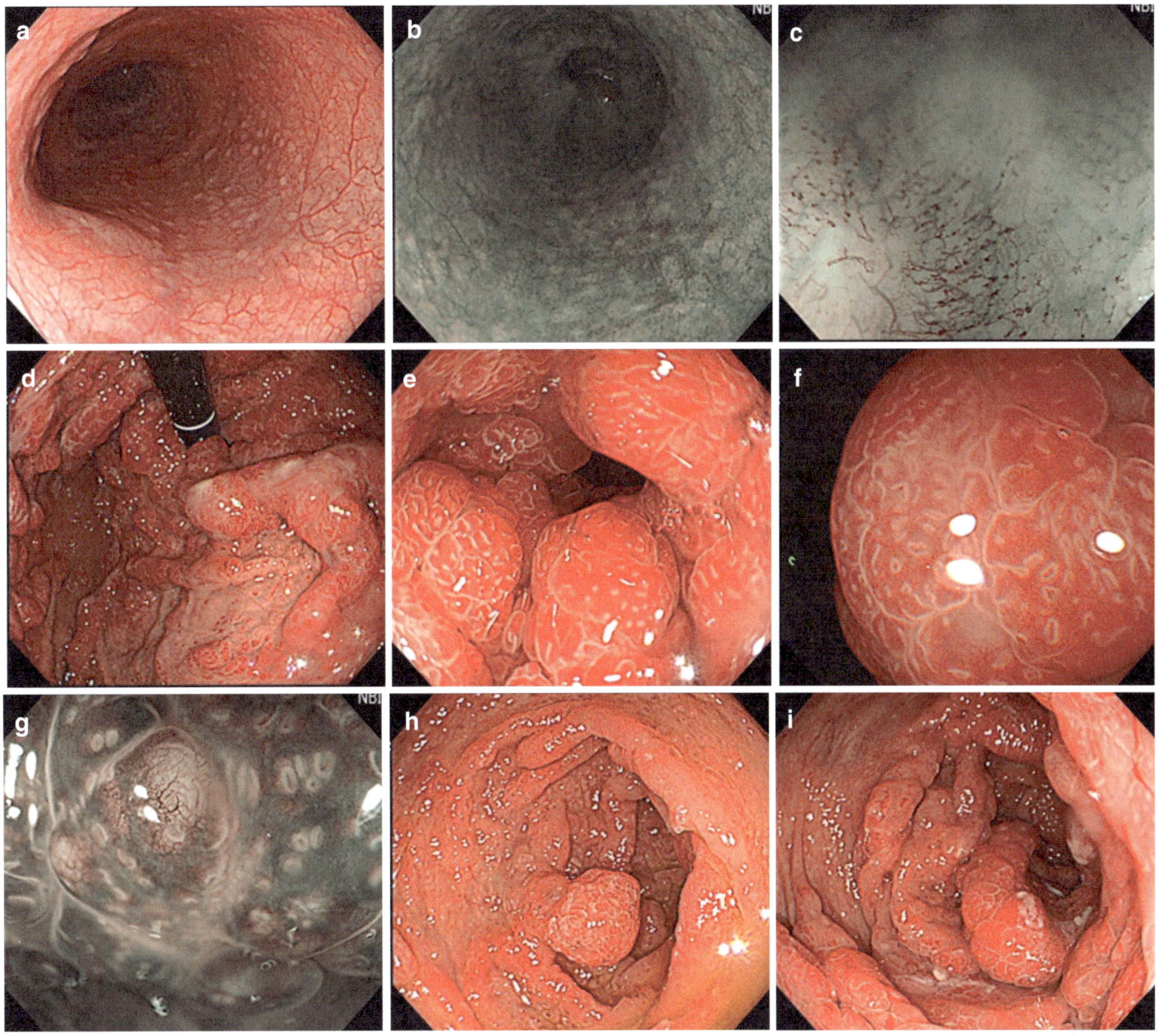

Fig. 20 (**a**) Esophagus: Sparse type. Small, white flat elevations. (**b**) NBI observation of (**a**). (**c**) Magnified NBI observation of (**a**). (**d**) Gastric cardia: Confluent type. Medium, edematous, erythematous, erosive, and whitish mucus adhered polyps. (**e**) Gastric antrum: Confluent type. Erythematous polyps with dilated distance between pits. (**f**) Magnified observation of (**e**). (**g**) Magnified NBI observation of (**e**). (**h**) Duodenum: Semi-confluent type. Medium polyps. (**i**) Ascending colon: Confluent type. Large, edematous, erythematous, and whitish mucus adhered polyps. Normal mucosa and edematous mucosa with decreased vascular pattern were mixed. (**j**) Descending colon: Sparse type. Medium, erythematous polyps. (**k**) Magnified observation of (**j**). (**l**) Magnified NBI observation of (**j**). Opening of the pits was observed. There was no dilated distance between the pits. (**m**) Transverse colon: Lobulated polyps with erythematous and slightly white nodules. (**n**) Magnified observation with indigocarmine dyeing of (**m**). White nodules showed elongated glands like a cerebral convolution shape and contained white material. Pathological diagnosis: Tubular adenoma with high atypia

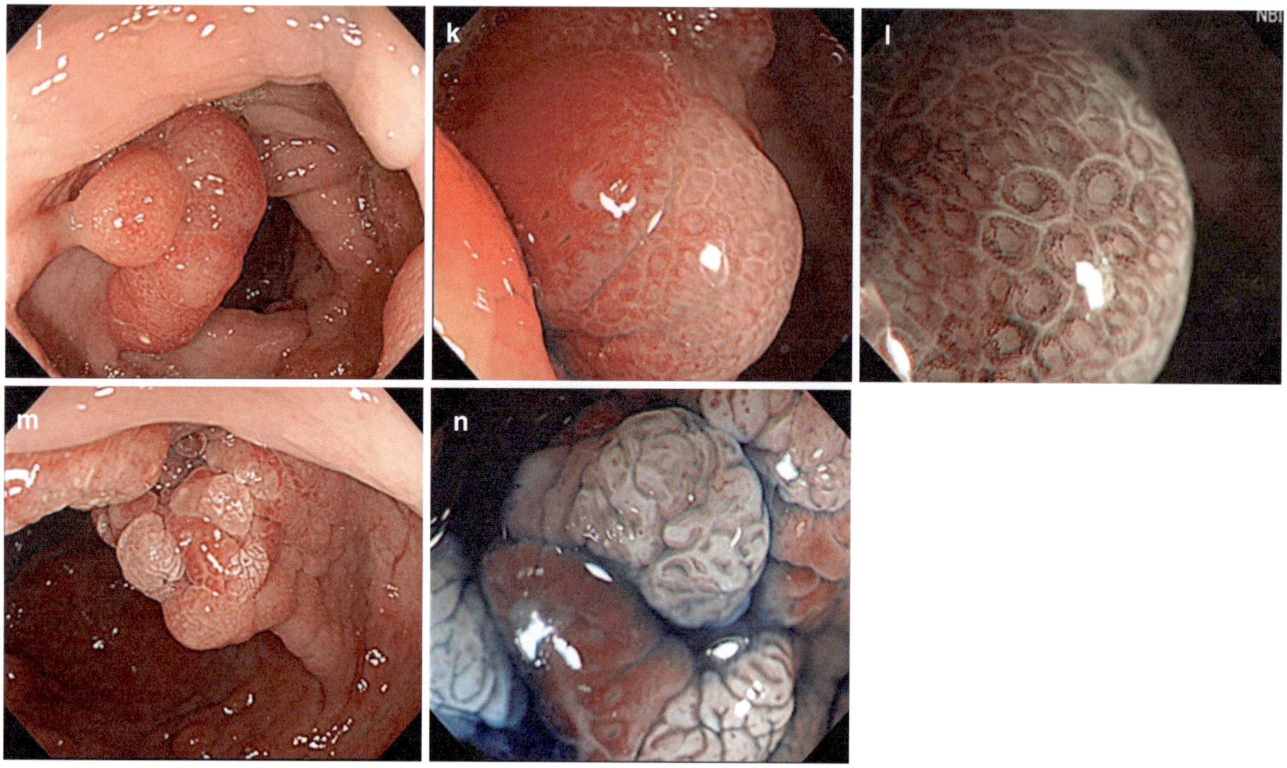

Fig. 20 (continued)

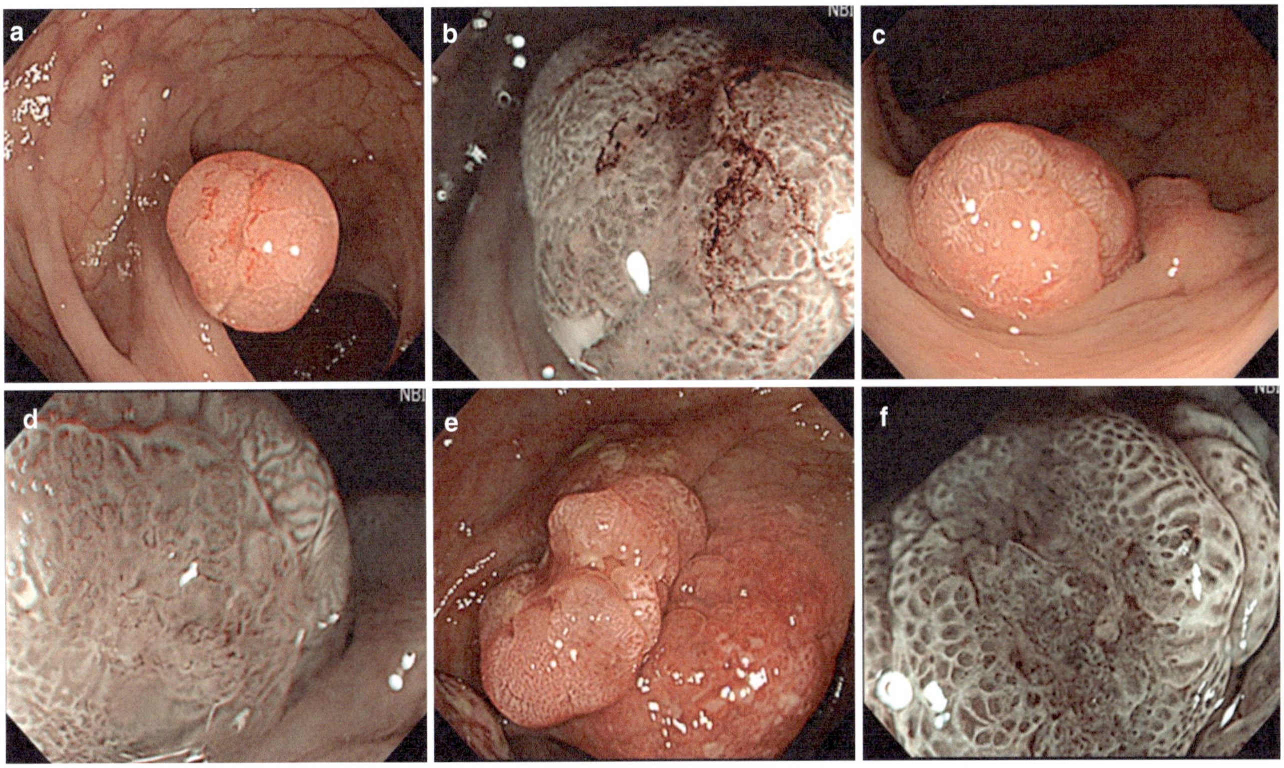

Fig. 21 (**a**) Sigmoid colon: Isp polyp. (**b**) Magnified NBI observation of (**a**). Pathological diagnosis: Tubular adenoma. (**c**) Transverse colon: Isp polyp. (**d**) Magnified NBI observation of (**c**). Pathological diagnosis: Tubular adenoma. (**e**) Ascending colon: Isp polyp. (**f**) Magnified NBI observation of (**e**). Pathological diagnosis: Tubular adenoma

Case 51: A case who was refractory to corticosteroid therapy and nourished by total parenteral nutrition

Provided by Keiichi Mitsuyama and Shinichiro Yoshioka

[Patient]

A 66-year-old male. CC: Diarrhea, melena.

[Clinical findings]

Alopecia (+), onychodystrophy (+), hyperpigmentation (+), dysgeusia (+).

[Laboratory findings]

Alb 3.6 mg/dL, CRP 0.28 mg/dL, Hb 15.9 g/dL.

[Endoscopic image] (Fig. 22)

[Clinical course]

Relapse-remitting type.

Initial treatment: unknown.

Maintenance dose: PSL 5 mg. TPN was temporally administered concurrently.

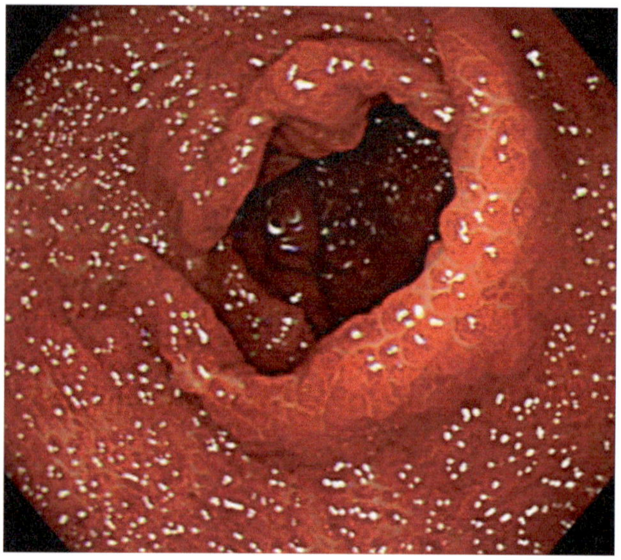

Fig. 22 Stomach: Confluent type. Small, edematous, erythematous, and erosive polyps

Case-Based Images: Cases Treated with Other Than Corticosteroids

Ryota Hokari, Tadakazu Hisamatsu, and Masaaki Higashiyama

Case 52: A case who had few digestive symptoms and achieved endoscopic remission by mesalazine

Provided by Katsuyuki Fukuda

[Patient]

A 70-year-old woman. CC: Anorexia.

[Clinical findings]

Alopecia (+), onychodystrophy (+), hyperpigmentation (+), dysgeusia (+).

[Laboratory findings]

3.0 mg/dL, CRP 4.05 mg/dL, Hb 13.8 g/dL.

[Endoscopic images 1] (Fig. 1a–d)

[Clinical course]

First attack type.

Initial treatment: Mesalazine 1500 mg continuously.

[Endoscopic images 2] (Fig. 2a–c)

EGD and CS after treatments.

All lesions achieved endoscopic remission.

R. Hokari (✉) · M. Higashiyama
Department of Internal Medicine, National Defense Medical College, Tokorozawa, Saitama, Japan
e-mail: ryota@ndmc.ac.jp; masaakih@ndmc.ac.jp

T. Hisamatsu
Department of Gastroenterology and Hepatology, Kyorin University School of Medicine, Mitaka, Tokyo, Japan

R. Hokari, T. Hisamatsu (eds.), *Atlas of Cronkhite-Canada Syndrome*, https://doi.org/10.1007/978-981-19-0652-7_9

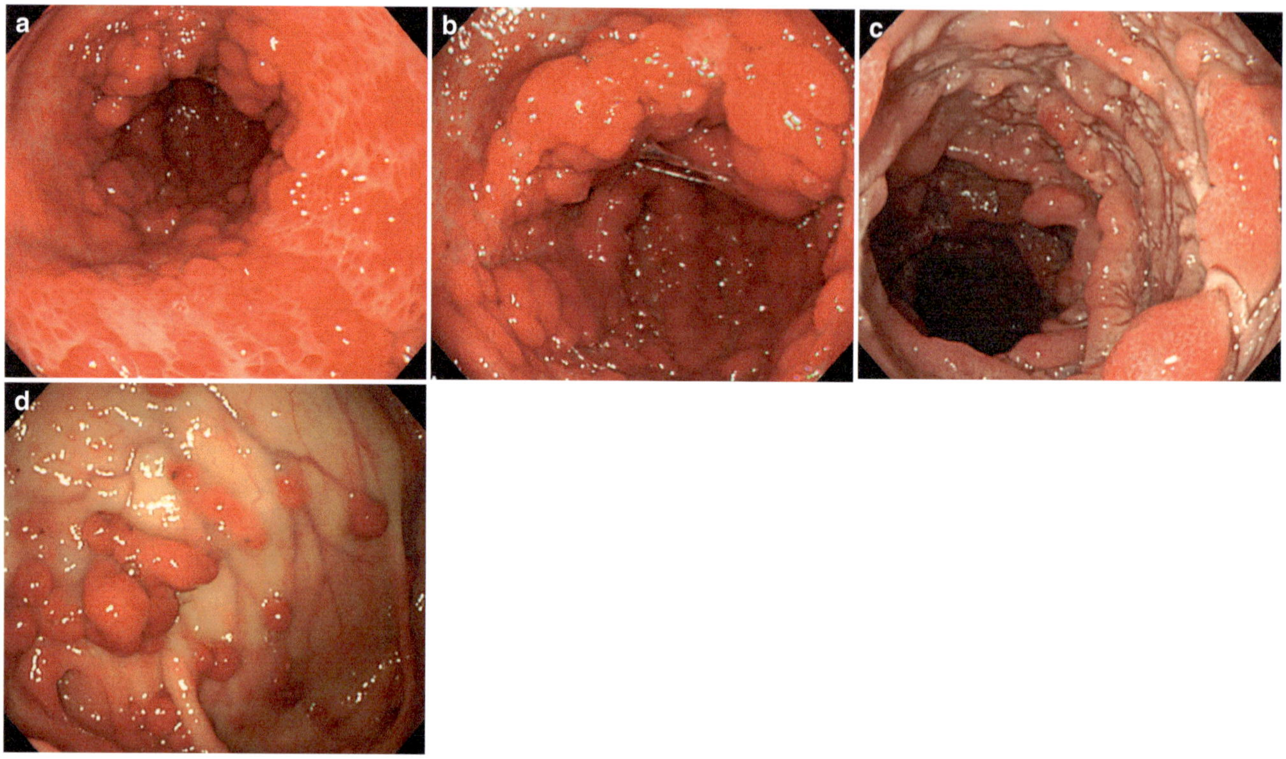

Fig. 1 (**a**), (**b**) Stomach: Confluent type. Medium, edematous, and erythematous polyps. (**c**) Duodenum: Fold thickening type with white villi. (**d**) Colon: Sparse type. Medium, edematous, and erythematous polyps

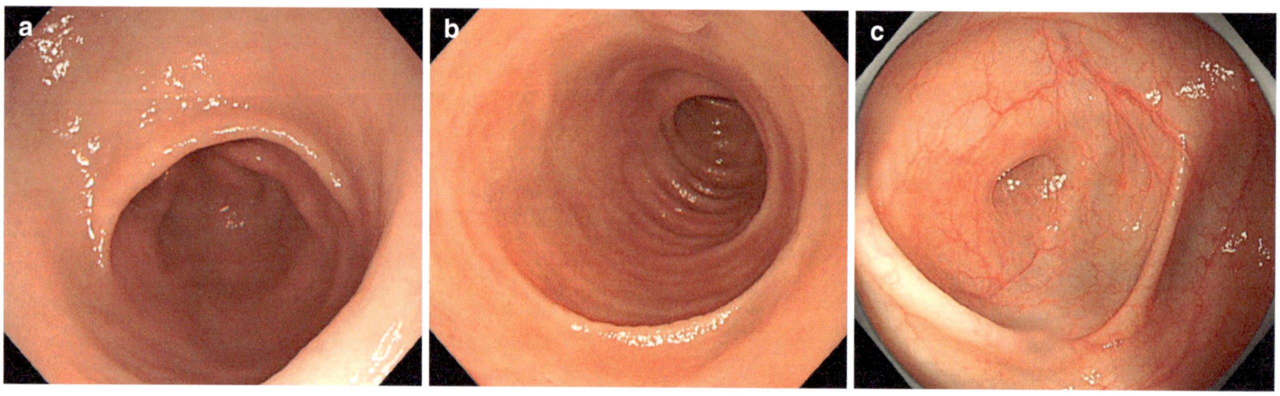

Fig. 2 (**a**) Stomach. (**b**) Duodenum. (**c**) Colon

Case 53: A case who had few digestive symptoms and achieved clinical remission by mesalazine

Provided by Kan Uchiyama

[Patient]

A 60-year-old woman. CC: Weight loss (54.3 kg → 46 kg in 5 months), alopecia, hyperonychia.

[Clinical findings]

Alopecia (+), onychodystrophy (+), hyperpigmentation (+), dysgeusia (+), defecation: 2 times/day.

[Laboratory findings]

Alb 3.9 mg/dL, CRP 0.10 mg/dL, Hb 13.5 g/dL.

[Cutaneous manifestations and endoscopic images 1] (Fig. 3a–i)

[Clinical course]

First attack type.

Initial treatment: Mesalazine (Pentasa®) 3000 mg/day. No PSL was administered. Remission was induced by mesalazine.

[Cutaneous manifestations and endoscopic images 2] (Fig. 4a–f)

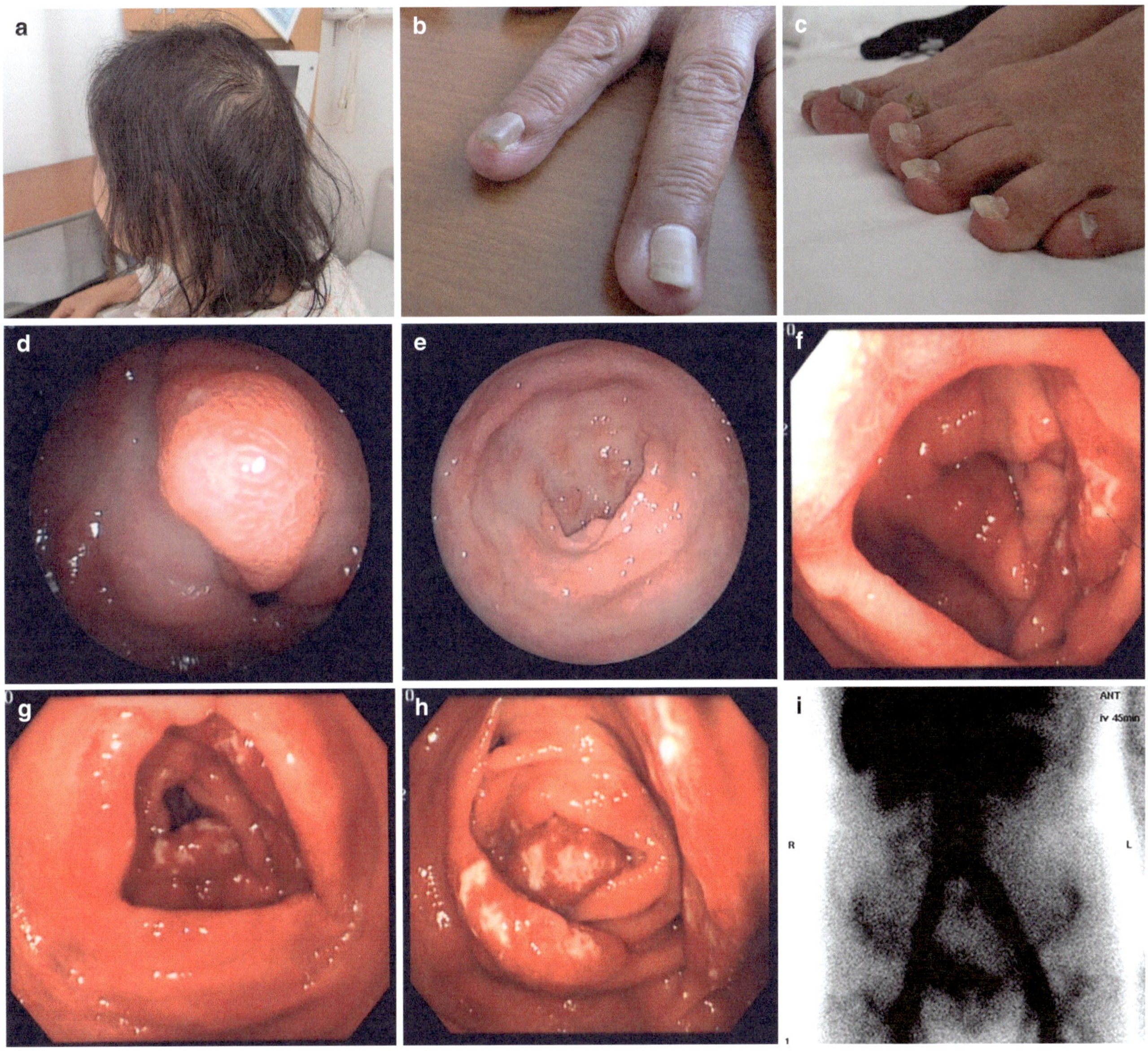

Fig. 3 (**a**) Head: Alopecia. (**b**) Fingers: Onychodystrophy. (**c**) Toes: Onychodystrophy. (**d**), (**e**) Stomach (EGD performed by a previous physician): Sparse type. Medium, edematous, and erosive polyps. (**f**) Cecum: Semi-confluent type. Large, edematous, erythematous, and erosive polyps. (**g**), (**h**) Colon: Semi-onfluent type. Large, edematous, erythematous, and erosive polyps. (**i**) 99Tc-human serum albumin scintigraphy: Abnormal leakage from the intestine

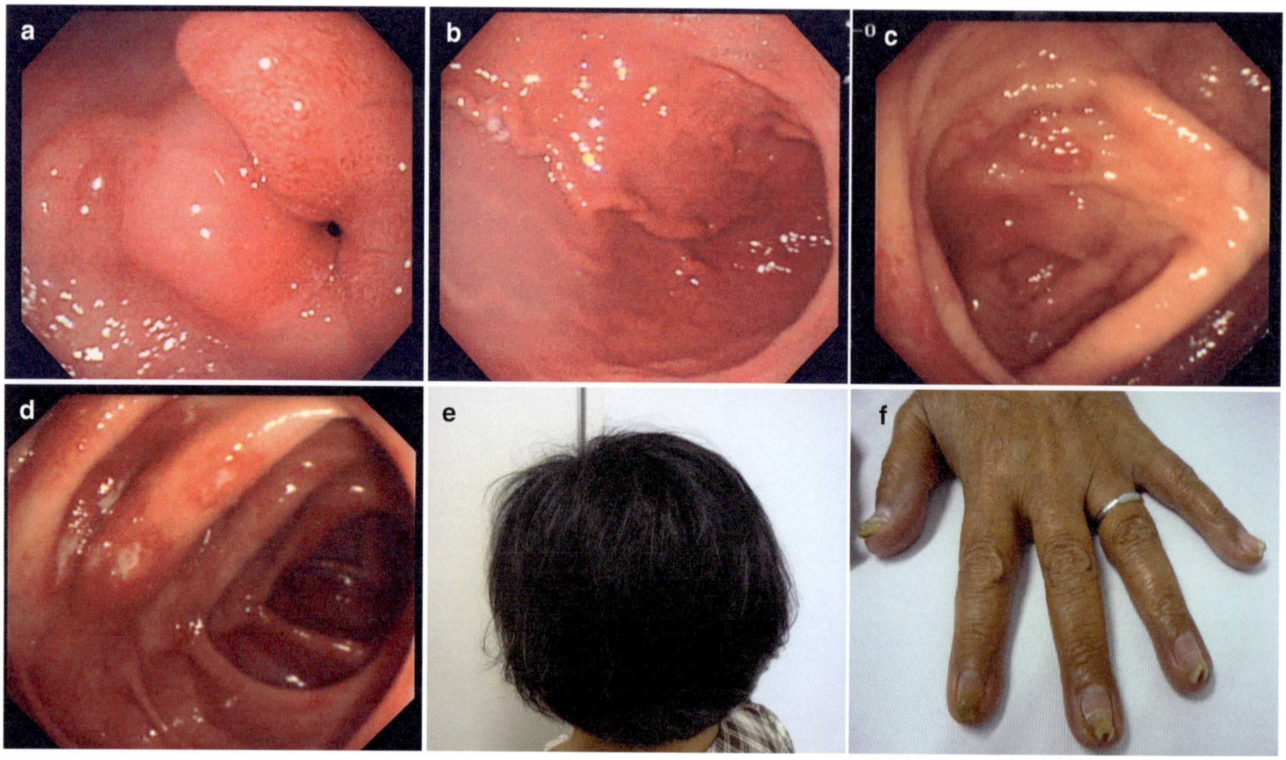

Fig. 4 (**a**), (**b**) Stomach (6 months after the treatment): Gastric polyps were reduced and mucosal findings improved. (**c**), (**d**) Colon (1 year after the treatment): Some polyps remained. Erythema and erosions became mild. (**e**) Head (1 year after the treatment): Alopecia markedly improved. (**f**) Fingers (1 year after the treatment): Deformed nail plates remained in the distal side, but nail plates were normalized in the proximal side

Case 54: A case who had few digestive symptoms and was observed carefully without treatments

Provided by Mari Hayashida

[Patient]

A 43-year-old male. CC: Positive fecal occult blood.

[Clinical findings]

Alopecia (+), onychodystrophy (+), hyperpigmentation (+), dysgeusia (+), defecation: 1 time/day.

[Laboratory findings]

Alb 4.0 mg/dL, CRP 0.01 mg/dL, Hb 16.0 g/dL.

[Endoscopic images] (Fig. 5)

[Clinical course]

Chronic continuous type. Follow-up without treatments.

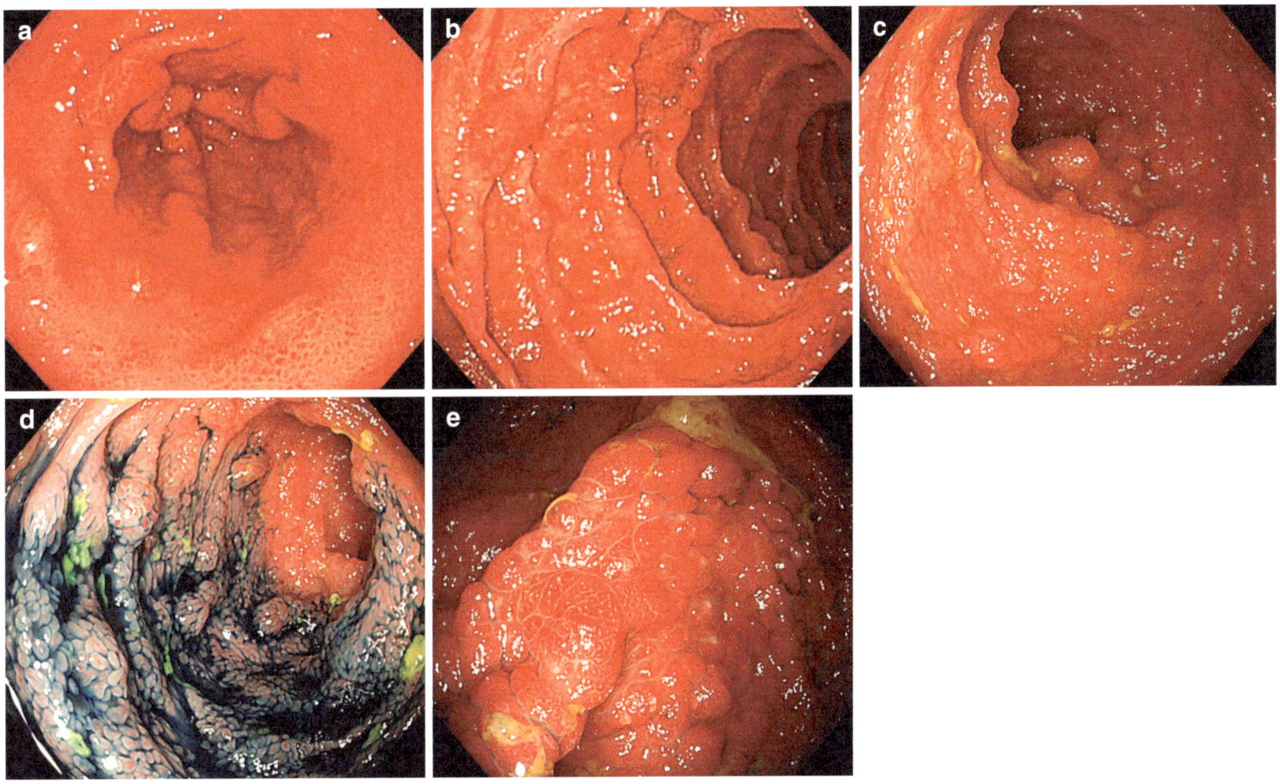

Fig. 5 (**a**) Stomach: Semi-confluent type. Medium, edematous, erythematous, and erosive polyps. (**b**) Duodenum: Fold thickening type with small polyps. (**c**) Terminal ileum: Fold thickening type with small polyps. (**d**) Indigocarmine dyeing of (**c**). (**e**) Colon: Semi-confluent type. Medium, edematous, erythematous, and erosive polyps

Case 55: A case who could not take corticosteroids due to poor general condition and died in spite of total parenteral nutrition

Provided by Keiichi Mitsuyama and Shinichiro Yoshioka

[Patient]

A 67-year-old male. CC: Anorexia, diarrhea.

[Clinical findings]

Alopecia (+), onychodystrophy (+), hyperpigmentation (+), dysgeusia (−), severe edema.

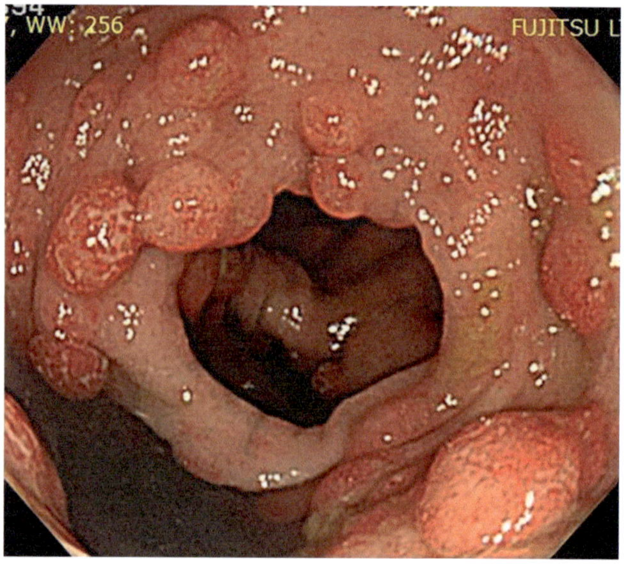

Fig. 6 Colon: Semi-confluent type. Medium, erythematous, hemorrhagic, and whitish mucus adhered polyps

[Laboratory findings]

Alb 1.7 mg/dL, CRP 0.98 mg/dL, Hb 9.3 g/dL.

[Endoscopic images] (Fig. 6)

[Clinical course]

Chronic continuous type. He had been treated for chronic renal failure. Due to shunt malfunction in hemodialysis several times, PSL was not administered. Despite the combined use of TPN and enteral feeding, hypoalbuminemia did not improve and the patient died.

Case-Based Images: Cases with Atypical Clinical Symptoms/Possible Cases

Ryota Hokari, Tadakazu Hisamatsu, and Masaaki Higashiyama

Case 56: An atypical case without diarrhea, whose symptoms were improved by corticosteroids and steroid-free clinical remission was maintained

Provided by Noriko Kamata

[Patient]

A 47-year-old woman. CC: Anorexia, stomach discomfort, dysgeusia, weight loss, onycodystrophy, alopecia, hyperpigmentation.

[Clinical findings]

Alopecia (+), onychodystrophy (+), hyperpigmentation (+), dysgeusia (+), defecation: 1 time/day.

[Laboratory findings]

Alb 3.0 mg/dL, CRP 0.22 mg/dL, Hb 11.7 g/dL.

[Endoscopic images 1] (Fig. 1a–d)

[Clinical course]

Relapse-remitting type.

Initial treatment: PSL 30 mg for 2 weeks.

Clinical response: 1 week.

Clinical remission: 1 week.

[Endoscopic images 2] (Fig. 2a, b)

Four months after the diagnosis.

R. Hokari (✉) · M. Higashiyama
Department of Internal Medicine, National Defense Medical College, Tokorozawa, Saitama, Japan
e-mail: ryota@ndmc.ac.jp; masaakih@ndmc.ac.jp

T. Hisamatsu
Department of Gastroenterology and Hepatology, Kyorin University School of Medicine, Mitaka, Tokyo, Japan

R. Hokari, T. Hisamatsu (eds.), *Atlas of Cronkhite-Canada Syndrome*, https://doi.org/10.1007/978-981-19-0652-7_10

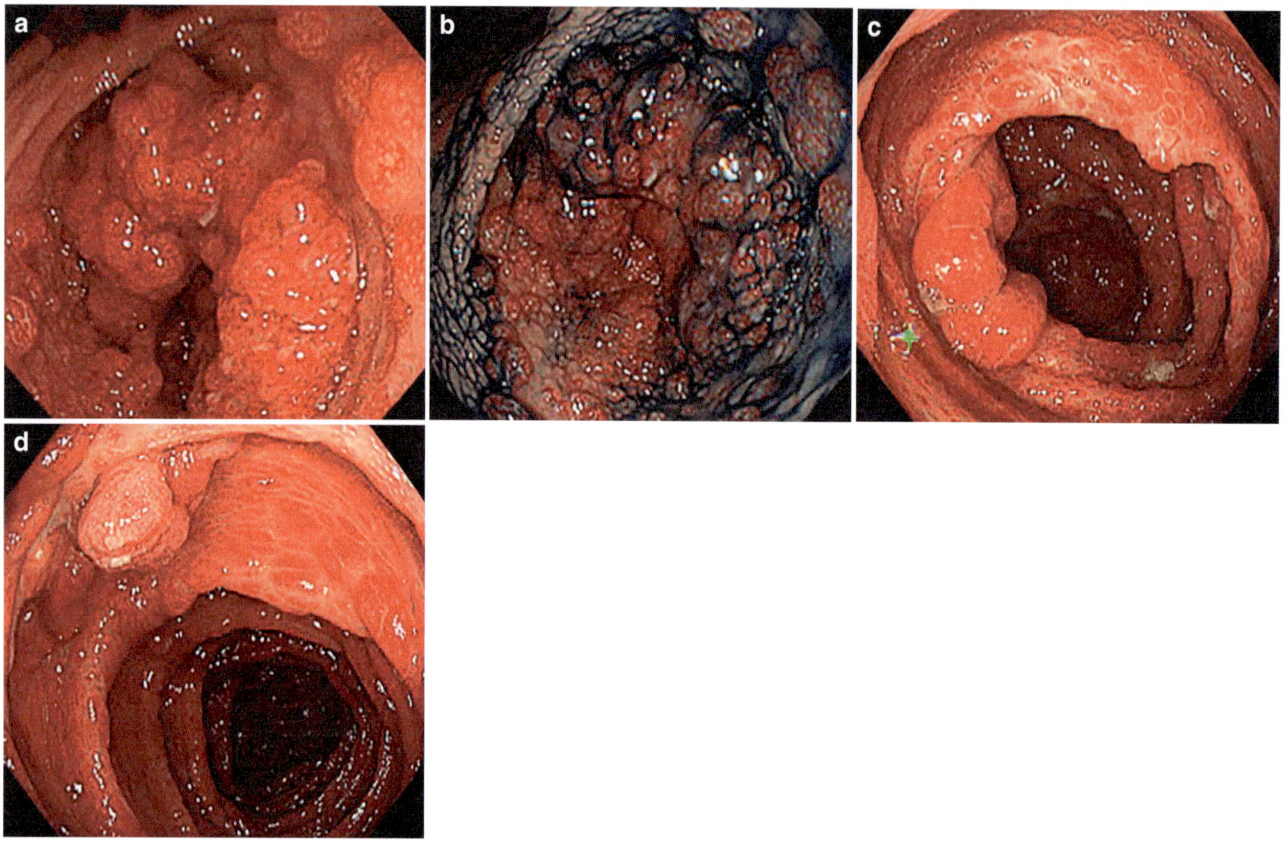

Fig. 1 (**a**) Stomach: Confluent type. Medium, edematous, erythematous, and hemorrhagic polyps. (**b**) Indigocarmine dyeing of (**a**). (**c**), (**d**) Colon: Confluent type. Medium, edematous, and erythematous polyps

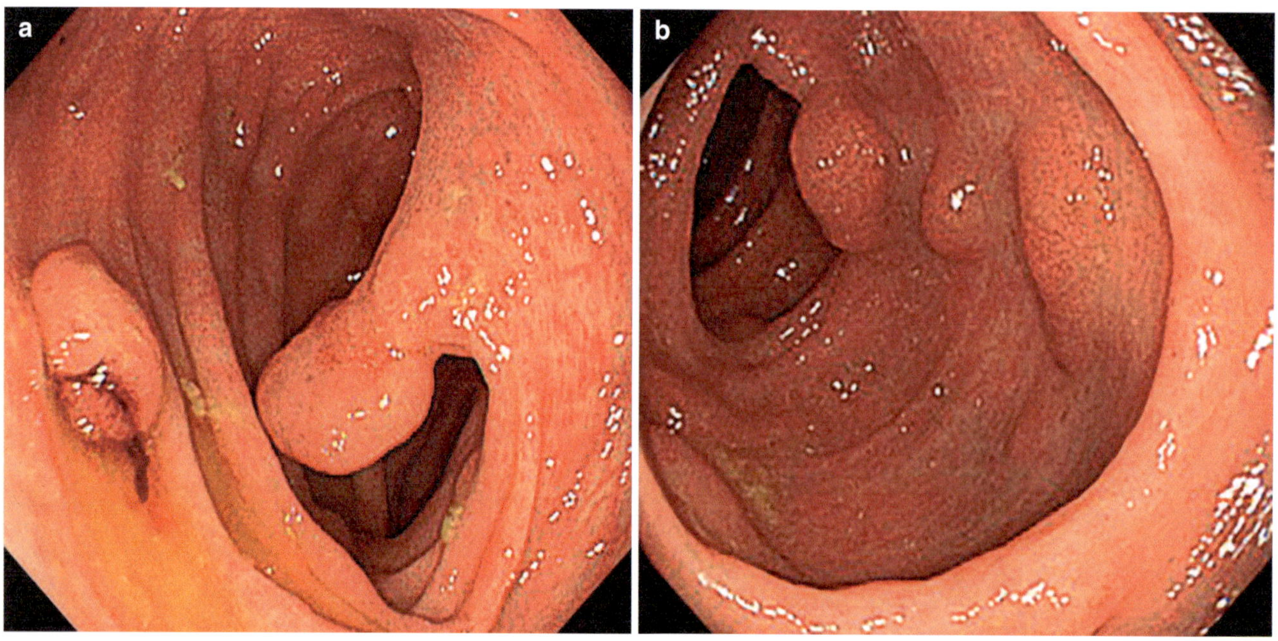

Fig. 2 (**a**), (**b**) Colon

Case 57: An asymptomatic case who was suspected by the gastric cancer screening

Provided by Teppei Omori

[Patient]

A 40-year-old male. CC: Abnormal findings pointed out in the barium X-ray radiography of the stomach of medical checkup.

[Clinical findings]

Onychodystrophy (−), hyperpigmentation (−), dysgeusia (−).

[Laboratory findings]

Hb 8.2 g/dL.

[Endoscopic images] (Fig. 3)

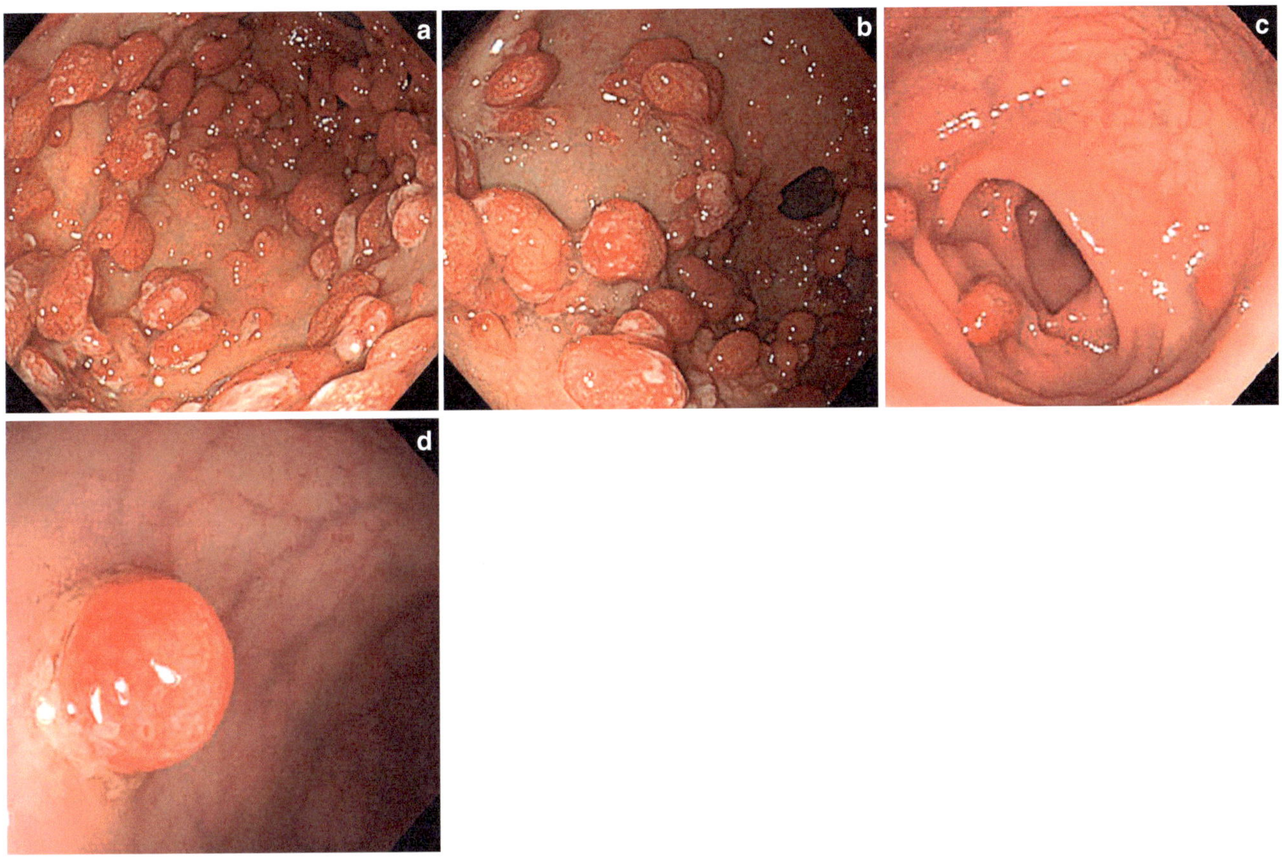

Fig. 3 (**a**), (**b**) Stomach: Semi-confluent type. Medium, erythematous polyps. Edematous intervening mucosa. (**c**), (**d**) Colon: Sparse type. Medium, edematous polyps

Case 58: A possible case complaining of dysgeusia and anorexia, who was treated with corticosteroids

Provided by Makoto Ooi and Yuzo Kodama

[Patient]

A 58-year-old male. CC: Anorexia, dysgeusia.

[Clinical findings]

Alopecia (−), onychodystrophy (−), hyperpigmentation (−), dysgeusia (+), edema (−). Weight loss: −5 kg/month.

[Laboratory findings]

Alb 3.4 mg/dL, CRP 0.03 mg/dL Hb 19.5 g/dL.

[Endoscopic images] (Fig. 4)

[Clinical course]

First attack type.

Initial treatment: PSL 40 mg for 2 weeks.

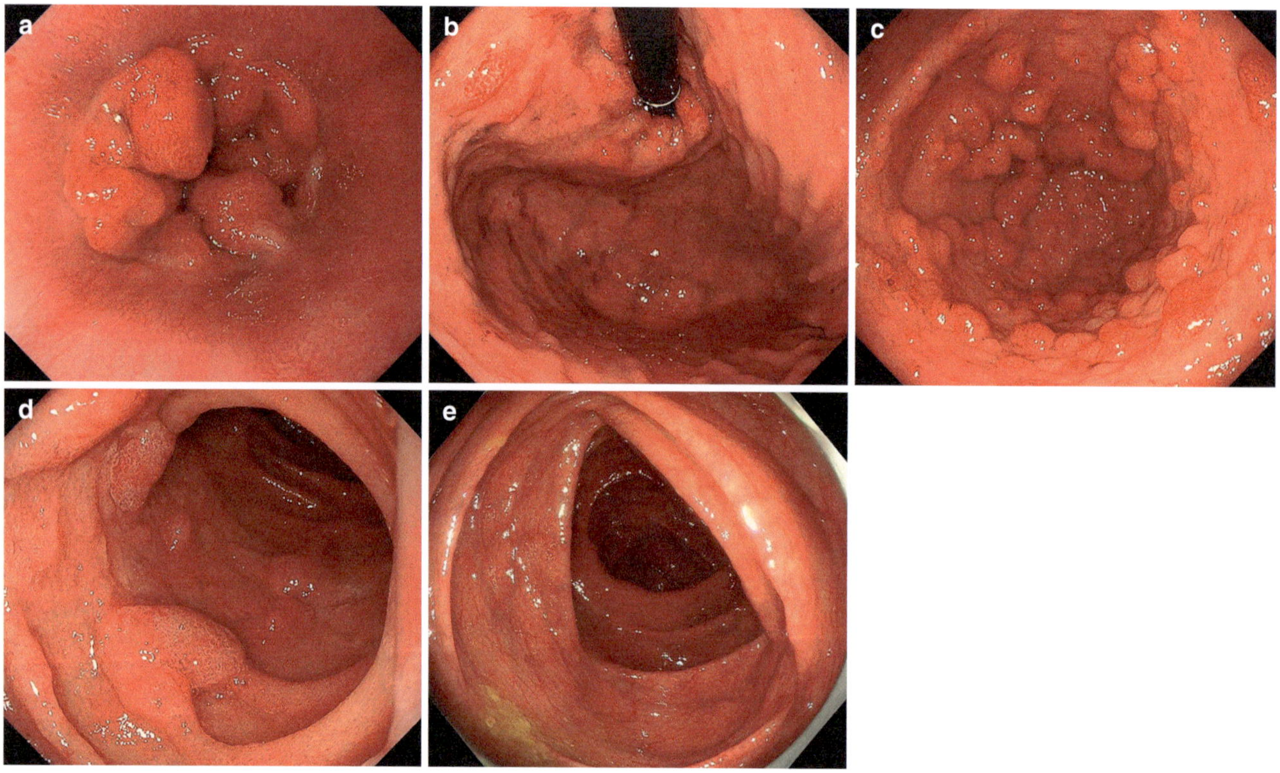

Fig. 4 (**a**) Esophagogastric junction: The esophageal mucosa was normal. The gastric mucosa showed multiple polyps. (**b**), (**c**) Stomach: Semi-confluent type. Medium, erythematous polyps. Edematous intervening mucosa. (**d**) Duodenum: Fold thickening type with medium polyps. (**e**) Colon: No abnormal findings

Case 59: A possible case who complained of postprandial abdominal discomfort and alopecia

Provided by Fukunori Kinjo and Tetsu Kinjo

[Patient]

A 56-year-old woman. CC: Abdominal discomfort after meal.

[Clinical findings]

Alopecia (+), hyperpigmentation (−), diarrhea (+).

[Laboratory findings]

Alb 3.5 mg/dL.

[Endoscopic images] (Fig. 5)

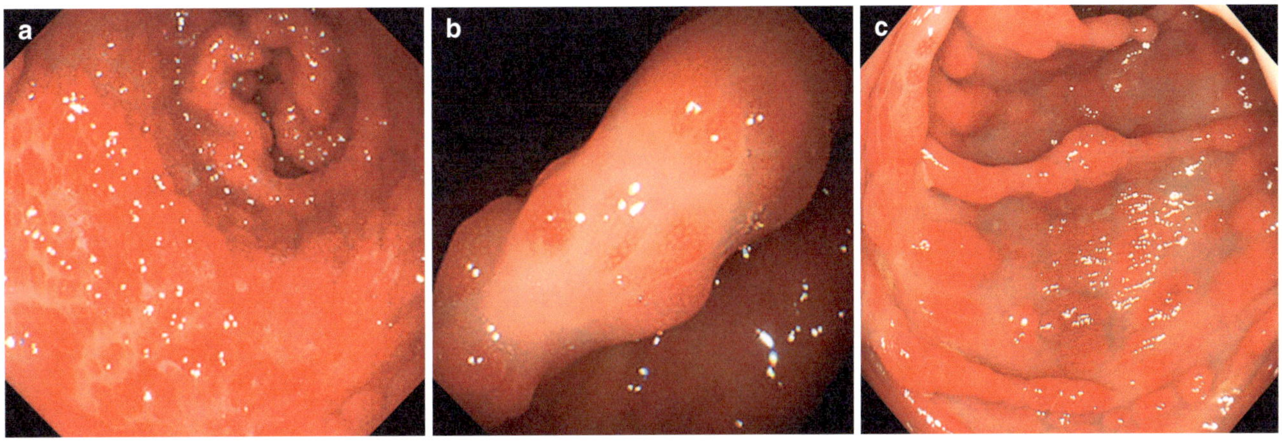

Fig. 5 (**a**), (**b**) Stomach: Confluent type. Small polyps. Edematous intervening mucosa. (**c**) Colon: Confluent type. Small polyps

Case 60: A possible case complaining of dysgeusia and weight loss, whose colonic mucosa showed yellowish-white mucus adherence and clinical remission was achieved by corticosteroids

Provided by Rintaro Moroi and Atsushi Masamune

[Patient]

An 83-year-old man. CC: Dysgeusia, weight loss.

[Clinical findings]

Alopecia (−), onychodystrophy (−), hyperpigmentation (−), frequency of defecation: unknown, mild edema.

[Laboratory findings]

Alb 2.0 mg/dL, CRP 0.69 mg/dL, Hb 10.4 g/dL.

[Endoscopic images 1] (Fig. 6a–e)

[Clinical course]

First attack type.

Initial treatment: PSL 30 mg for 1 week.

Clinical response: 2 weeks.

Clinical remission: 12 weeks.

Maintenance dose: PSL 0 mg.

[Endoscopic images 2] (Fig. 7a–c)

EGD and CS 1 month after the diagnosis.

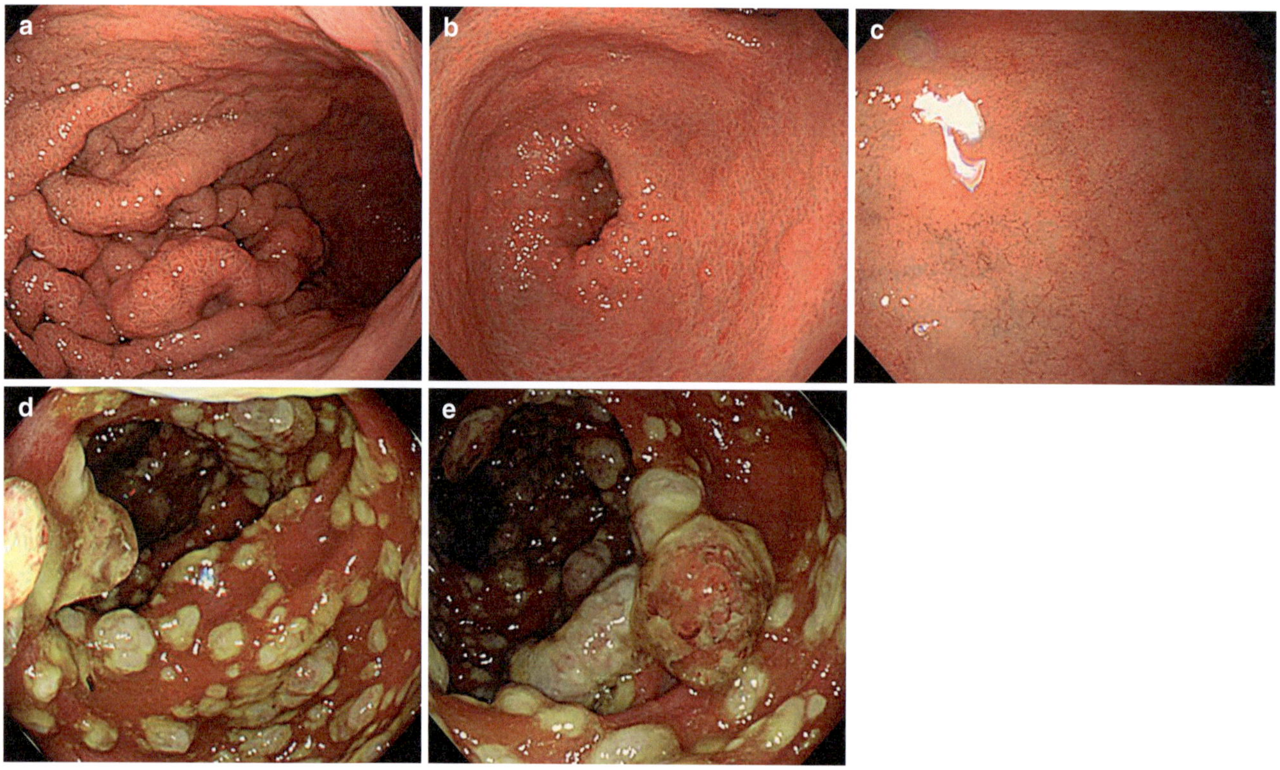

Fig. 6 (**a**), (**b**) Stomach: Semi-confluent type. Small to medium polyps. (**c**) Duodenum: normal. (**d**), (**e**) Colon: Semi-confluent type. Small to medium, whitish mucus adhered polyps

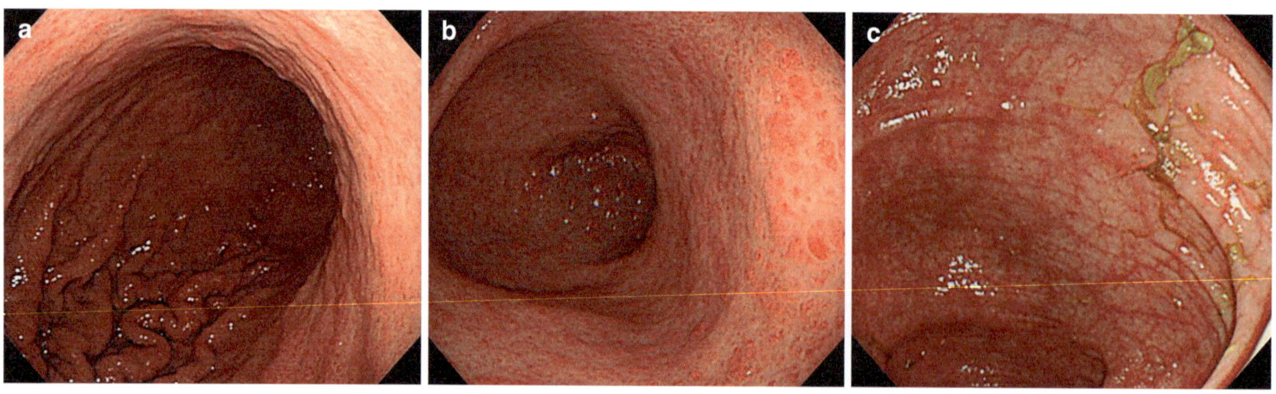

Fig. 7 (**a**), (**b**) Stomach: Only a slight improvement compared with previous findings. (**c**) Colon: Remarkable decrease in polyps contrary to stomach findings

Case 61: An atypical case whose digestive symptom included bloody stool

Provided by Masanao Nakamura and Mitsuhiro Fujishiro

[Patient]

A 65-year-old male. CC: Edema of lower limbs, bloody stool.

[Clinical findings]

Alopecia (+), onychodystrophy (+), hyperpigmentation (+), dysgeusia (+), defecation: 5 times/day, mild edema.

[Laboratory findings]

Alb 3.9 mg/dL, CRP 0.14 mg/dL, Hb 11.1 g/dL.

99Tc-human serum albumin scintigraphy: Negative study.

[Endoscopic images] (Fig. 8)

[Clinical course]

First attack type.

Initial treatment: PSL 30 mg for 6 weeks.

Clinical response: 6 weeks.

Maintenance dose: PSL 10 mg.

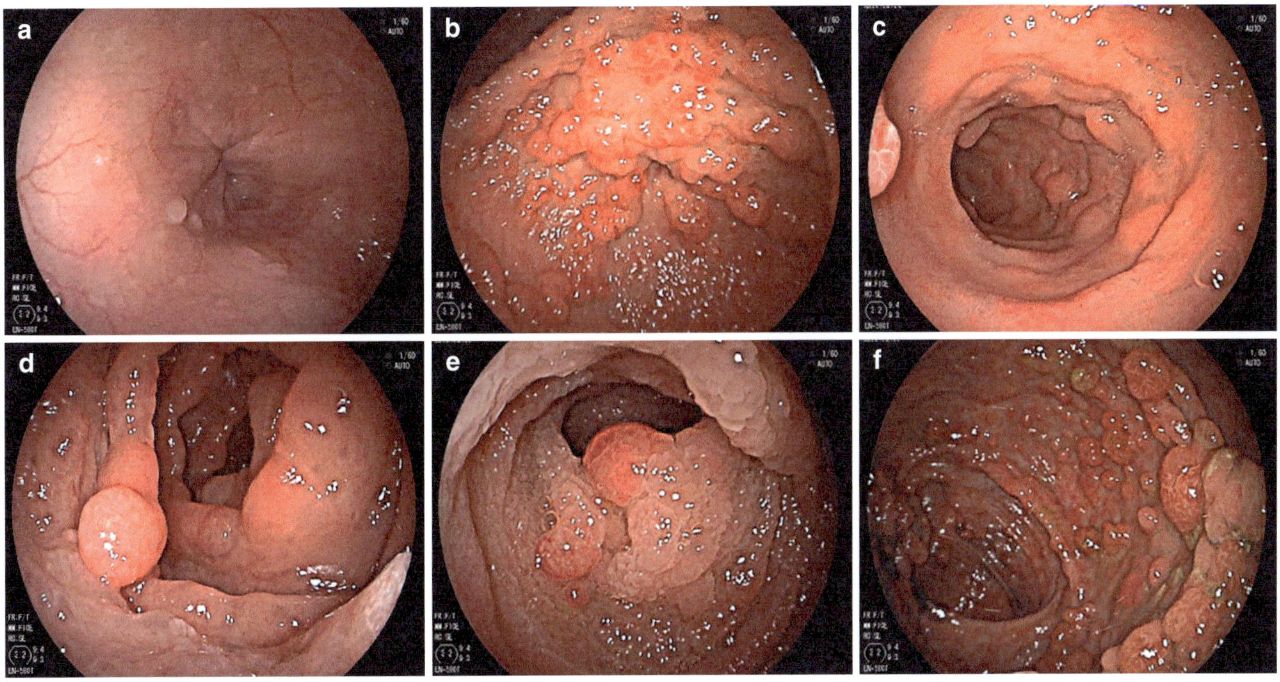

Fig. 8 (**a**) Esophagus: Sparse type. Small, flat to hemispherical, edematous polyps. (**b**) Stomach: Semi-confluent type. Medium, edematous, erythematous, and hemorrhagic polyps. (**c**) Duodenum: Fold thickening type with scattered medium polyps. (**d**) Jejunum: Fold thickening type with scattered small to medium polyps. (**e**) Ileum: Fold thickening type with erythematous polyps. (**f**) Colon: Semi-confluent type. Small, edematous and erythematous polyps

Case 62: An atypical case without diarrhea, who responded to corticosteroids and maintained clinical remission with PSL 2.5 mg

Provided by Takehiro Torisu and Junji Umeno

[Patient]

A 55-year-old male. CC: Anorexia, hyperpigmentation on the face, onychodystrophy.

[Clinical findings]

Alopecia (−), onychodystrophy (+), hyperpigmentation (+), dysgeusia (−), defecation: 2 times/day.

[Laboratory findings]

Alb 4.3 mg/dL, CRP 0.01 mg/dL, Hb 9.4 g/dL.

Fecal alpha1-antitrypsin clearance test: 24.5 mL/day.

[Endoscopic images] (Fig. 9)

[Clinical course]

First attack type.

Initial treatment: PSL 30 mg for 2 weeks.

Clinical response: 1 week.

Clinical remission: 7 weeks.

Maintenance dose: PSL 2.5 mg.

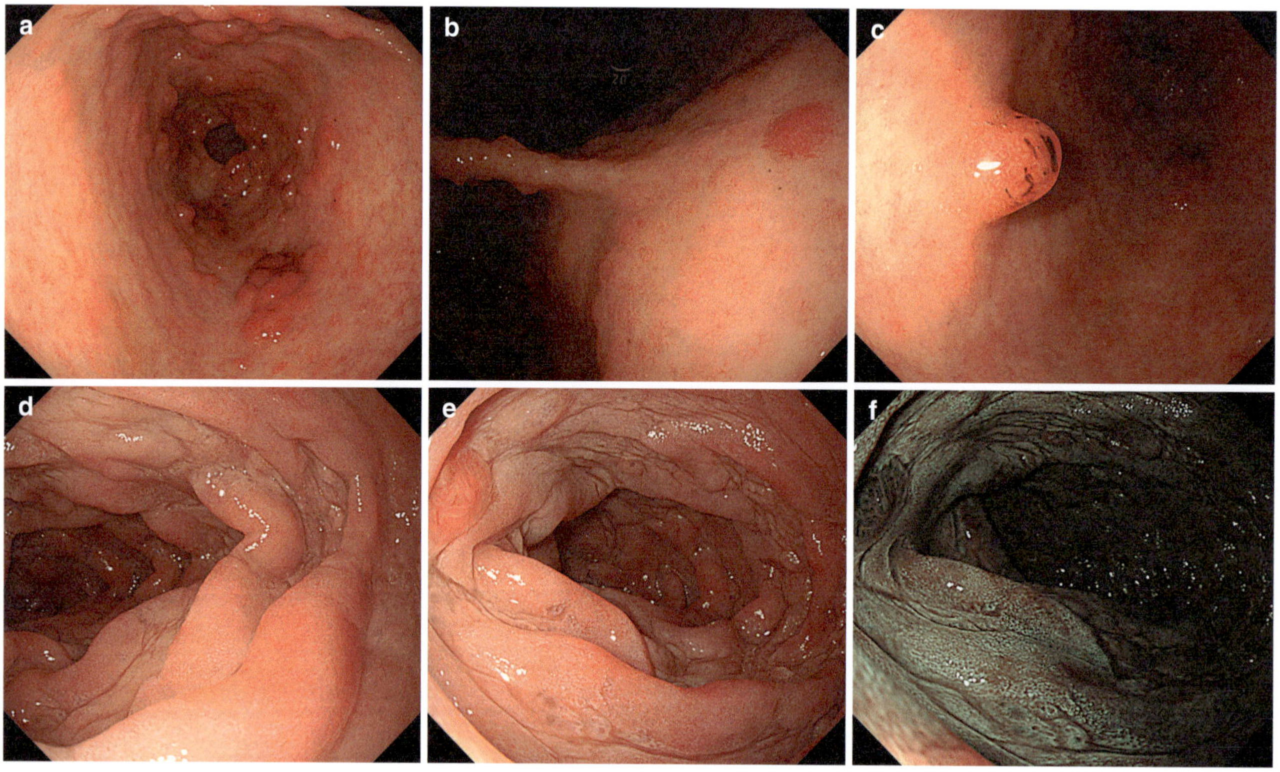

Fig. 9 (**a**), (**b**), (**c**) Stomach: Sparse type (some flat elevations were partially confluent). Medium, erythematous polyps. (**d**), (**e**), (**f**) Duodenum: Fold thickening type. Villi were flattened

Case 63: An atypical case without diarrhea, who responded markedly to corticosteroid and achieved PSL-free clinical remission.

Provided by Ken Sugimoto

[Patient]

A 61-year-old woman. CC: Dysgeusia, weight loss.

[Clinical findings]

Alopecia (+), onychodystrophy (+), hyperpigmentation (+), dysgeusia (+), defecation: 1 time/day.

[Laboratory findings]

Alb 3.7 mg/dL, CRP 0.37 mg/dL, Hb 14.3 g/dL.

[Endoscopic images 1] (Fig. 10a–g)

[Clinical course]

First attack type.

Initial treatment: PSL 30 mg for 1 week.

Clinical response: 1 week.

Clinical remission: 4 weeks.

Maintenance dose: PSL 0 mg.

[Endoscopic images 2] (Fig. 11a, b)

SBCE during treatments.

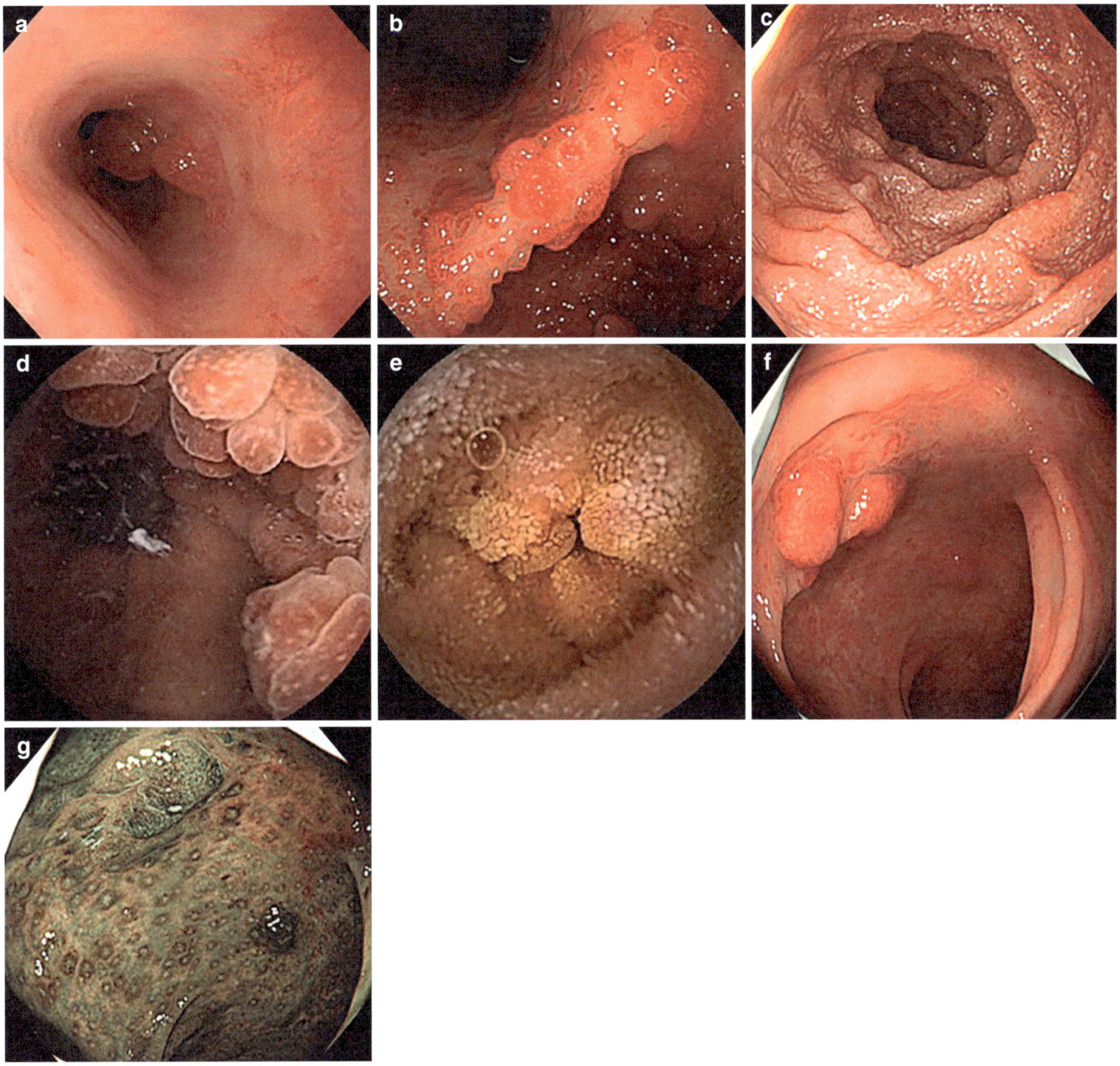

Fig. 10 (**a**) Esophagus: Sparse type. Medium, edematous polyps. (**b**) Stomach: Semi-confluent type. Medium, edematous, and erythematous polyps. (**c**) Duodenum: Fold thickening type with edematous villi. (**d**), (**e**) Jejunum (SBCE): Semi-confluent type. Small polyps and white villi. (**f**) Colon: Semi-confluent type. Small to medium, edematous polyps. (**g**) NBI observation of (**f**)

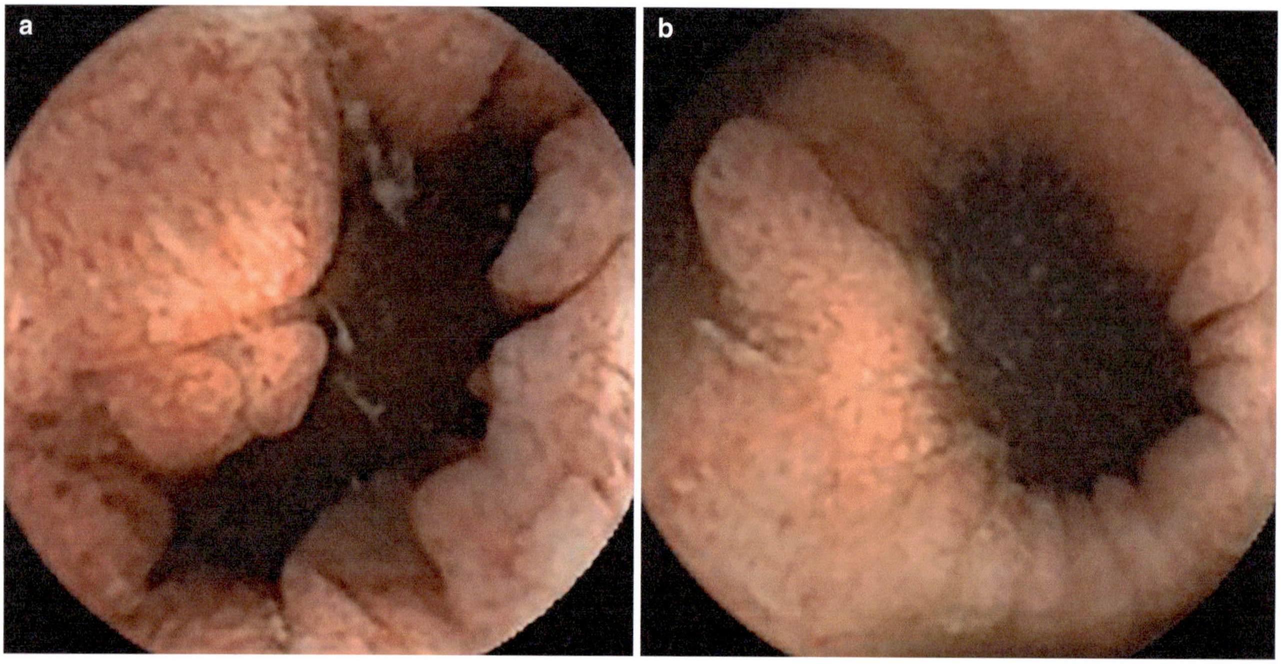

Fig. 11 (**a**), (**b**) Jejunum: Polyps decreased

Case 64: An atypical case without diarrhea, who responded to corticosteroid and maintained clinical remission with PSL 10 mg.

Provided by Naoki Hosoe and Takanori Kanai

[Patient]

A 61-year-old male. CC: Loose stool.

[Clinical findings]

Alopecia (+), onychodystrophy (+), hyperpigmentation (−), dysgeusia (+), defecation: 1 time/day.

[Laboratory findings]

Alb 3.7 mg/dL, CRP 0.51 mg/dL, Hb 15.2 g/dL.

[Cutaneous findings and endoscopic images] (Fig. 12)

[Clinical course]

First attack type.

Initial treatment: PSL 40 mg for 4 weeks.

Clinical response: 4 weeks.

Clinical remission: 12 weeks.

Maintenance dose: PSL 10 mg.

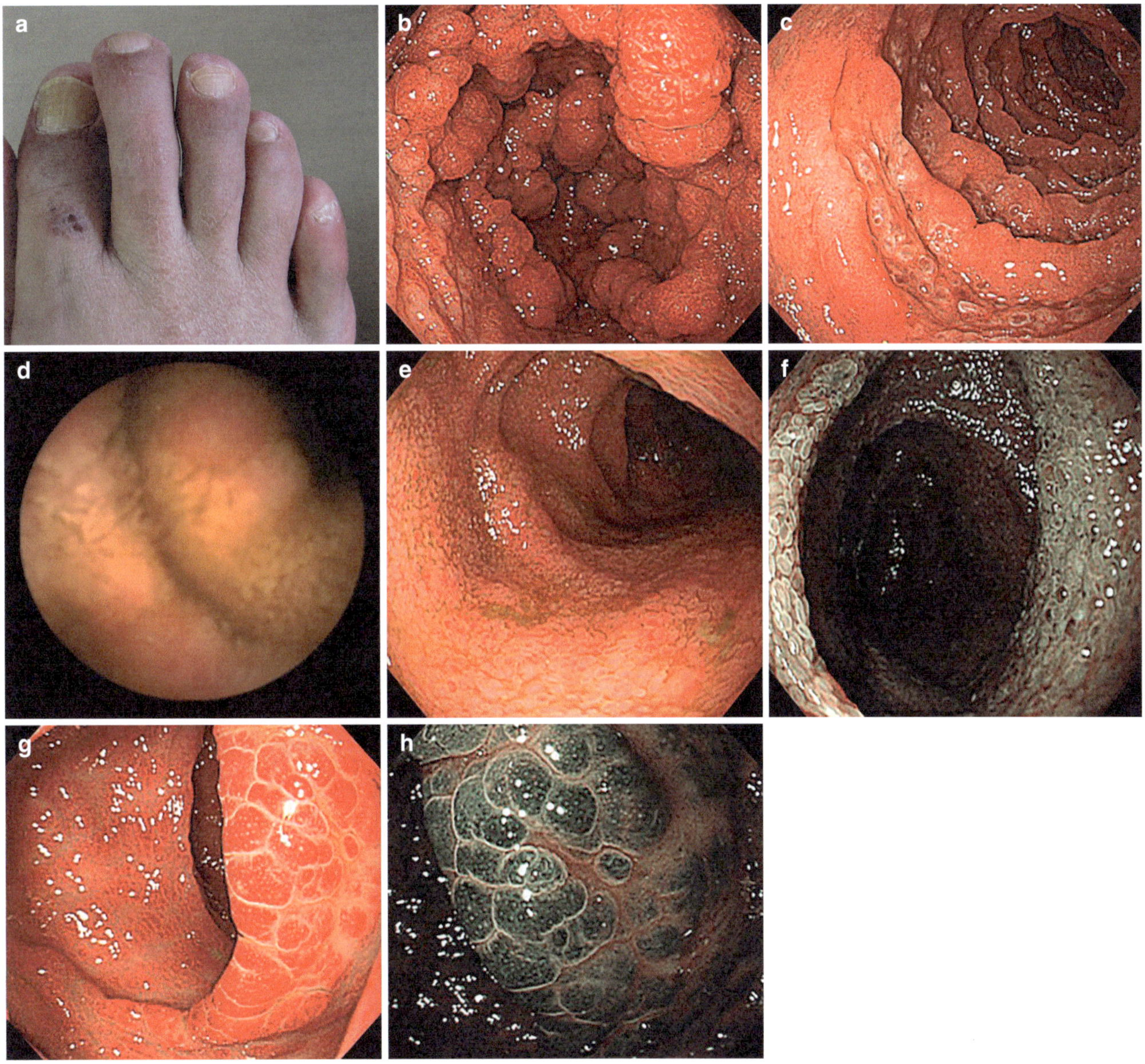

Fig. 12 (**a**) Toes: Onychdystrophy. (**b**) Stomach: Confluent type. Large, edematous, erythematous, and whitish mucus adhered polyps. (**c**) Duodenum: Fold thickening type with white villi. (**d**) Ileum (SBCE): Fold thickening type with some erythematous inflammatory polyps. (**e**) Terminal ileum: Swollen villi. (**f**) NBI observation of (**e**). (**g**) Colon: Confluent type. Medium, edematous, and erythematous polyps. (**h**) NBI observation of (**g**)

Case 65: An atypical case without diarrhea, who responded to corticosteroid, leading to almost complete disappearance of polyps

Provided by Kan Uchiyama

[Patient]

A 65-year-old woman. CC: Positive fecal occult blood.

[Clinical findings]

Alopecia (+), onychodystrophy (+), hyperpigmentation (−), dysgeusia (+), defecation: 1 time/day.

[Laboratory findings]

Alb 3.2 mg/dL, CRP 0.10 mg/dL, Hb 13.3 g/dL.

[Endoscopic images 1] (Fig. 13a–e)

[Clinical course]

First attack type.

Initial treatment: PSL 30 mg for 2 weeks.

Clinical response: 6 weeks.

Clinical remission: 14 weeks.

Maintenance dose: PSL 0 mg.

[Endoscopic images 2] (Fig. 14a–e)

EGD and CS in remission 2 years after the diagnosis.

Remarkable improvements of mucosal findings in all the lesions.

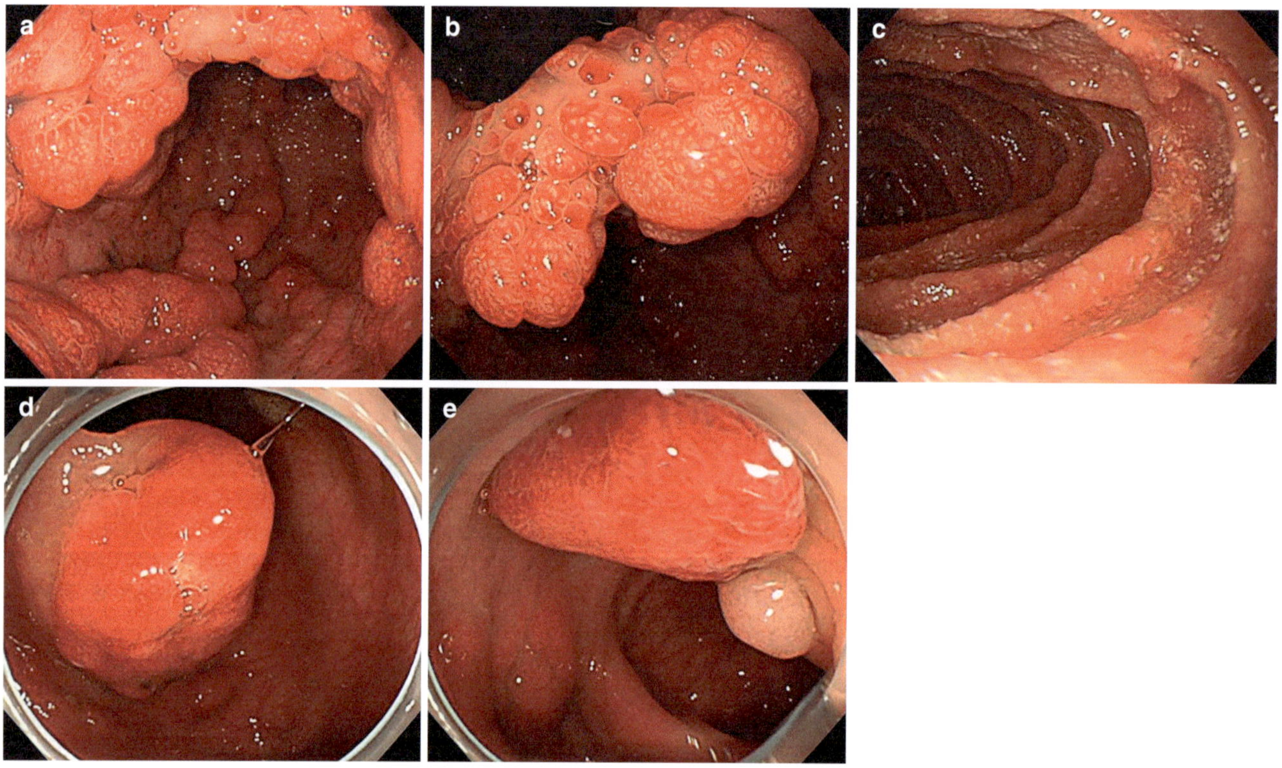

Fig. 13 (**a**), (**b**) Stomach: Confluent type. Medium, edematous, and erosive polyps. (**c**) Duodenum: Fold thickening type with small white patches. (**d**), (**e**) Colon: Sparse type. Large, erythematous polyps. Some polyps were discolored. The intervening mucosa was almost normal and well demarcated

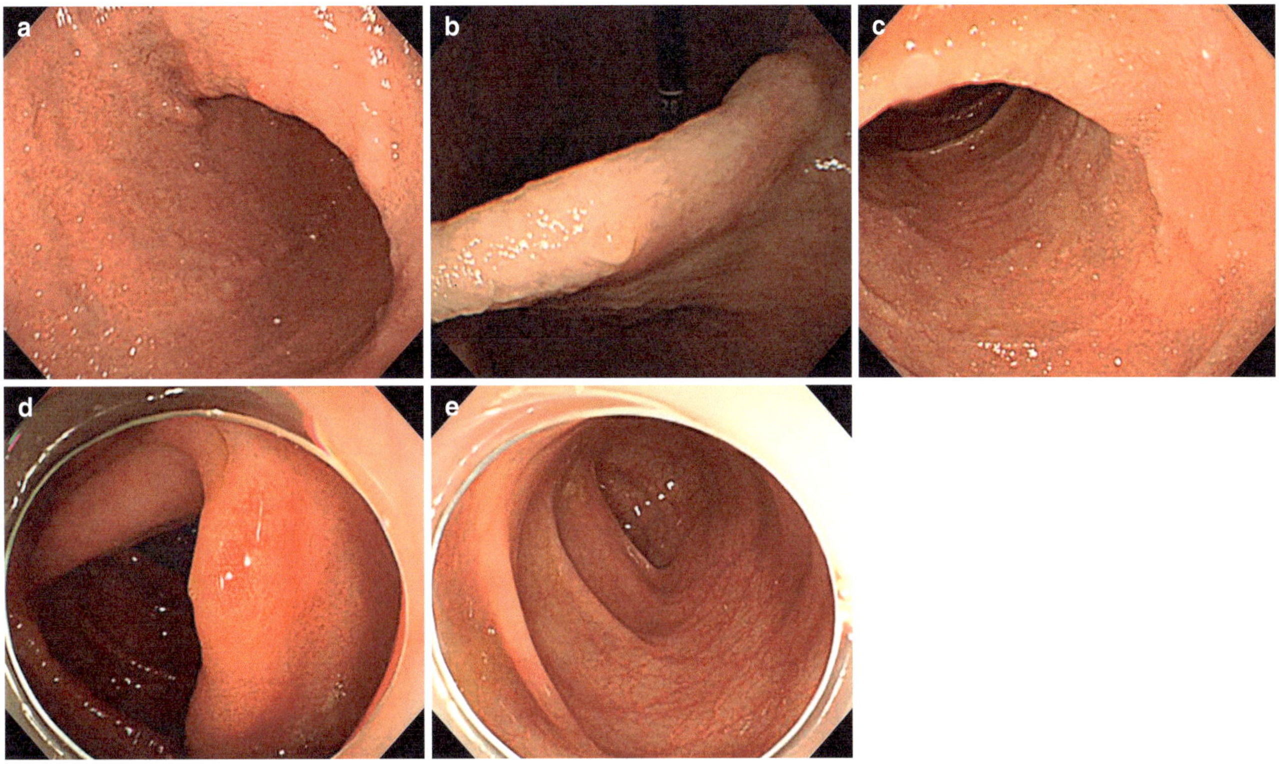

Fig. 14 (**a**), (**b**) Stomach. (**c**) Duodenum. (**d**), (**e**) Colon

Case 66: An atypical case with few digestive symptoms, who responded markedly to corticosteroids and achieved endoscopic remission

Provided by Takayuki Matsumoto and Shunichi Yanai

[Patient]

A 63-year-old woman. CC: dysgeusia

[Clinical findings]

Alopecia (+), onychodystrophy (+), skin pigmentation (+), defecation: 2 times/day.

[Laboratory findings]

Alb 3.6 mg/dL, CRP <0.10 mg/dL, Hgb 13.1 g/dL.

[Endoscopic images 1] (Fig. 15a–d)

[Clinical course]

First attack type.

Initial treatment: PSL 40 mg for 2 weeks.

Clinical response: 2 weeks.

Clinical remission: 8 weeks.

Maintenance dose: PSL 5 mg.

[Endoscopic images 2] (Fig. 16a, b)

EGD after treatments.

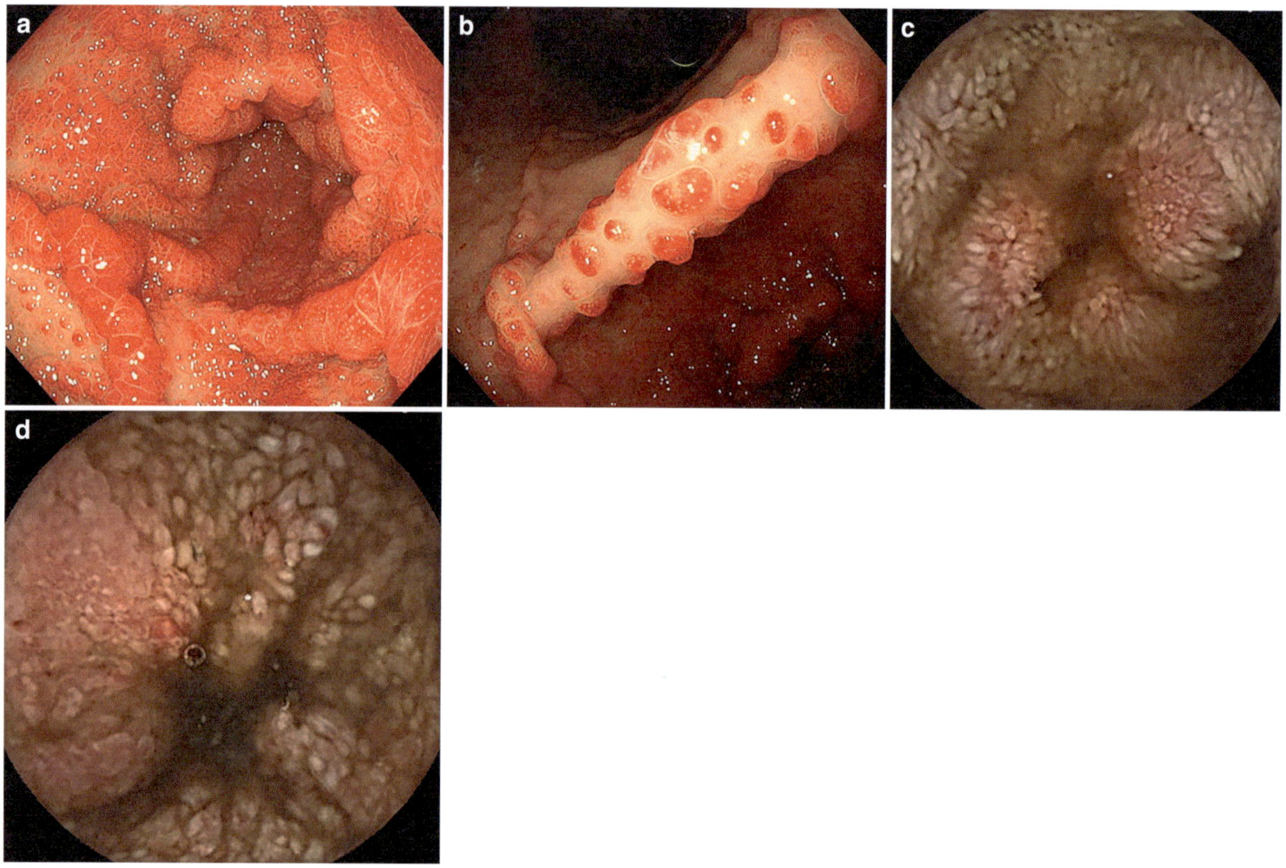

Fig. 15 (**a**), (**b**) Stomach: Semi-confluent type. Small, edematous, and erythematous polyps with fold thickening in the antrum. (**c**), (**d**) Small intestine (SBCE): Fold thickening type with granular, erythematous mucosa and white villi

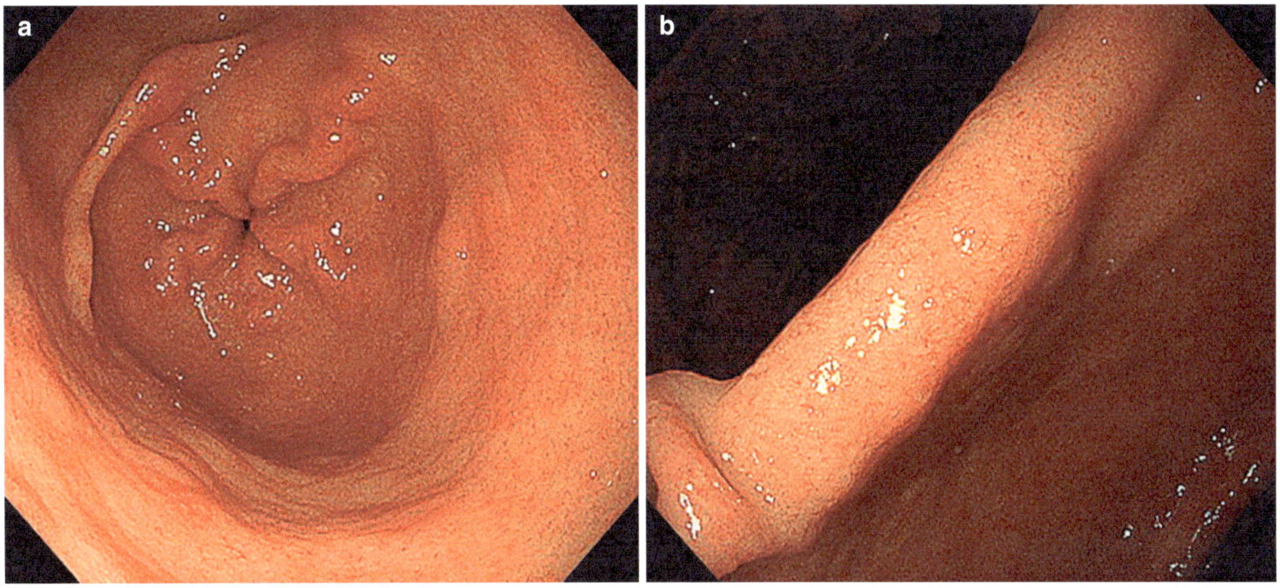

Fig. 16 (**a**), (**b**) Stomach: Polyps disappeared

Case 67: An atypical case with no digestive symptoms, who responded markedly to corticosteroids and had only a few residual polyps

Provided by Makoto Ooi and Yuzo Kodama

[Patient]

A 50-year-old woman. CC: Dysgeusia, hyperpigmentation, alopecia, edema.

[Clinical findings]

Alopecia (+), onychodystrophy (+), hyperpigmentation (+), moderate edema.

[Laboratory findings]

Alb 2.8 mg/dL, CRP 0 mg/dL, Hb 12.8 g/dL.

[Endoscopic images 1] (Fig. 17a–e)

[Clinical course]

First attack type.

Initial treatment: PSL 40 mg for 2 weeks.

Endoscopic response: 1 month.

Endoscopic remission: 42 months.

Maintenance dose: PSL 0 mg.

[Endoscopic images 2] (Fig. 18a–e)

EGD and CS 42 months after the initial treatment.

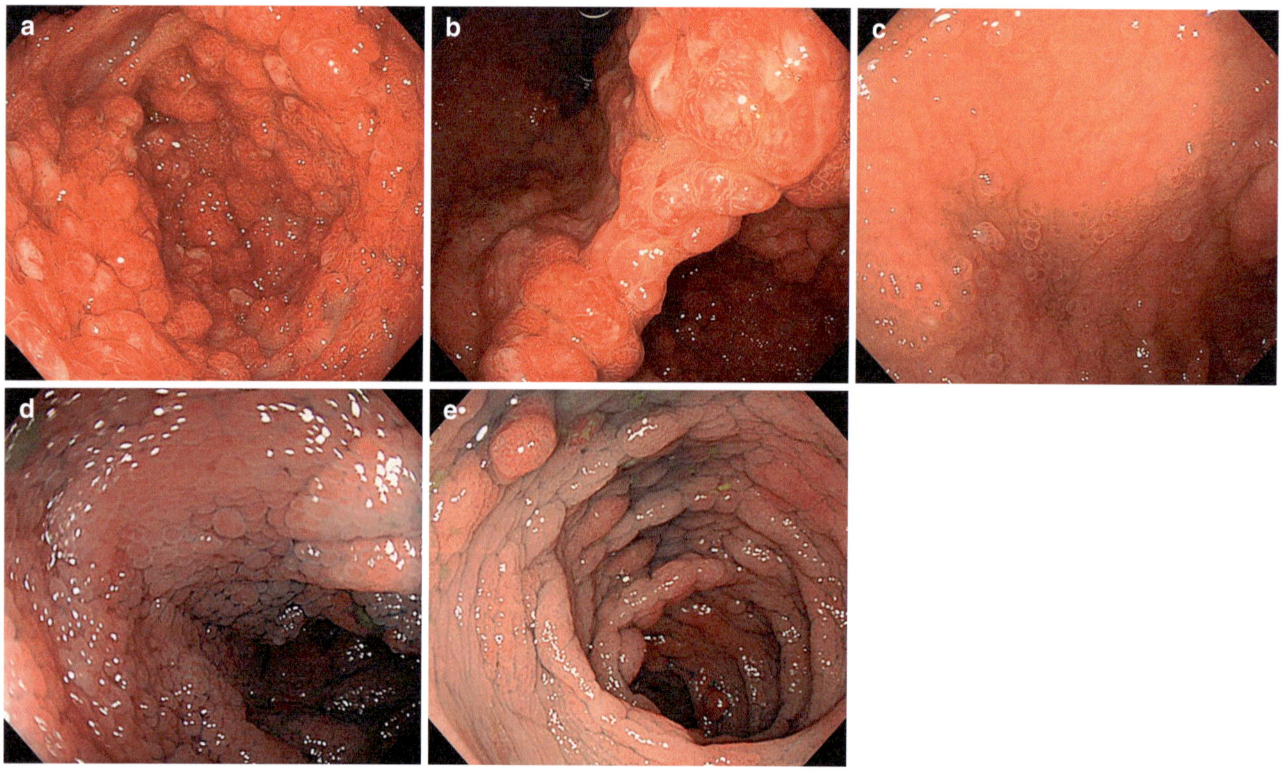

Fig. 17 (**a**), (**b**) Stomach: Confluent type. Small, edematous, and erythematous polyps. Edematous intervening mucosa. (**c**) Duodenum: Fold thickening type with small polyps. (**d**) Terminal ileum: Fold thickening type with small polyps. (**e**) Colon: Semi-confluent type. Medium, edematous polyps

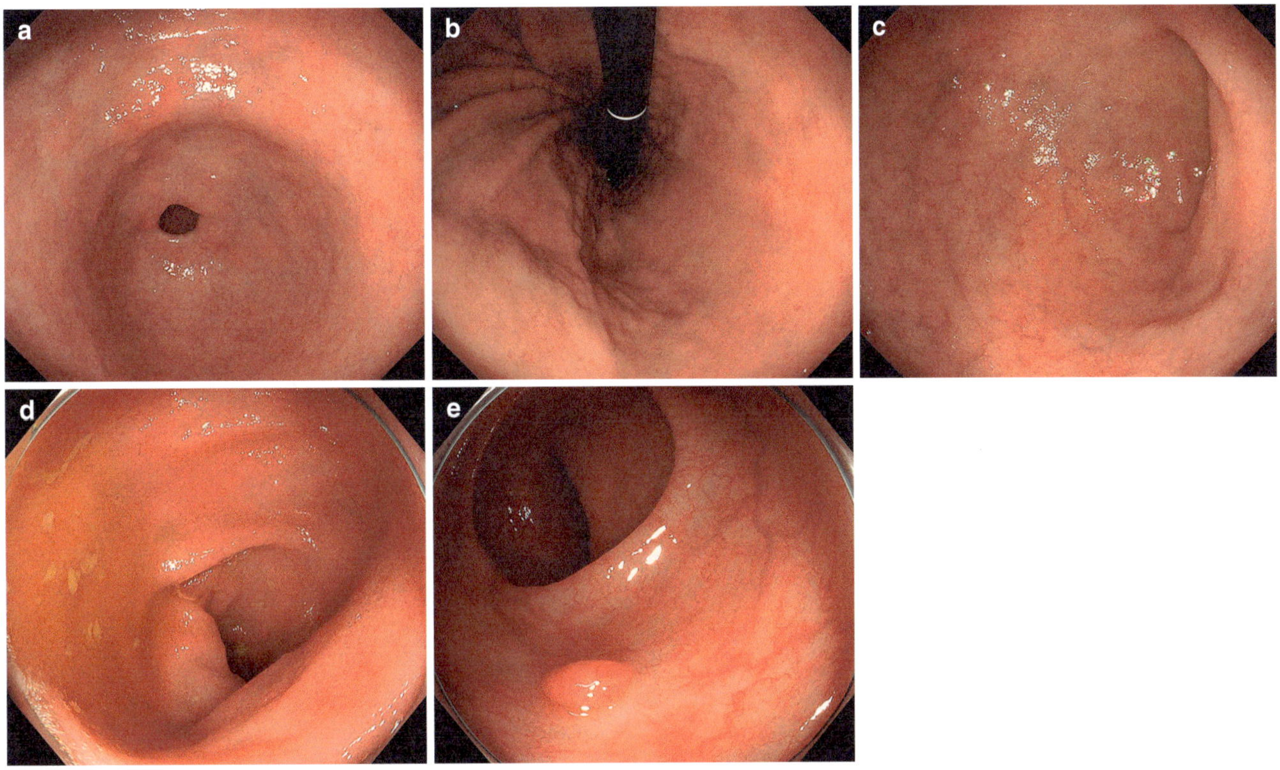

Fig. 18 (**a**), (**b**) Stomach: Gastric polyps markedly disappeared. (**c**) Duodenum: Endoscopic findings improved. (**d**) Terminal ileum: Polyps disappeared, and edematous villi improved. (**e**) Colon: Only a few polyps remained

Case 68: An atypical case without diarrhea, whose early-stage colorectal cancer was detected at the first examination and resected endoscopically

Provided by Makoto Ooi and Yuzo Kodama

[Patient]

A 64-year-old male. CC: Hyperpigmentation, dysgeusia, anorexia, onychodystrophy.

[Clinical findings]

Alopecia (+), onychodystrophy (+), hyperpigmentation (+), dysgeusia (+), defecation: 1 time/day.

[Laboratory findings]

Alb 4.2 mg/dL, CRP 0.15 mg/dL, Hb 15.4 g/dL.

[Endoscopic images 1] (Fig. 19a–e)

[Clinical course]

First attack type.

Initial treatment: PSL 40 mg for 2 weeks.

Clinical response: 2 weeks.

Clinical remission: 8 weeks.

Maintenance dose: PSL 0 mg.

[Endoscopic images 2] (Fig. 20a–c)

EGD and CS during remission 2 years after the diagnosis.

Marked reduction or almost disappearance of polyps in all lesions.

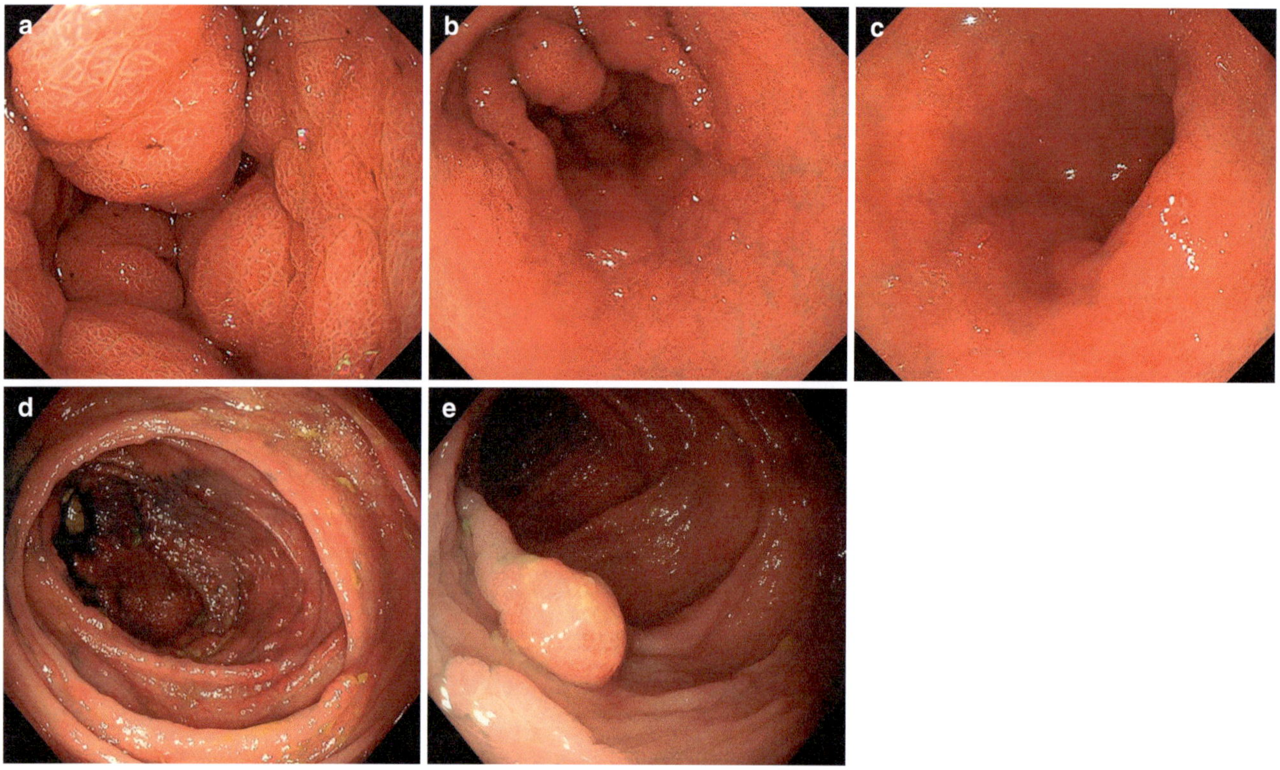

Fig. 19 (**a**), (**b**) Stomach: Confluent type. Medium, edematous, and erythematous polyps. Edematous intervening mucosa. (**c**) Duodenum: Fold thickening type with scattered, small polyps. (**d**) Colon: Sparse type. Medium, edematous, and erythematous polyps. Edematous intervening mucosa. (**e**) Colon: Colonic tumors endoscopically resected were diagnosed as tub1, pTis(M), ly0, v0, pHM0, pVM0

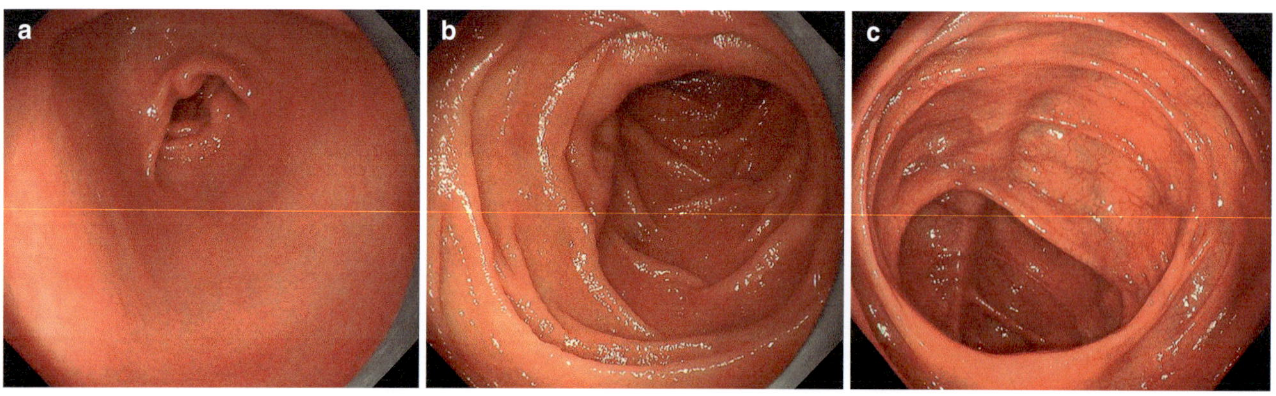

Fig. 20 (**a**) Stomach. (**b**) Duodenum. (**c**) Colon

Case 69: A possible case who had cutaneous manifestations but were free from diarrhea

Provided by Tomonori Yano and Hironori Yamamoto

[Patient]

A 73-year-old woman. CC: Anorexia, general malaise, cystitis-like symptom, nail discoloration and peeling, alopecia, hand tremor.

[Clinical findings]

Alopecia (+), onychodystrophy (+), hyperpigmentation (−), dysgeusia (−), defecation: 1 time/day.

[Laboratory findings]

Alb 3.8 mg/dL, CRP 0.01 mg/dL, Hb 12.8 g/dL.

[Endoscopic images] (Fig. 21)

[Clinical course]

First attack type

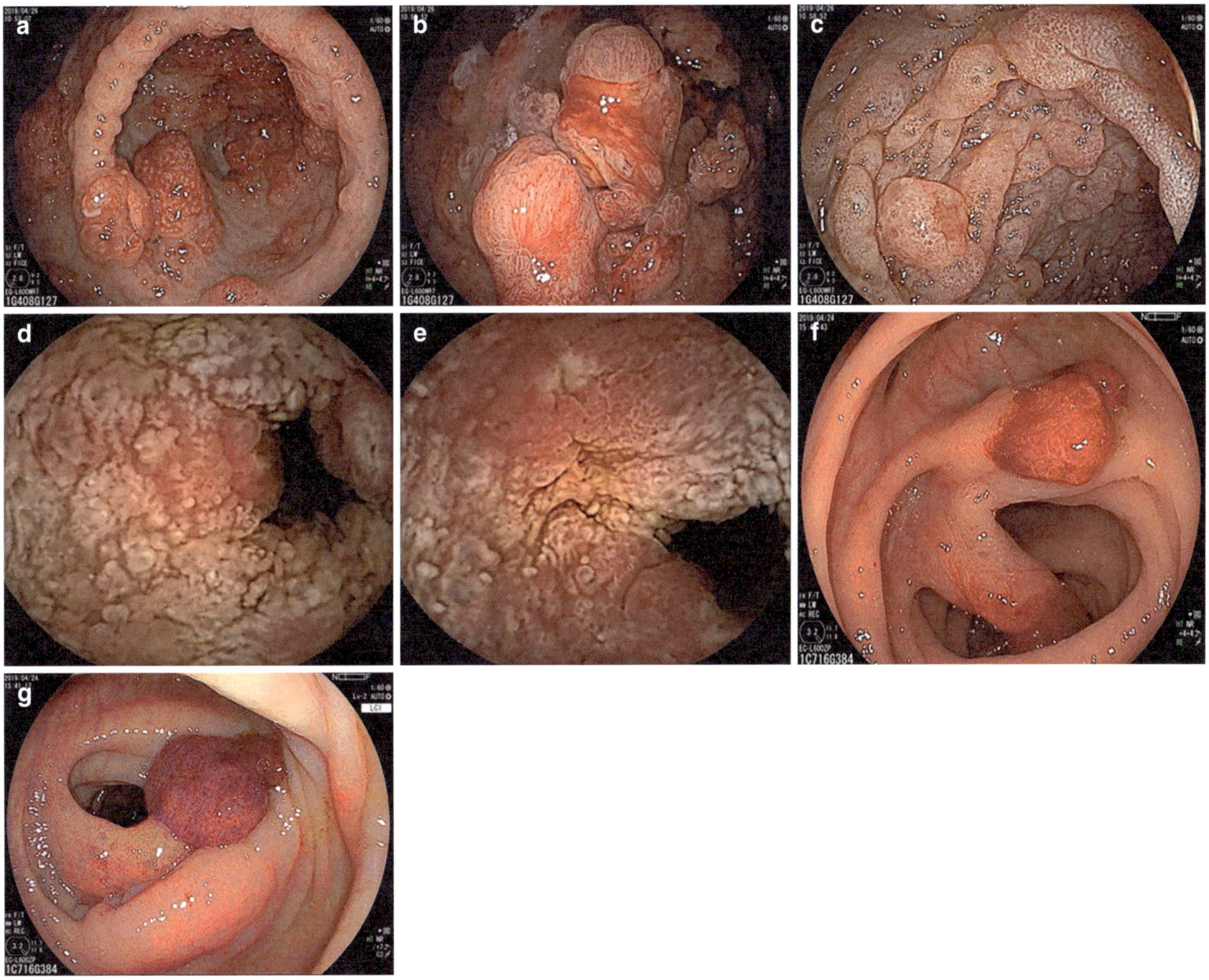

Fig. 21 (**a**), (**b**) Stomach: Confluent type. Medium, edematous, hemorrhagic, and whitish mucus adhered polyps. (**c**) Duodenum: Folid thickening type with edematous polyps. (**d**), (**e**) Small intestine (SBCE): Fold thickening type with white villi and erosion. (**f**) Colon: Sparse type. Large, erythematous polyps. (**g**) LCI observation of (**f**)

Case 70: An atypical case whose onset was abdominal discomfort after meal

Provided by Fukunori Kinjo and Tetsu Kinjo

[Patient]

A 56-year-old woman. CC: Abdominal discomfort after meal.

[Clinical findings]

Alopecia (+), hyperpigmentation (−), diarrhea (+).

[Laboratory findings]

Alb 3.5 mg/dL.

[Endoscopic images] (Fig. 22)

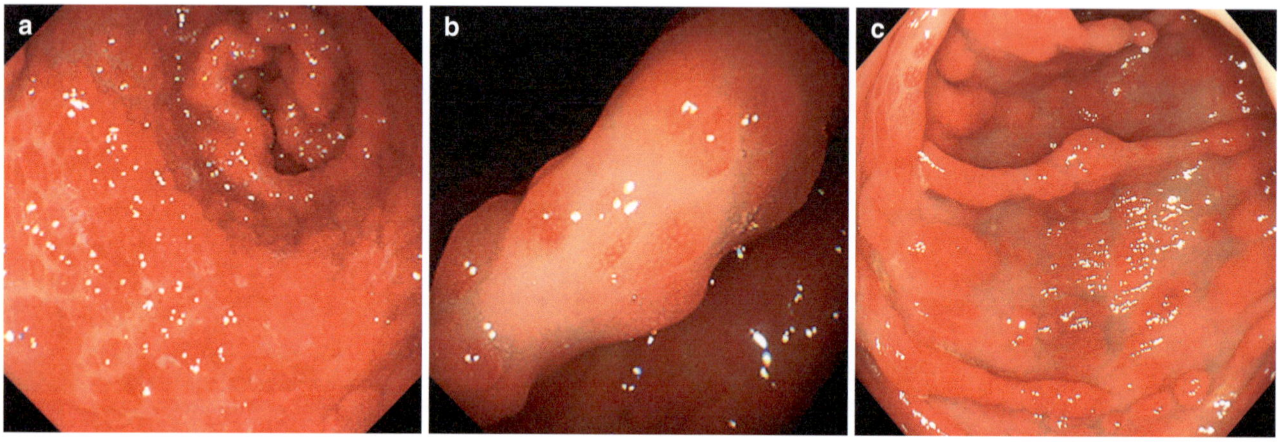

Fig. 22 (**a**), (**b**) Stomach: Confluent type. Small, erythematous polyps. Edematous intervening mucosa. (**c**) Colon: Confluent type. Small, erythematous polyps

Case 71: A case suffering from weight loss and dysgeusia with sustained serum albumin level

Provided by Tomonori Yano and Hironori Yamamoto

[Patient]

A 75-year-old male. CC: Weight loss, dysgeusia, nail deformity, bloody stool, diarrhea.

[Clinical findings]

Alopecia (−), onychodystrophy (+), hyperpigmentation (−), dysgeusia (+), weight loss: −10 kg/3 months.

[Laboratory findings]

Alb 3.5 mg/dL, CRP 0.2 mg/dL, Hb 16.1 g/dL.

[Endoscopic images] (Fig. 23)

[Clinical course]

First attack type

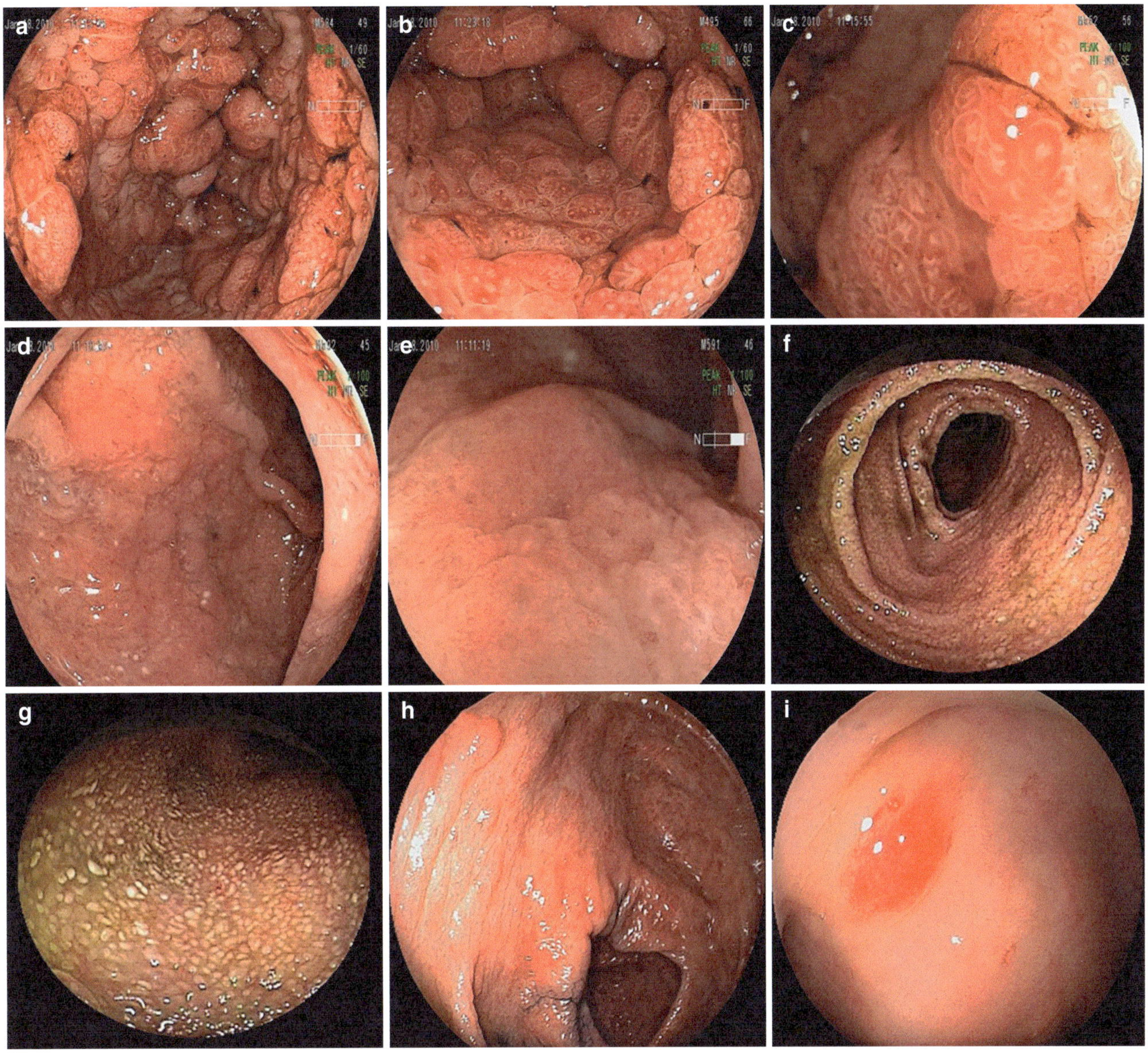

Fig. 23 (**a**), (**b**), (**c**) Stomach: Confluent type. Large, edematous, erythematous, and whitish mucus adhered polyps. (**d**), (**e**) Duodenum: Fold thickening type. Small polyps with white villi. (**f**), (**g**) Small intestine (BAE): Fold thickening type with white villi. (**h**), (**i**) Colon: Sparse type. Medium, edematous, and erythematous polyps

Case 72: A possible case whose gastric lesions were detected by screening endoscopy

Provided by Masakazu Nagahori

[Patient]

A 68-year-old male. CC: Abnormal findings detected in screening EGD.

[Clinical findings]

Alopecia (−), onychodystrophy (+), hyperpigmentation (+), dysgeusia (−), defecation: 1 time/day.

[Laboratory findings]

Alb 4.0 mg/dL, CRP 0.2 mg/dL, Hb 12.4 g/dL.

[Endoscopic images] (Fig. 24)

[Clinical course]

First attack type. No additional data obtained.

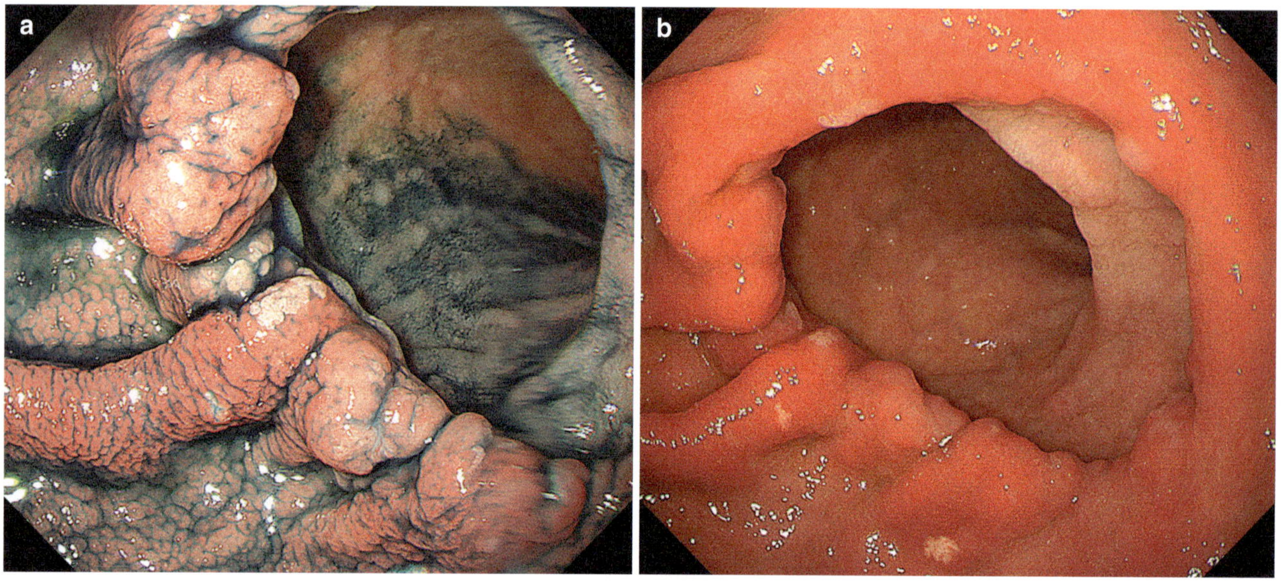

Fig. 24 (**a**), (**b**) Gastric anastomosis after gastric ulcer perforation (pyloric gastrectomy). Mucosal edema and scattered small polyps

Case-Based Images: Cases with Coincident Esophageal Lesions/ Coincident Tumor

Ryota Hokari, Tadakazu Hisamatsu, and Masaaki Higashiyama

1 Cases with Coincident Esophageal Lesions

Case 73: A case with esophageal papilloma-like lesions, which shrunk and disappeared after treatments along with regression of gastric polyps

{Reprinted with permission from A Tanaka et al. Digestive and Liver Disease. 2020; 352: 52(3)}

Provided by Shuji Kanmura

[Patient]

A 62-year-old male. CC: Dysgeusia, diarrhea, weight loss.

[Clinical findings]

Alopecia (+), onychodystrophy (+), hyperpigmentation (+), dysgeusia (+), defecation: 5 times/day

[Laboratory findings]

Alb 3.5 mg/dL, CRP 0.09 mg/dL, Hb 16.1 g/dL.

[Endoscopic images 1] (Fig. 1a–f)

[Clinical course]

Relapse-remitting type.

Initial treatment: PSL 40 mg for 2 weeks.

Clinical response: 1 week.

Clinical remission: 4 weeks.

Maintenance dose: PSL 5 mg.

Therapeutic dose at relapse: PSL 40 mg.

[Endoscopic images 2] (Fig. 2a–e)

The polyps in the stomach disappeared and the villous-like structures of the esophageal lesions shrunk in remission.

R. Hokari (✉) · M. Higashiyama
Department of Internal Medicine, National Defense Medical College, Tokorozawa, Saitama, Japan
e-mail: ryota@ndmc.ac.jp; masaakih@ndmc.ac.jp

T. Hisamatsu
Department of Gastroenterology and Hepatology, Kyorin University School of Medicine, Mitaka, Tokyo, Japan

R. Hokari, T. Hisamatsu (eds.), *Atlas of Cronkhite-Canada Syndrome*, https://doi.org/10.1007/978-981-19-0652-7_11

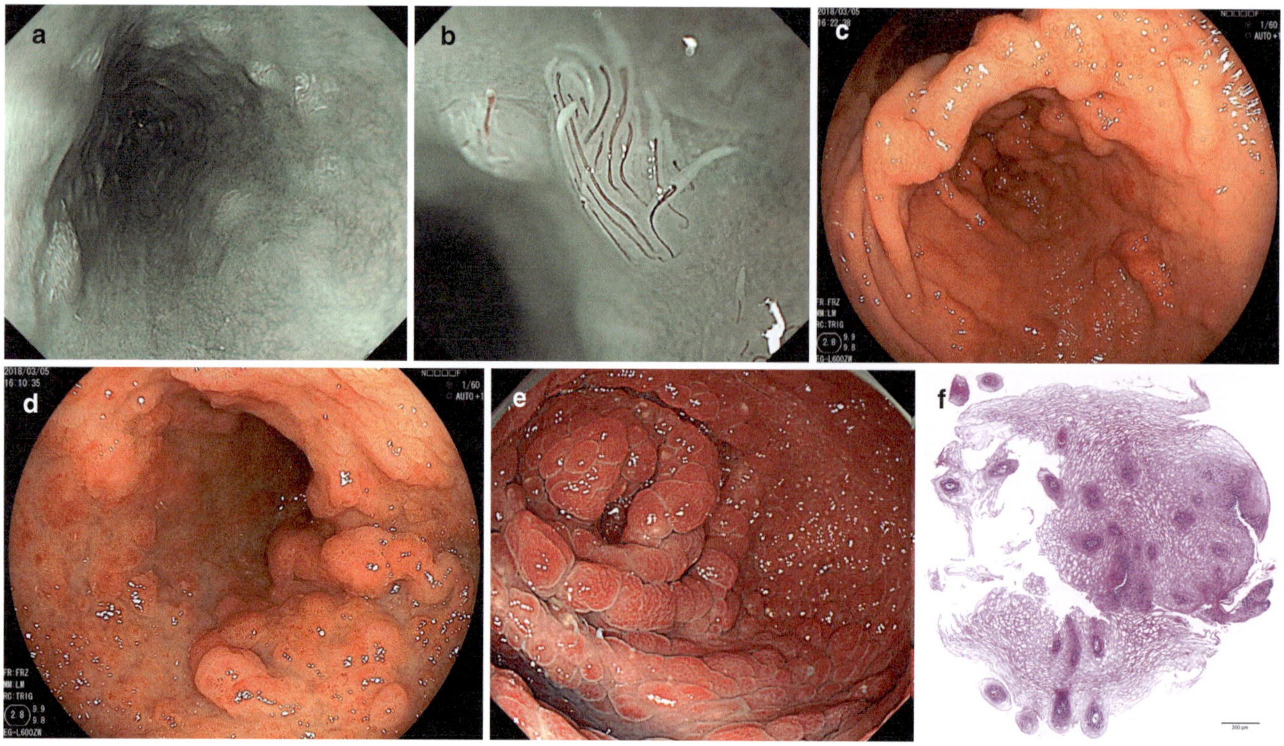

Fig. 1 (**a**), (**b**) Esophagus: Sparse type. Small papilloma-like lesions were sparsely present. (**c**) Stomach: Semi-confluent type. Medium, edematous, and erythematous polyps. (**d**) Duodenum: Fold thickening type with edematous and erythematous mucosa. (**e**) Colon: Confluent type. Medium, edematous, erythematous, and hemorrhagic polyps. (**f**) Pathological diagnosis of esophageal lesions. Villous hyperplasia of multilayered squamous epithelium without edematous changes or inflammatory cell infiltrates

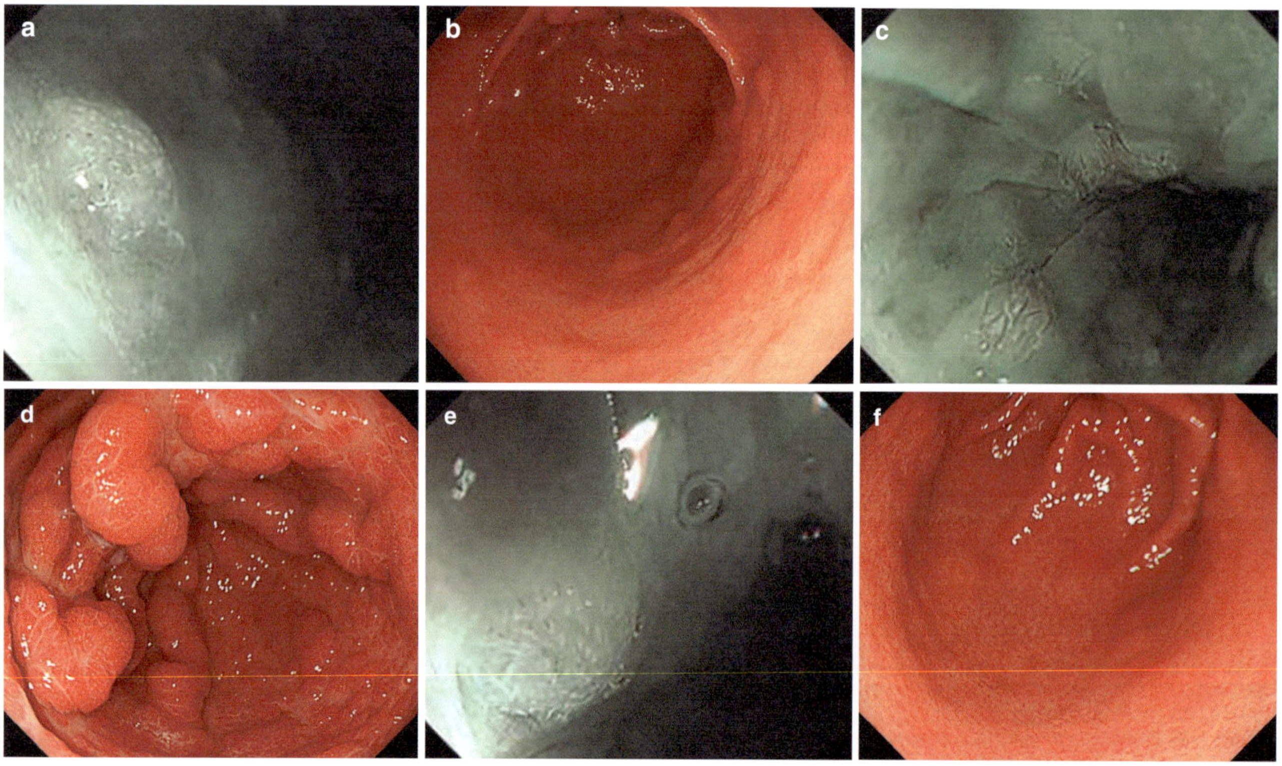

Fig. 2 (**a**), (**c**), (**e**): Esophageal lesions (NBI observation). (**b**), (**d**), (**f**): Gastric antrum. (**a**), (**b**): After initial PSL treatment. (**c**), (**d**): At relapse. (**e**), (**f**): After second PSL treatment

2 Cases with Coincident Tumor

Case 74: A case whose gastric and colorectal cancers were simultaneously detected 3 months after the initial treatment and were resected surgically and endoscopically

Provided by Ichiro Hirata, Kazuki Kakimoto and Kazuhide Higuchi

[Patient]

A 46-year-old male. CC: Diarrhea, dysgeusia, alopecia.

[Clinical findings]

Alopecia (+), onychodystrophy (+), hyperpigmentation (+), dysgeusia (+), defecation: 4 times/day, mild edema.

[Laboratory findings]

Alb 3.2 mg/dL, CRP 0.72 mg/dL, Hb 14.2 g/dL.

[Cutaneous manifestations and endoscopic images 1] (Fig. 3a–e)

[Clinical course]

First attack type.

Initial treatment: PSL 50 mg for 2 weeks.

Clinical response: 2 weeks.

Clinical remission: 12 weeks.

Endoscopic response: 3 months.

Endoscopic remission: 12 months.

Maintenance dose: PSL 3 mg.

[Endoscopic images 2] (Fig. 4a–d)

EGD 3 months after the treatment.

[Endoscopic images 3] (Fig. 5a–c)

CS 3 months after the onset.

[Endoscopic images 4] (Fig. 6a–c)

CS 21 years after treatments.

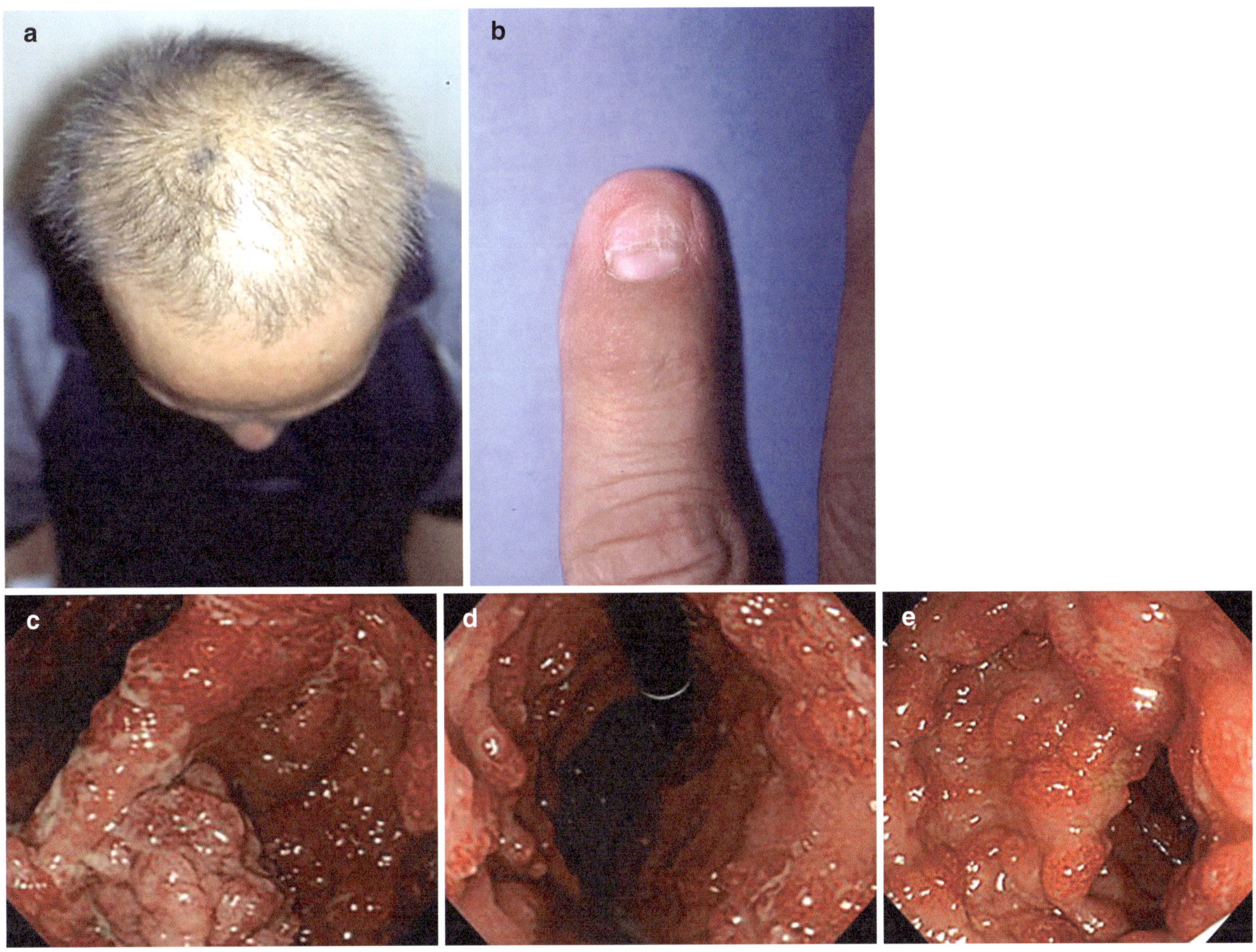

Fig. 3 (**a**) Head. Hyperpigmentation on the forehead in addition to alopecia. (**b**) Hand. Onychodystrophy. (**c**), (**d**) Stomach: Confluent type. Medium, erythematous, and whitish mucus adhered polyps. Edematous intervening mucosa. (**e**) Colon: Confluent type. Small, erythematous polyps

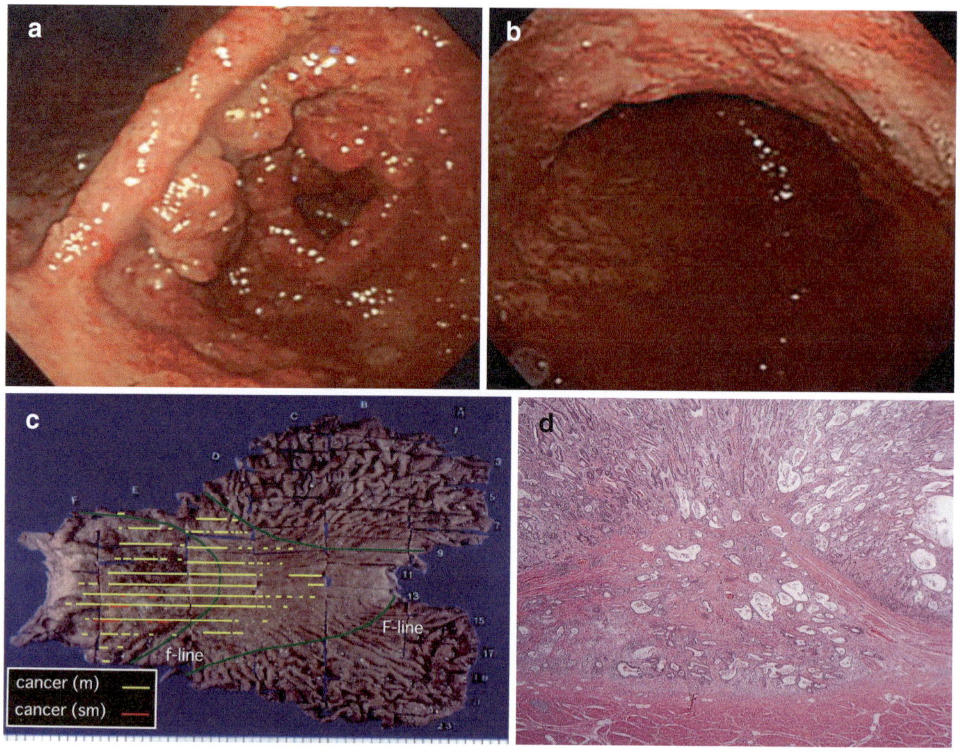

Fig. 4 (**a**) Although the polyps showed a tendency to shrink, a biopsy from the antral polyp showed moderately differentiated adenocarcinoma. (**b**) A biopsy from erythematous mucosa at the body lesser curvature showed poorly differentiated adenocarcinoma, but it was difficult to identify the extent of the disease endoscopically. (**c**) Surgical specimen: Superficially extending adenocarcinoma mainly through the mucosal layer from the upper part of the body to the antral polyps. 150 × 95 mm in diameter, cType0 I+IIa+IIb, tub2 > por, sig, sm2, ly0, v0, n0, Stage IA. (**d**) Pathological image of the antral polyps. Proliferation of moderately differentiated adenocarcinoma predominantly in the mucosa

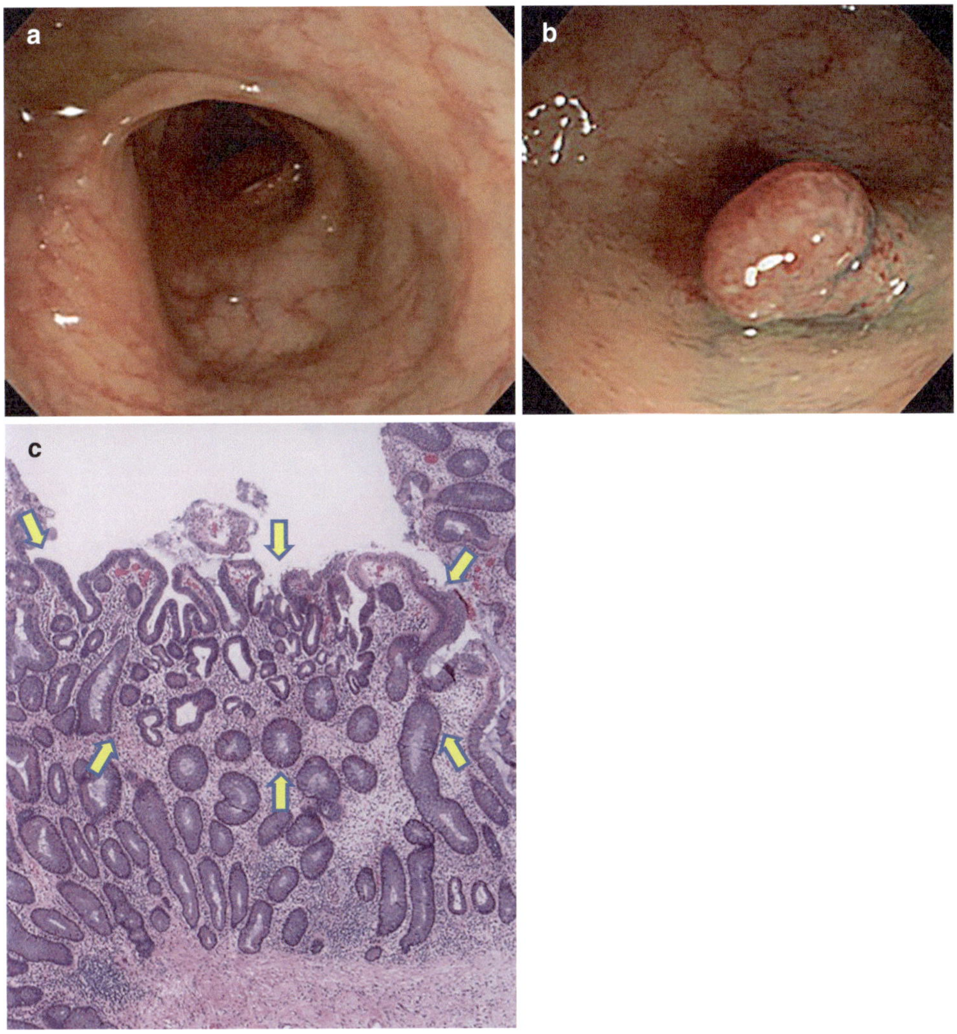

Fig. 5 (**a**) Polyps were reduced through the entire colon. (**b**) A 6-mm-diameter Isp polyp in the middle part of the descending colon. (**c**) Pathological image of (**b**). The majority of the polyp was mainly formed by cystically dilated hyperplastic glands and edematous stroma, but a small lesion of well-differentiated adenocarcinoma with low grade atypia was detected at the apex (within the arrows)

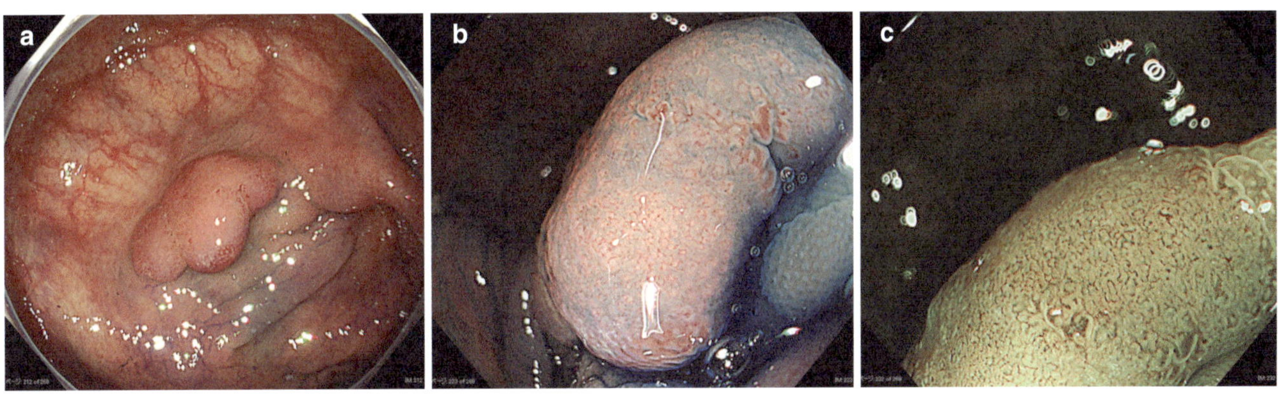

Fig. 6 (**a**) Endoscopic remission was maintained but 10-mm Isp polyp was detected, which was pathologically diagnosed as colorectal adenoma. (**b**) Magnified observation with indigocarmine dyeing of (**a**). (**c**) Magnified NBI observation of (**a**)

Case 75: A case whose early gastric cancer was detected 8 months after the diagnosis and resected endoscopically

Provided by Makoto Ooi and Yuzo Kodama

[Patient]

A 72-year-old male. CC: Epigastralgia, anorexia, weight loss, diarrhea, alopecia, dysgeusia

[Clinical findings]

Alopecia (+), onychodystrophy (+), hyperpigmentation (+), dysgeusia (+), defecation: 10 times/day.

[Laboratory findings]

Alb 3.8 mg/dL, Hb 14.1 g/dL.

[Endoscopic images 1] (Fig. 7a–e)

[Clinical course]

First attack type.

Initial treatment: PSL 30 mg for 2 weeks.

Clinical remission: 4 weeks.

Maintenance dose: PSL 0 mg.

[Endoscopic images 2] (Fig. 8a–f)

[Endoscopic images 3] (Fig. 9a–e)

EGD and CS 3 years after the diagnosis. Remission was maintained.

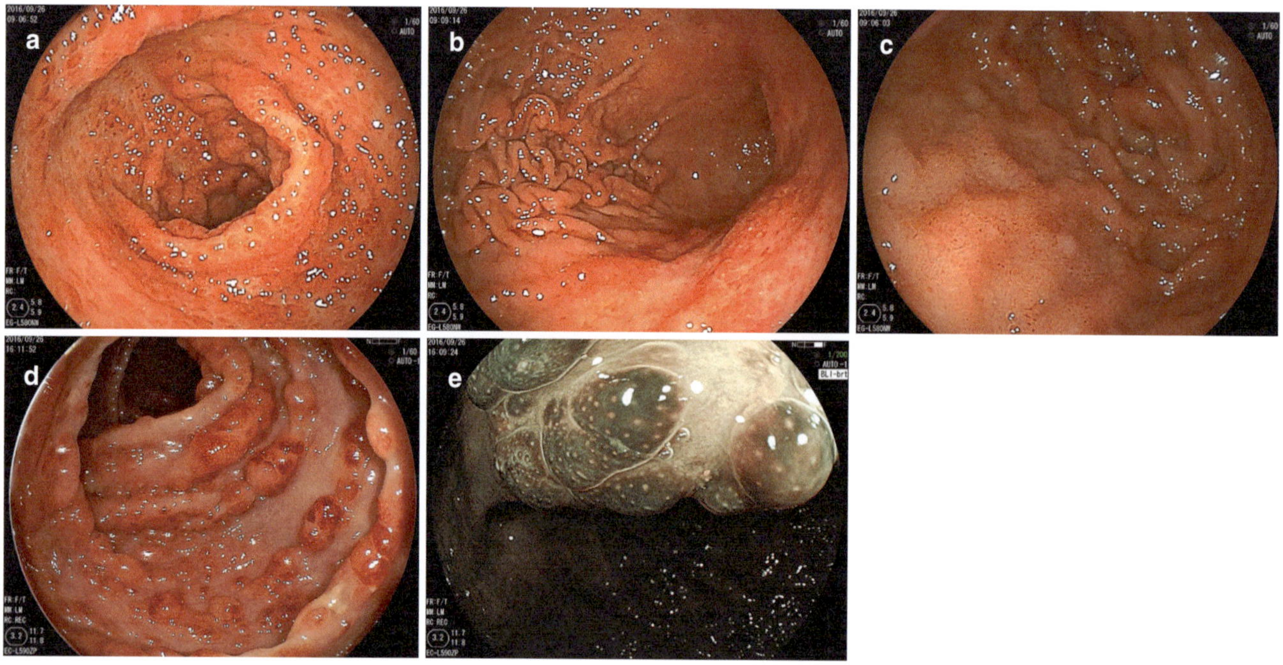

Fig. 7 (**a**), (**b**) Stomach: Semi-confluent type. Small, erythematous polyps. Edematous intervening mucosa. (**c**) Duodenum: Fold thickening type with small polyps. (**d**) Colon: Semi-confluent type. Medium, erythematous polyps. (**e**) BLI observation of (**d**)

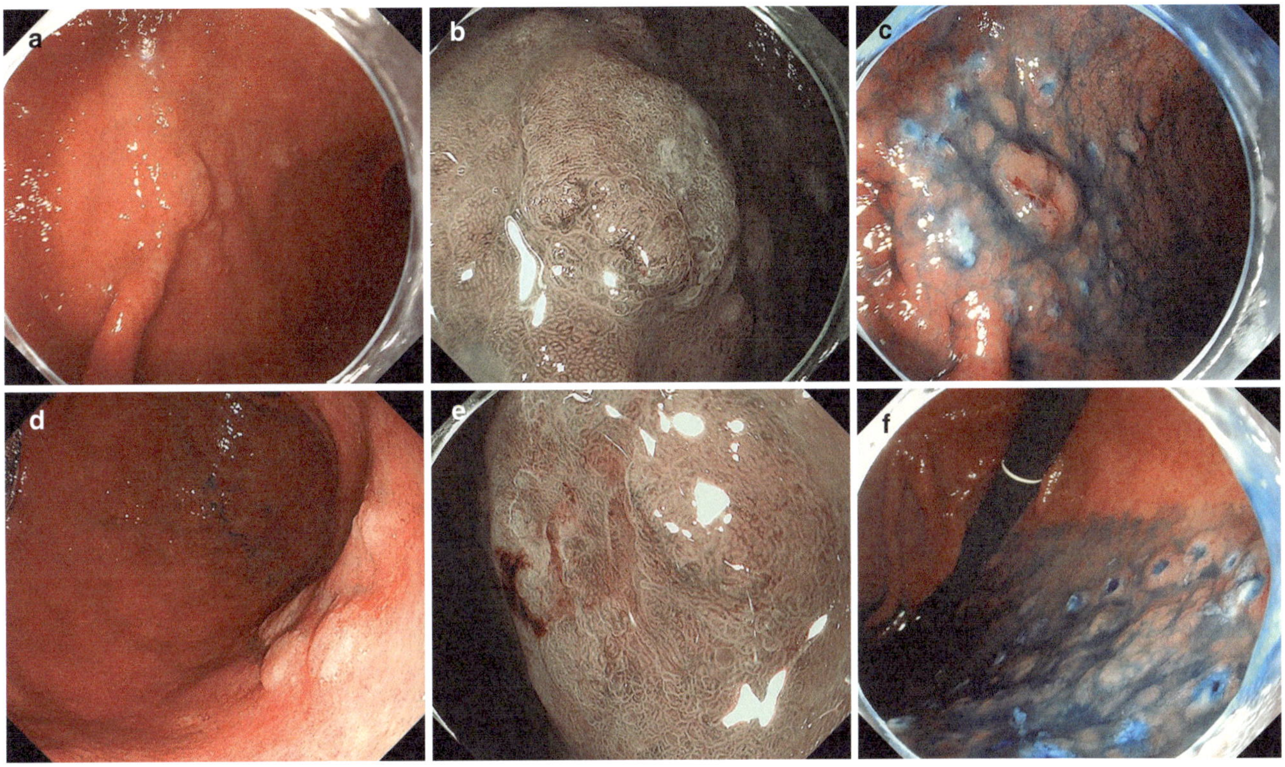

Fig. 8 (**a**), (**b**), (**c**) EGD 6 months after the diagnosis. Early gastric cancer in the anterior wall of lower gastric body, which was resected by endoscopic submucosal dissection (ESD). (**d**), (**e**), (**f**) EGD 8 months after the diagnosis. Another early gastric cancer (0-IIa) in the posterior wall of lower gastric body was resected by ESD. Pathological diagnosis: Adenocarcinoma (tub1) in both lesions

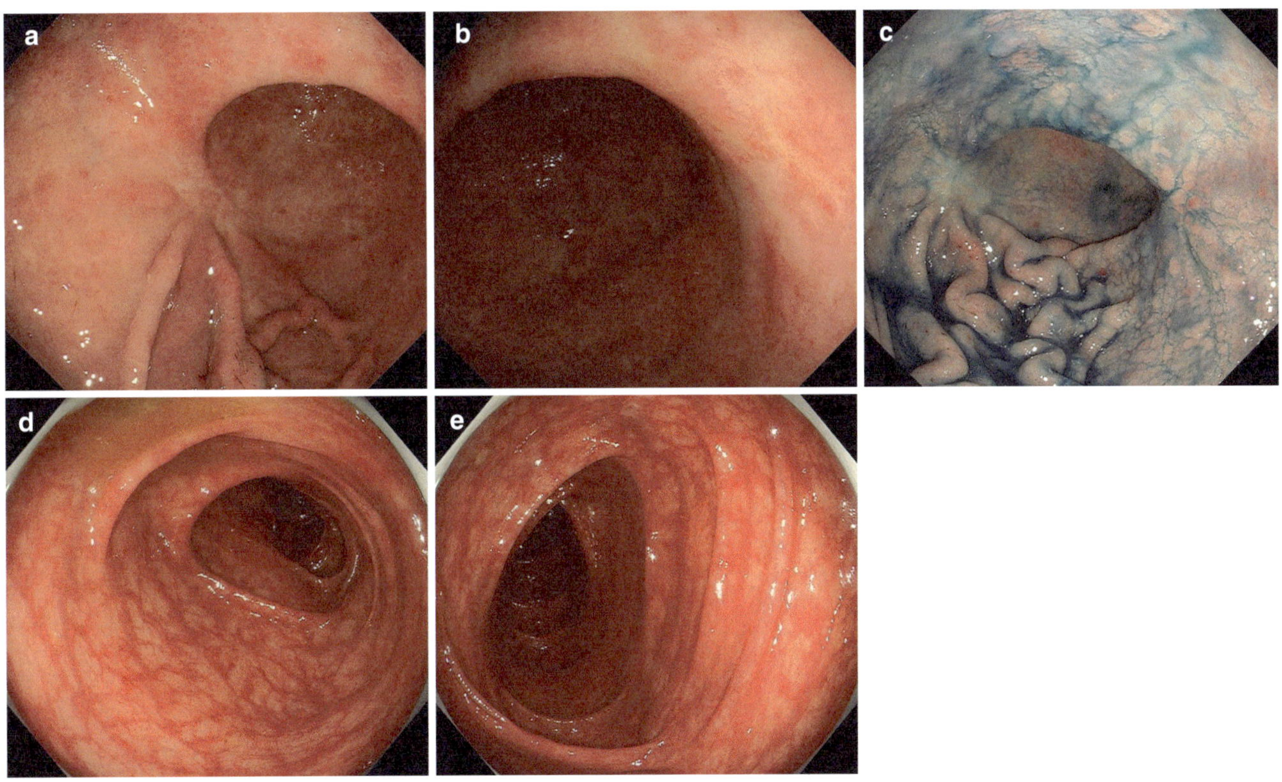

Fig. 9 (**a**), (**b**), (**c**) Stomach. (**d**), (**e**) Colon

Case 76: A case whose multiple gastric cancers were detected simultaneously at the diagnosis and resected surgically before administration of corticosteroids

Provided by Keiichi Mitsuyama and Shinichiro Yoshioka

[Patient]

A 64-year-old woman. CC: Diarrhea, weight loss, alopecia, onychodystrophy, hyperpigmentation.

[Clinical findings]

Alopecia (+), onychodystrophy (+), hyperpigmentation (+), dysgeusia (+)

[Laboratory findings]

Alb 3.1 mg/dL, Hb 7.0 g/dL.

[Endoscopic images] (Fig. 10a–e)

[Clinical course]

First attack type.

The patient received total gastrectomy followed by administration of PSL and achieved remission (details regarding dose of PSL were not obtained).

[Resected gastric specimen] (Fig. 11)

*(b)~(e) are corresponding to Fig. 10b–e.

(b), (c), (d) Gastric cancer, tubular adenocarcinoma, well-differentiated type, pT1a(m), int, Ly0(D2-40), v0(EVG)

(e) Gastric cancer, tubular adenocarcinoma, well-differentiated type, 44 × 24 mm, pT1b2(SM2), int, INFα, Ly1(D2-40), v0(EVG), pPM0, pDM0

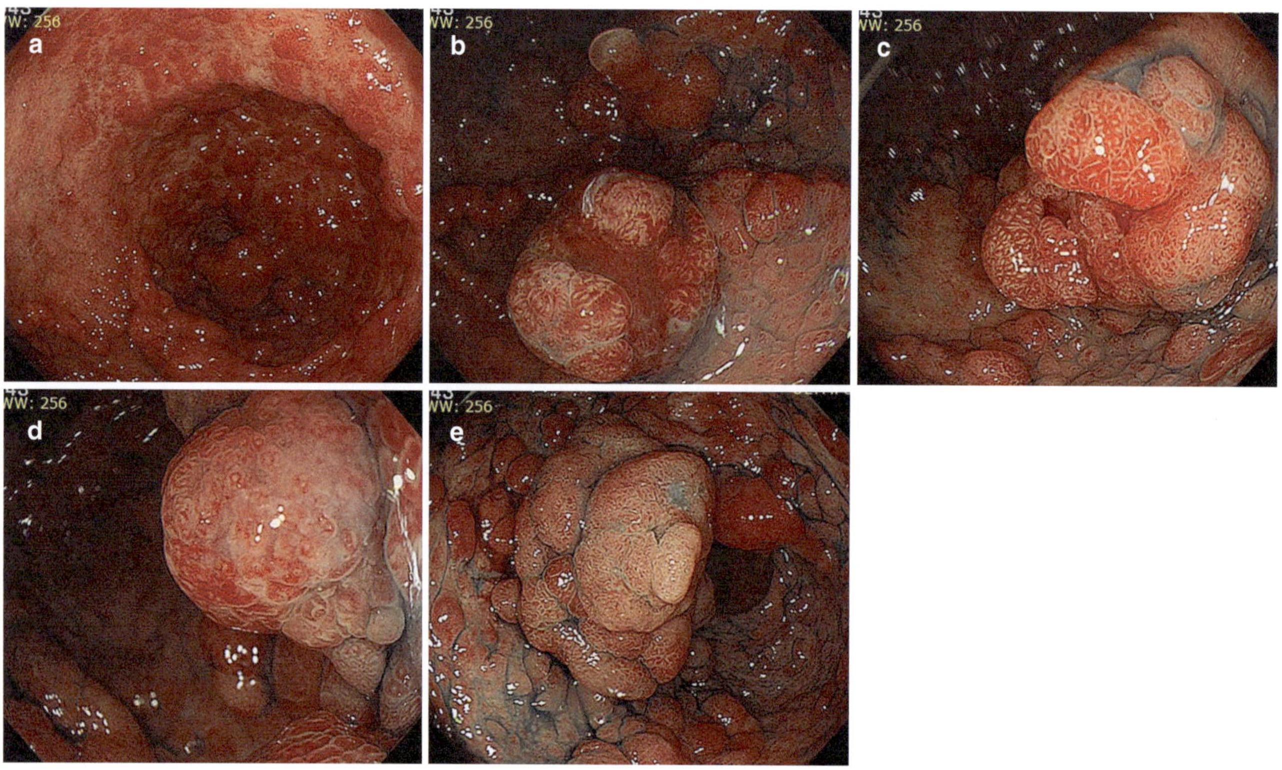

Fig. 10 (**a**) Stomach: Confluent type. Large, edematous, erythematous, and hemorrhagic polyps. (**b**) Stomach: 0-I (15 mm) at the lesser curvature of the angle. (**c**) Stomach: 0-I + IIc (30 mm) at the lesser curvature of the antrum. (**d**) Stomach: 0-I (15 mm) at the posterior wall of the antrum. (**e**) Stomach: 0-I (25 mm) at the anterior wall of the pyloric ring

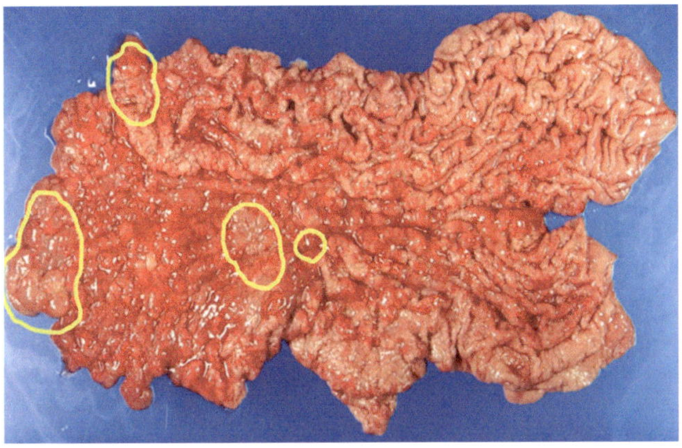

Fig. 11 Macroscopic view of the resected stomach

Case 77: A case whose gastric cancer was detected after the initial treatment and resected surgically

Provided by Rintaro Moroi and Atsushi Masamune

[Patient]

A 59-year-old male. CC: Anemia.

[Clinical findings]

Alopecia (−), onychodystrophy (+), hyperpigmentation (+), defecation: unknown., weight loss: −8 kg/6 months.

[Laboratory findings]

Alb 1.7 mg/dL, CRP 0.4 mg/dL, Hgb 9.1 g/dL.

[Endoscopic images 1] (Fig. 12a, b)

[Clinical course]

First attack type.

Initial treatment: PSL 40 mg for 1 week.

Clinical response: 1 week.

Clinical remission: 12 weeks.

Maintenance dose: PSL 0 mg.

[Endoscopic images 2] (Fig. 13a, b)

EGD 3 months after the diagnosis.

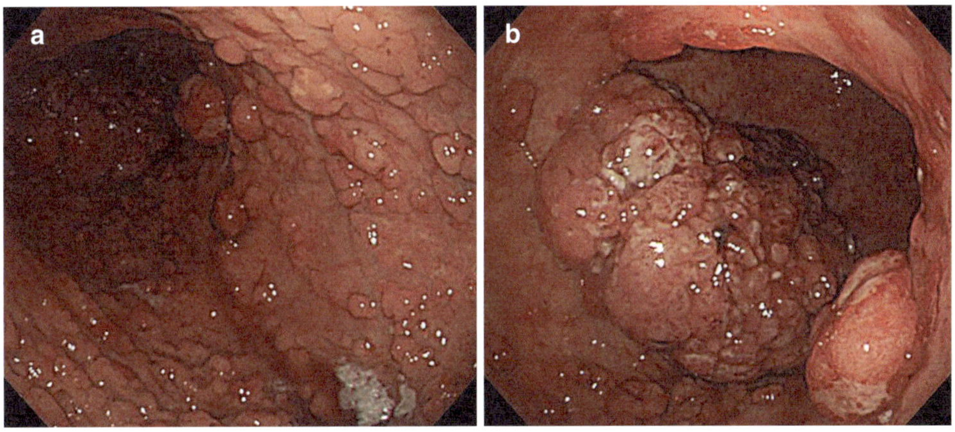

Fig. 12 (**a**) Gastric body: Confluent type. Small, edematous, and erythematous polyps. (**b**) Greater curvature of the gastric angle: Large, edematous, and hemorrhagic polyps

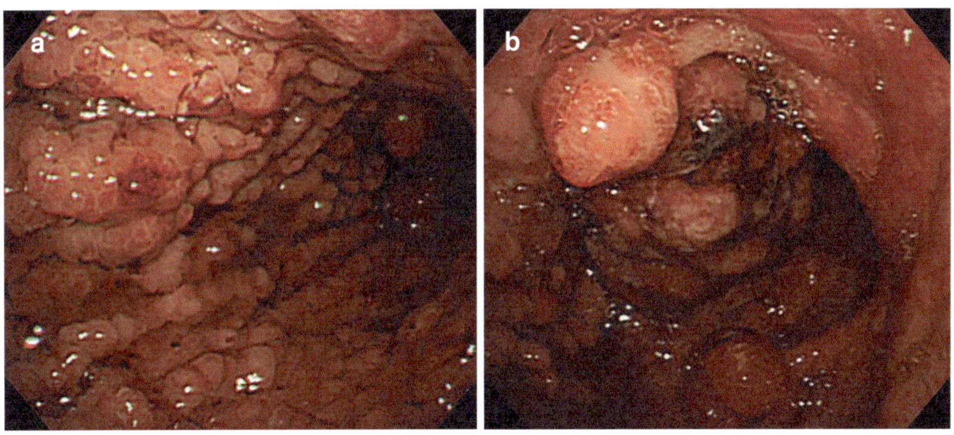

Fig. 13 (**a**) Polyps shrunk after the treatment, but endoscopic remission was not achieved. (**b**) The lesions at the greater curvature of gastric angle shrunk, but an irregularly elevated lesion became apparent, which was diagnosed as gastric cancer and resected by total gastrectomy

Case 78: A case whose gastric cancer was detected at the diagnosis and resected endoscopically

Provided by Tadayuki Oshima, Jiro Watari and Hiroto Miwa

[Patient]

A 74-year-old male. CC: Diarrhea, disturbance of consciousness.

[Clinical findings]

Alopecia (+), onychodystrophy (+), hyperpigmentation (+), dysgeusia (+), defecation: 12 times/day, mild edema.

[Laboratory findings]

Alb 2.3 mg/dL, CRP 10.8 mg/dL, Hb 15.6 g/dL.

[Endoscopic images] (Fig. 14)

[Clinical course]

Chronic continuous type.

Initial treatment: PSL 60 mg for 1 week.

Clinical response: 2 weeks.

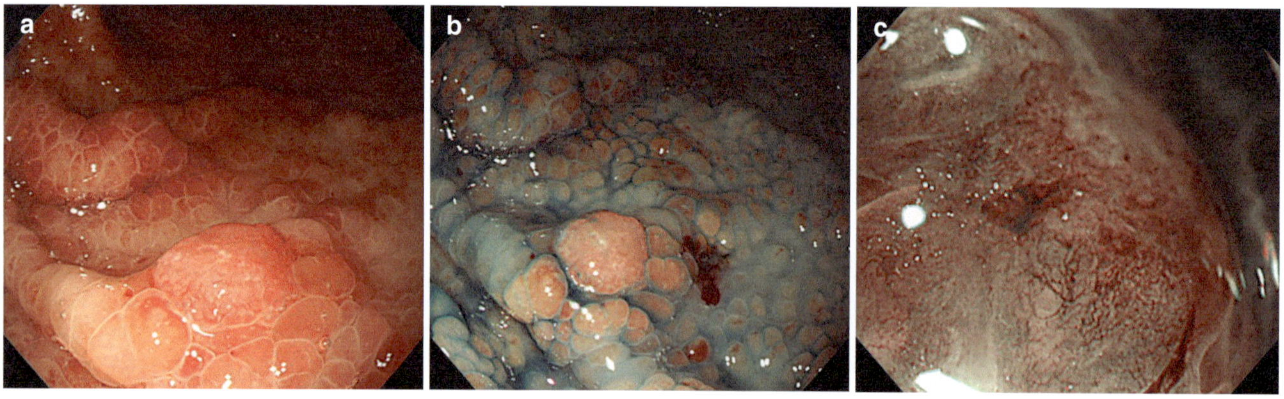

Fig. 14 (**a**), (**b**), (**c**) Stomach: Confluent type. Small, edematous, erythematous, and whitish mucus adhered polyps. (**b**) Indigocarmine dyeing of (**a**). 0-IIa at the greater curvature of the lower body was detected. (**c**) Magnified NBI observation of 0-IIa showed irregular microvascular pattern. The lesion was resected by ESD. Pathological diagnosis: Intramucosal well-differentiated tubular adenocarcinoma (7 × 6 mm)

Case 79: A case whose duodenal carcinoma of Vater papilla was detected after the initial treatment

Provided by Takehiro Torisu and Junji Umeno

[Patient]

A 66-year-old male. CC: Dysgeusia

[Clinical findings]

Alopecia (+), onychodystrophy (+), hyperpigmentation (+), defecation: 2 times/day, mild edema.

[Laboratory findings]

Alb 2.5 mg/dL, CRP 0.04 mg/dL, Hb 15.6 g/dL.

[Endoscopic images 1] (Fig. 15a–e)

[Clinical course]

First attack type.

Initial treatment: PSL 60 mg for 1 week.

Clinical response: 8 weeks.

Clinical remission: 16 weeks.

Maintenance dose: PSL 5 mg.

[Endoscopic images 2] (Fig. 16a, b)

Duodenal carcinoma of Vater papilla was detected after the treatment.

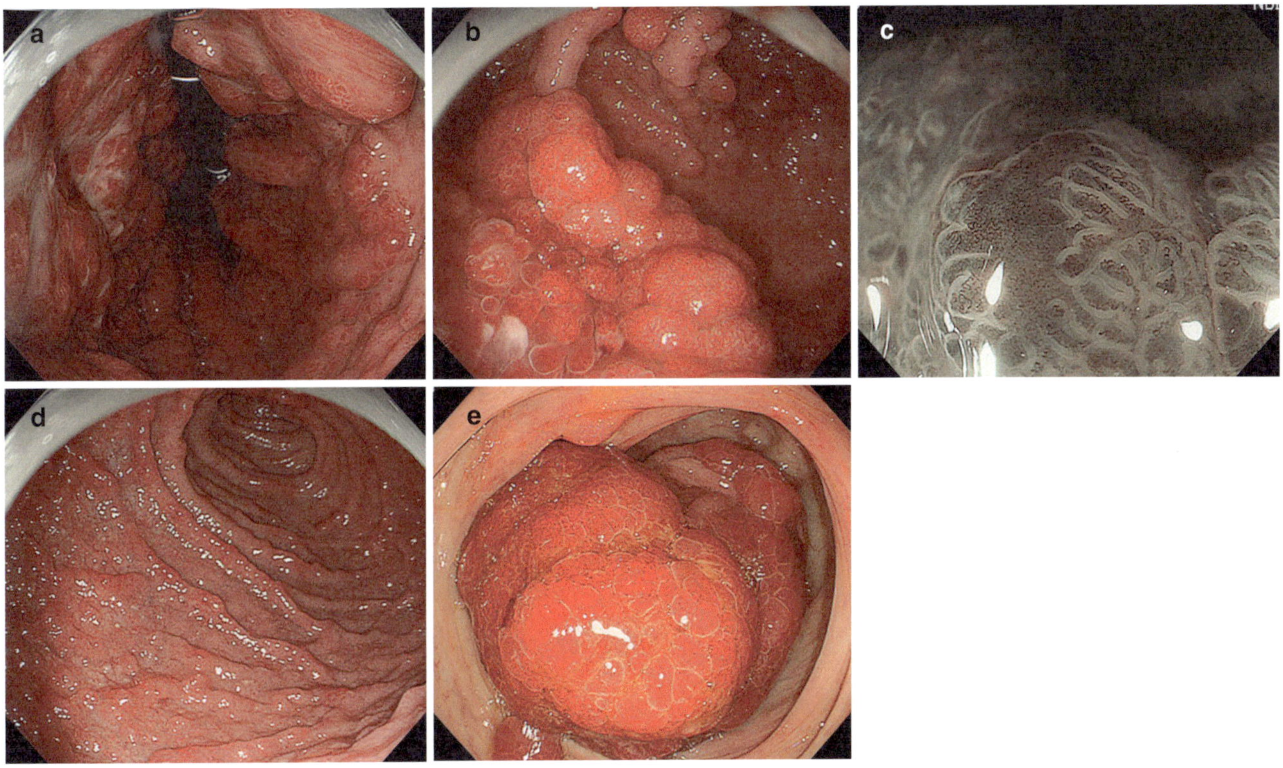

Fig. 15 (**a**), (**b**) Stomach: Confluent type. Medium, edematous polyps. (c) Magnified NBI observation of gastric polyps. (**d**) Duodenum: Fold thickening type with small, edematous polyps. (**e**) Colon: Sparse type. Large, edematous polyps

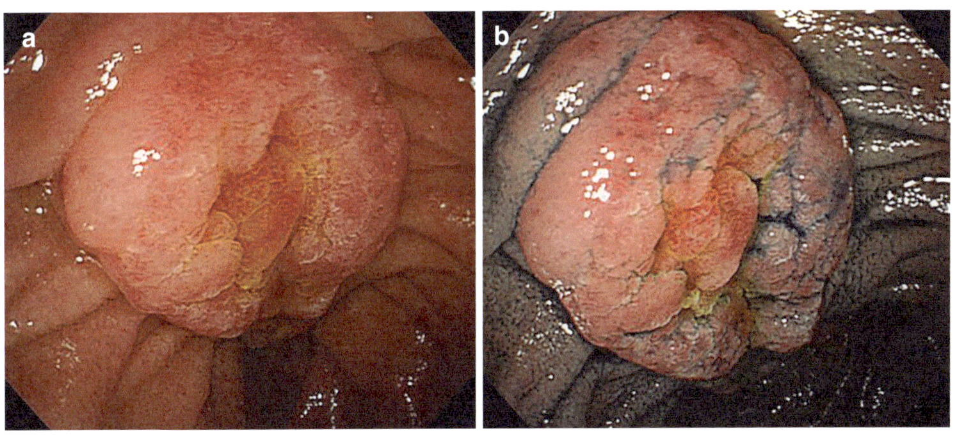

Fig. 16 (**a**) An irregularly elevated lesion on the duodenal papilla. (**b**) Indigocarmine dyeing of (**a**)

Case 80: A case whose colon carcinoma was detected at the diagnosis and resected surgically

Provided by Teppei Omori

[Patient]

A 75-year-old woman. CC: Dysgeusia, alopecia.

[Clinical findings]

Alopecia (+), onychodystrophy (+), hyperpigmentation (+), dysgeusia (+).

[Laboratory findings]

Alb 3.0 mg/dL, CRP 0.17 mg/dL, Hb 13.6 g/dL.

[Endoscopic images] (Fig. 17)

[Clinical course]

Relapse-remitting type.

Initial treatment: PSL 20 mg for 2 weeks.

Clinical response: 2 weeks.

Clinical remission: 2 weeks.

Therapeutic dose at relapse: PSL 20 mg.

Maintenance dose: PSL 10 mg.

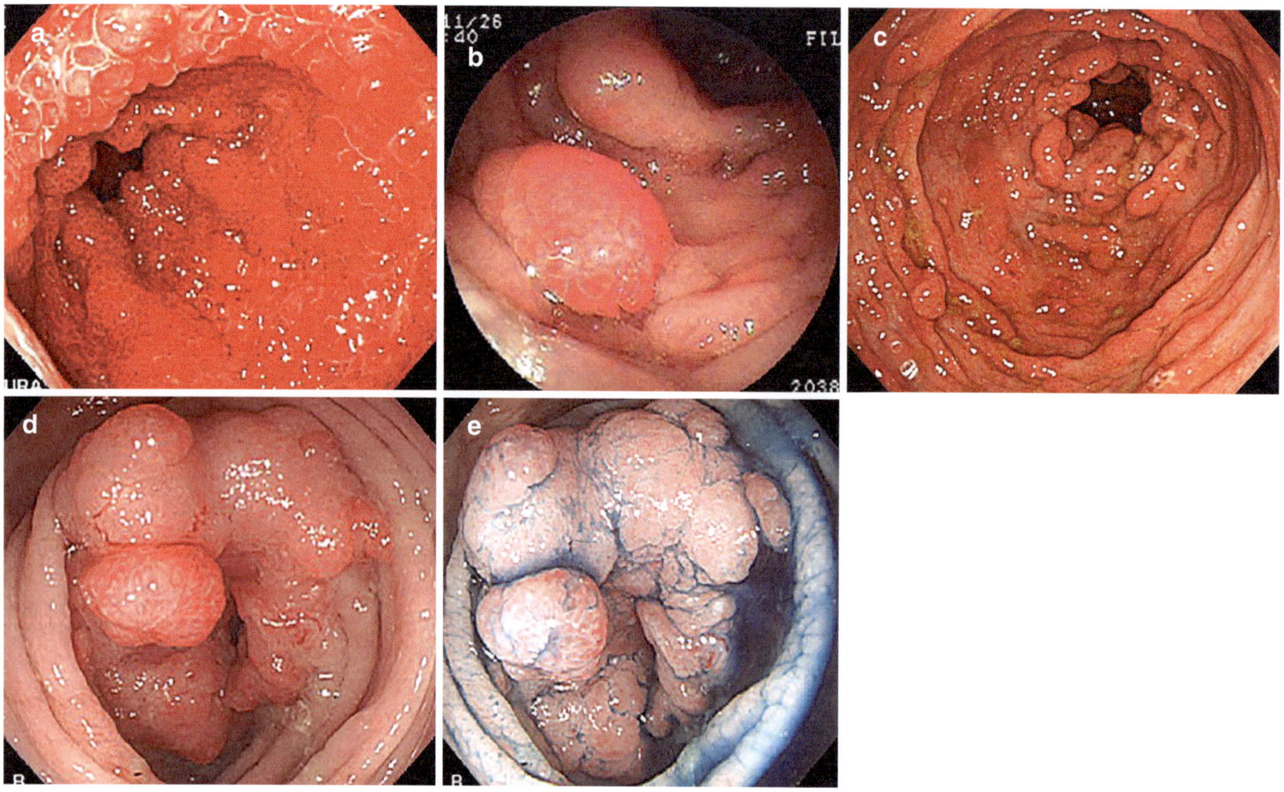

Fig. 17 (**a**) Stomach: Confluent type. Small, edematous, and erythematous polyps. (**b**) Ileum (BAE): Semi-confluent type. Medium polyps. (**c**) Colon: Semi-confluent type. Medium, edematous, and erythematous polyps. (**d**) Ascending colon carcinoma was surgically resected. Pathological diagnosis: Well-differentiated adenocarcinoma. (**e**) Indigocarmine dyeing of (**d**)

Case 81: A colonic carcinoma complicated case who was not eligible for surgery due to severe malnutrition and received treatment with single-agent cetuximab and corticosteroids, leading to tumor shrinkage as well as improved nutritional status, and successful surgical resection of colonic carcinoma

Provided by Tsukasa Yamakawa and Hiroshi Nakase

[Patient]

A 68-year-old woman. CC: Diarrhea, weight loss.

[Clinical findings]

Alopecia (+), onychodystrophy (+), hyperpigmentation (−), dysgeusia (−), defecation: 20 times, moderate edema.

[Laboratory findings]

Alb 1.7 mg/dL, CRP <0.10 mg/dL, Hgb 10.9 g/dL.

[Endoscopic images] (Fig. 18a–e)

[Clinical course]

Initial treatment: PSL 40 mg for 2 weeks.

Clinical response: 4 weeks.

Maintenance dose: PSL 0 mg.

Mesalazine was additionally administered, but remission was not achieved. This patient was complicated with rectal carcinoma at the diagnosis of CCS and surgery was desirable, but difficult due to poor nutritional status. After administration of single-agent cetuximab and corticosteroids, the rectal carcinoma shrunk and the patient's general condition improved, leading to surgical resection of rectal carcinoma.

[Endoscopic images 2] (Fig. 19a–c)

EGD and CS 1.5 years after the diagnosis.

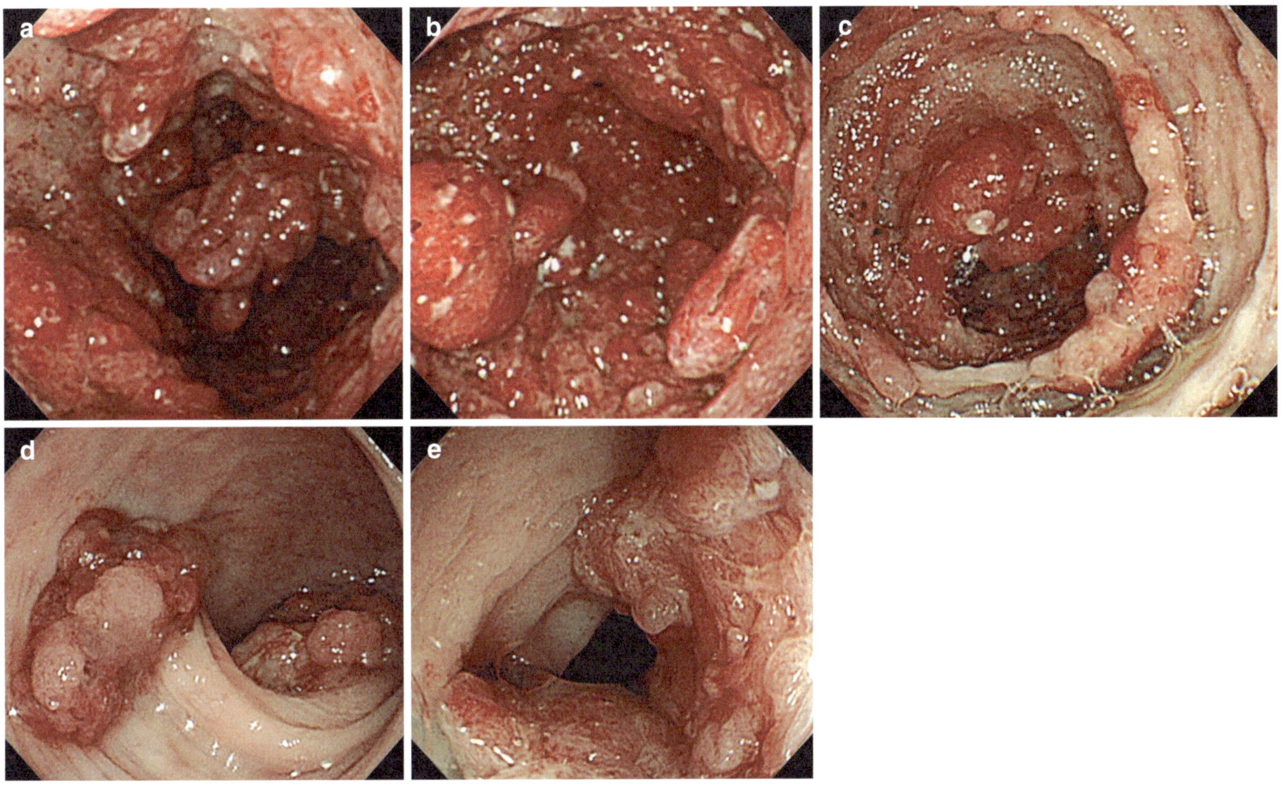

Fig. 18 (**a**), (**b**) Stomach: Confluent type. Medium to large, flat to semipedunculated, edematous, and erythematous polyps. Edematous intervening mucosa with unclear demarcation line (H. pylori: Positive). (**c**) Duodenum: Sparse type. Small polyps. (**d**) Colon: Sparse type. Medium to large, lobulated semipedunculated polyps. Normal intervening mucosa. (**e**) Coincidence of rectal carcinoma

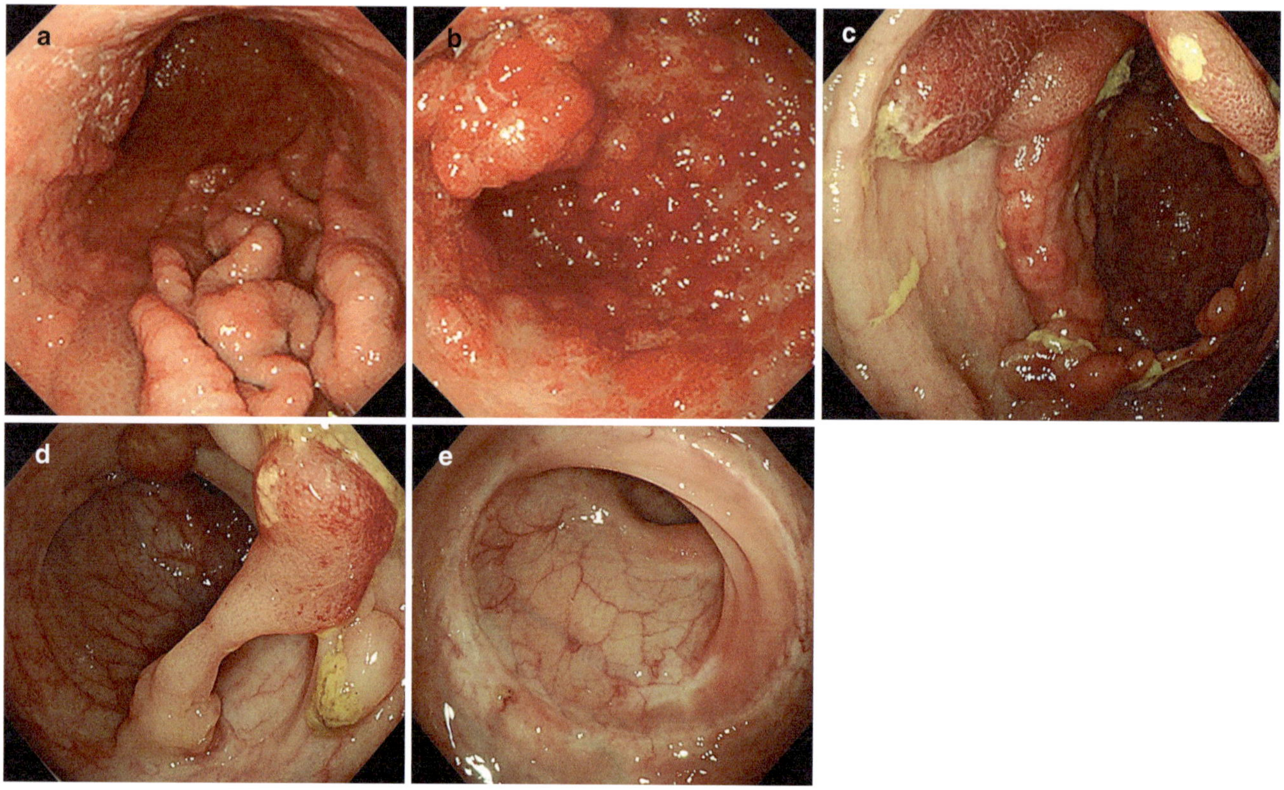

Fig. 19 (**a**), (**b**) Stomach: Confluent type. Small, flattened to hemispherical, edematous, and erythematous polyps. Edematous intervening mucosa. Polyps decreased compared to the first exam. (**c**), (**d**) Colon: Sparse type. Large, hemispherical, and stalked polyps. (**e**) Colon: Postoperative scarring of rectal carcinoma

Case 82: A case whose colonic carcinoma was detected 1.5 years after the diagnosis and received right hemi-colon cancer surgery, subsequently diagnosed to have distant metastasis 3 years after the surgery

Provided by Tomonori Yano and Hironori Yamamoto

[Patient]

A 74-year-old male. CC: Alopecia (head hair, axillary hair, leg hair, etc.), onycholysis, hyperpigmentation, diarrhea, leg edema

[Clinical findings]

Alopecia (+), onychodystrophy (+), hyperpigmentation (+), dysgeusia (−), defecation: 10 times/day, moderate edema.

[Laboratory findings]

Alb 1.5 mg/dL, CRP 0.17 mg/dL, Hb 10.6 g/dL.

[Endoscopic images 1] (Fig. 20a–h)

[Clinical course]

Relapse-remitting type.

Initial treatment: PSL 30 mg for 1 week.

Clinical response: 1 week.

Combined use of azathioprine 50 mg was not effective.

Therapeutic dose at relapse: PSL 30 mg.

Maintenance dose: PSL 0 mg.

[Endoscopic images 2] (Fig. 21a–e)

EGD and CS 1.5 years after the diagnosis.

Right hemi-colon was resected for transverse colon cancer 1.5 years after the diagnosis of CCS. However, distant metastases to the liver and bone were detected 3 years after the surgery.

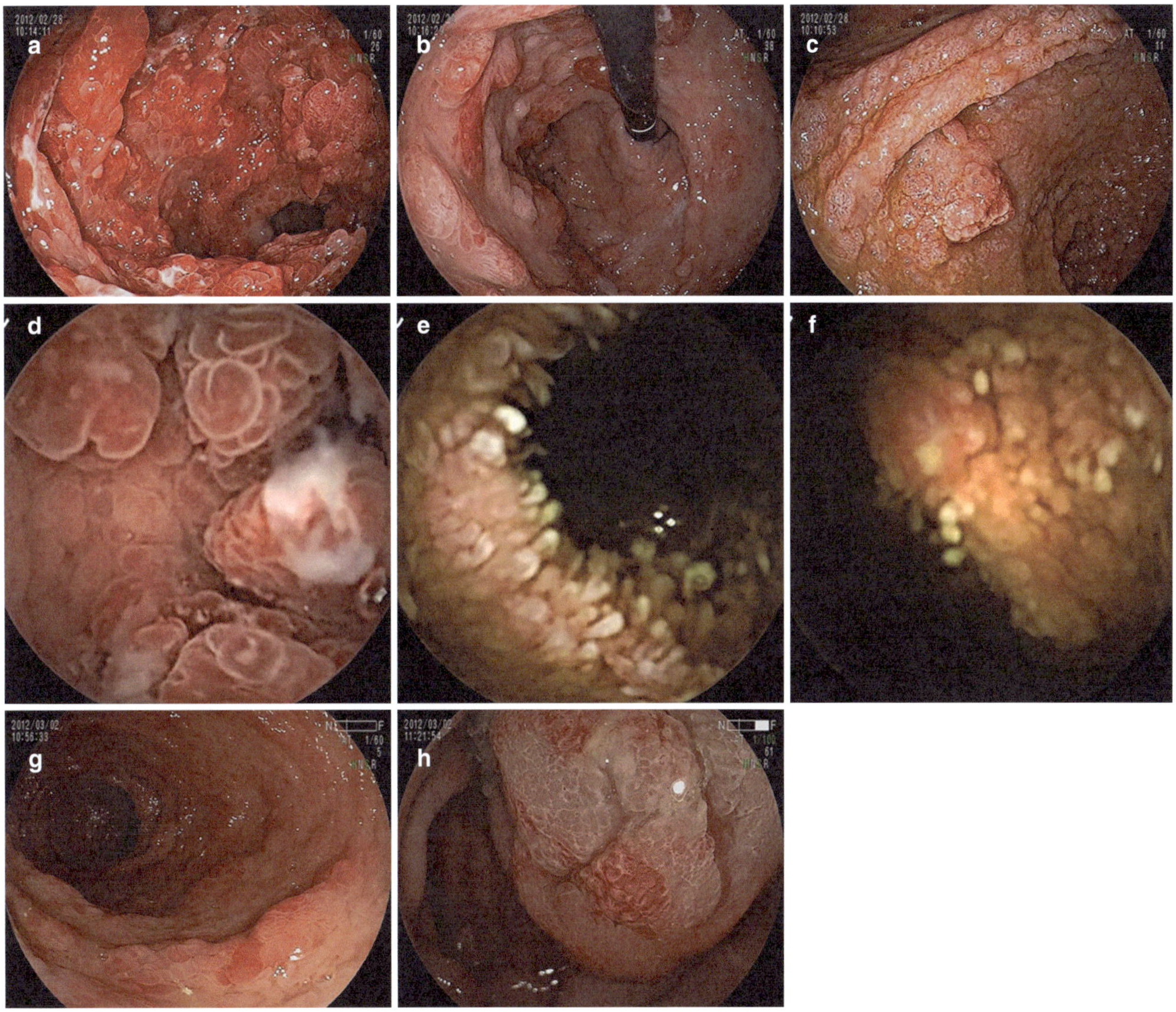

Fig. 20 (**a**), (**b**) Stomach: Confluent type. Large, edematous, erythematous, and whitish mucus adhered polyps. (**c**) Duodenum: Fold thickening type with small polyps. (**d**) Jejunum (SBCE): Sparse type. Small polyps. (**e**), (**f**) Ileum (SBCE): Long, enlarged white villi with erosion through the entire small intestine. (**g**), (**h**) Colon: Semi-confluent type. Large, edematous, and whitish mucus adhered polyps

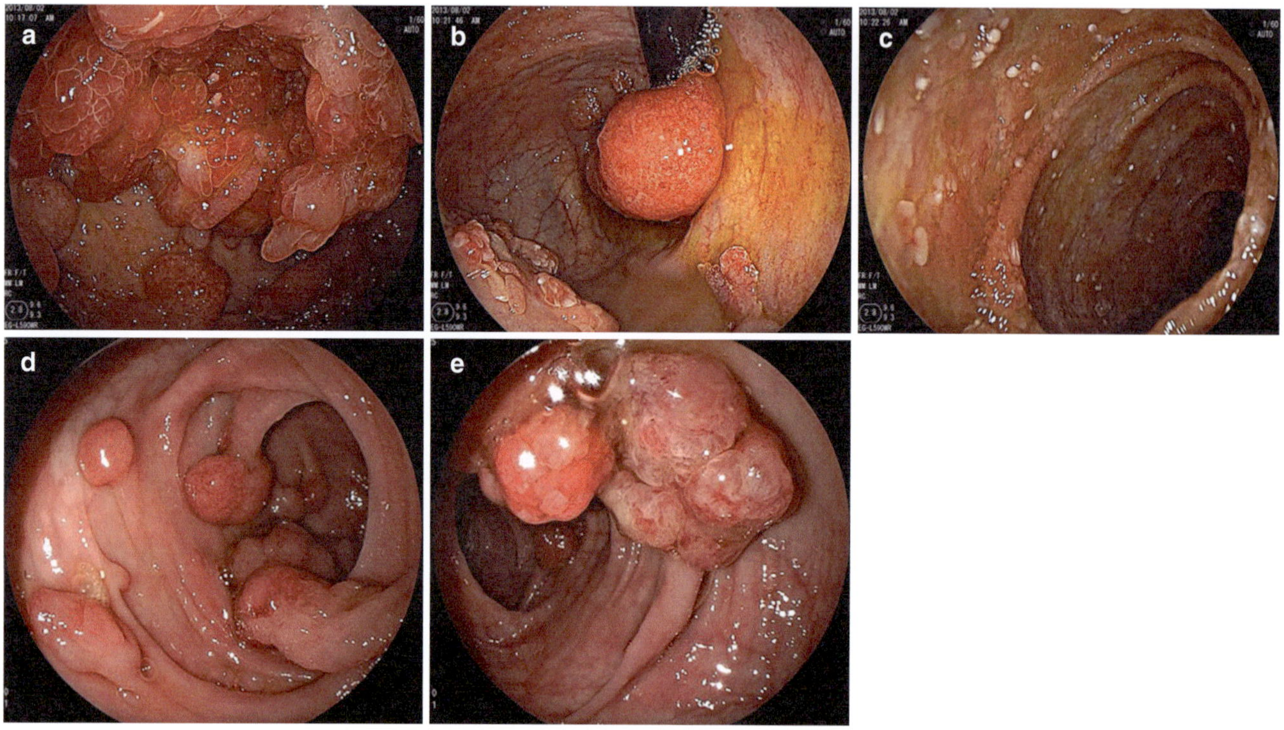

Fig. 21 (**a**), (**b**) Stomach. (**c**) Duodenum. (**d**), (**e**) Colon. Some polyps and inflammation remained after the treatment

Case 83: A case whose advanced transverse colon carcinoma was detected at the diagnosis

Provided by Takehiro Torisu and Junji Umeno

[Patient]

A 75-year-old male. CC: Anorexia, weight loss.

[Clinical findings]

Alopecia (+), onychodystrophy (−), hyperpigmentation (−), defecation: 20 times/day, mild edema.

[Laboratory findings]

Alb 1.6 mg/dL, CRP 0.42 mg/dL, Hb 13.5 g/dL.

[Endoscopic images] (Fig. 22a–h)

[Clinical course]

First attack type.

Initial treatment: PSL 50 mg for 8 weeks.

Clinical response: 2 weeks.

Clinical remission: 8 weeks.

Maintenance dose: PSL 2.5 mg.

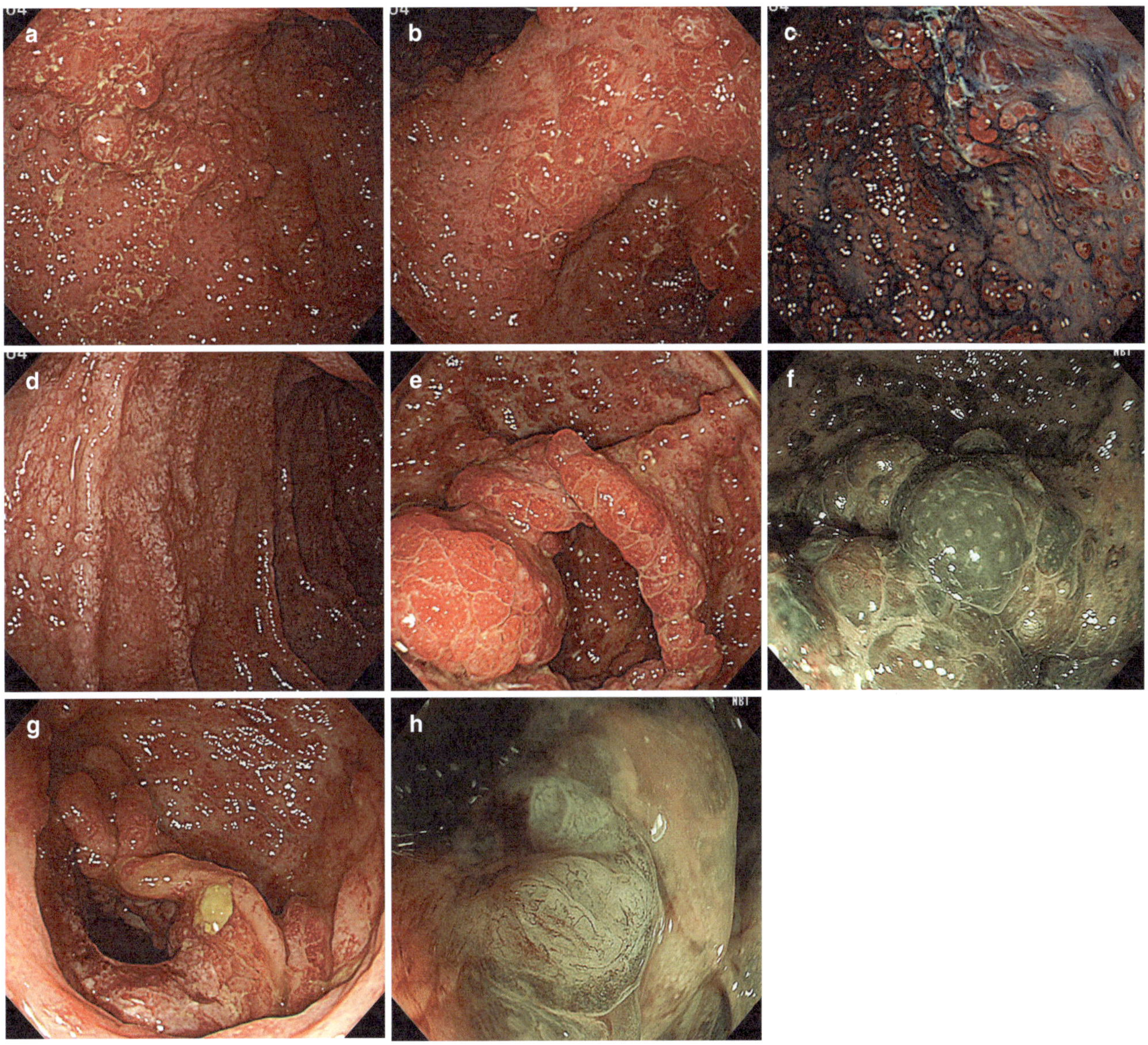

Fig. 22 (**a**), (**b**), (**c**) Stomach: Confluent type. Small, erythematous, and hemorrhagic polyps. Indigocarmine dyeing in (**c**). (**d**) Duodenum: Fold thickening type with white villi. (**e**), (**f**) Colon: Confluent type. Large, edematous, erythematous, and hemorrhagic polyps. NBI observation in (**f**). (**g**) Coincidence of transverse colon carcinoma. (**h**) Magnified NBI observation of (**g**)

Case 84: A case whose advanced sigmoid colon carcinoma was detected at the diagnosis
Provided by Kingo Hirasawa and Reiko Kunisaki
[Patient]

A 76-year-old man. CC: Narrow stool.

[Clinical findings]

Alopecia (+), onychodystrophy (+), hyperpigmentation (−), dysgeusia (−), defecation: 2 times/day, mild edema.

[Laboratory findings]

Alb 3.5 mg/dL, CRP 0.96 mg/dL, Hb 12.3 g/dL.

[Endoscopic images] (Fig. 23a–j)

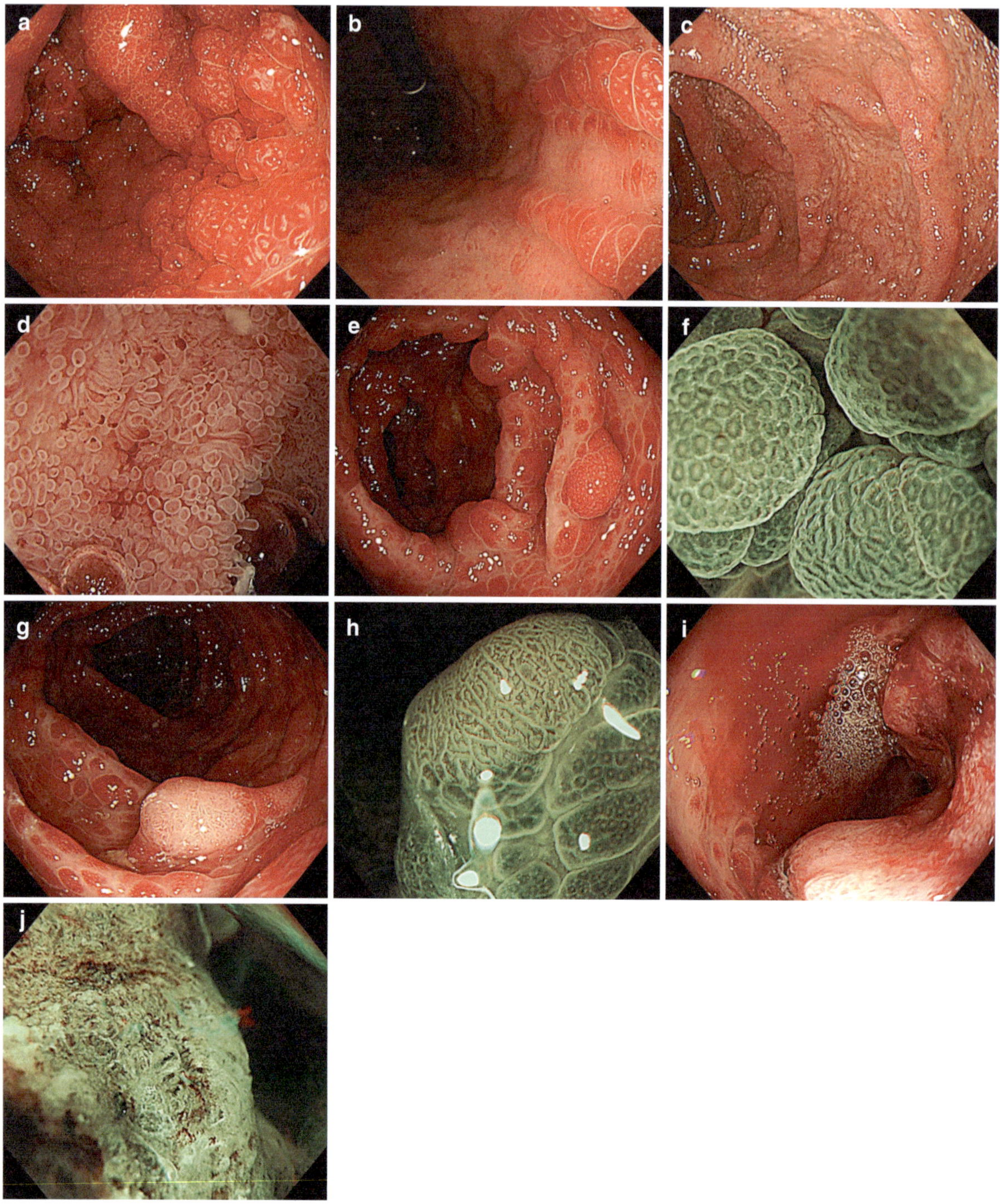

Fig. 23 (**a**) Stomach: Confluent type. Small, edematous, and erythematous polyps. (**b**) Stomach: Polyps at the lesser curvature were aligned on red streaks. (**c**) Duodenum: Fold thickening type with white villi. (**d**) Small intestine: Enlarged villi and small erosions. (**e**) Colon: Confluent type. Medium, edematous, and erythematous polyps. (**f**) Magnified NBI observation of (**e**). (**g**) Sigmoid colon: Is polyp with less erythematous surface than surrounding mucosa. (**h**) NBI observation of (**g**). Neoplastic vascular structures with subtle vascular caliber irregularities. JNET2A. pT1, tubular adenocarcinoma, well differentiated (tub 1). (**i**) Sigmoid colon: Type 2 tumor extending about half circumference of the lumen. (**j**) Magnified NBI observation of (**i**). JNET3. pT2N1M1a, tubular adenocarcinoma, well differentiated (tub 1)

Case 85: A case whose whole circumference elevated lesion in rectum was detected at the diagnosis and resected surgically, which turned out to be a benign tumor

Provided by Sakiko Hiraoka and Keita Harada

[Patient]

A 69-year-old male. CC: Dysgeusia, diarrhea.

[Clinical findings]

Alopecia (+), onychodystrophy (+), hyperpigmentation (−), dysgeusia (+), defecation: 5 times/day, mild edema.

[Laboratory findings]

Alb 3.4 mg/dL, CRP 0.79 mg/dL, Hb 12.3 g/dL.

[Endoscopic images 1] (Fig. 24a–f)

[Clinical course]

First attack type.

Initial treatment: PSL 40 mg for 1 week.

Clinical response: 1 week.

Clinical remission: 1 week.

Maintenance dose: PSL 0 mg.

[Endoscopic images 2] (Fig. 25a–h)

[Endoscopic images 3] (Fig. 26a–c)

SBCE 12 years after the treatment.

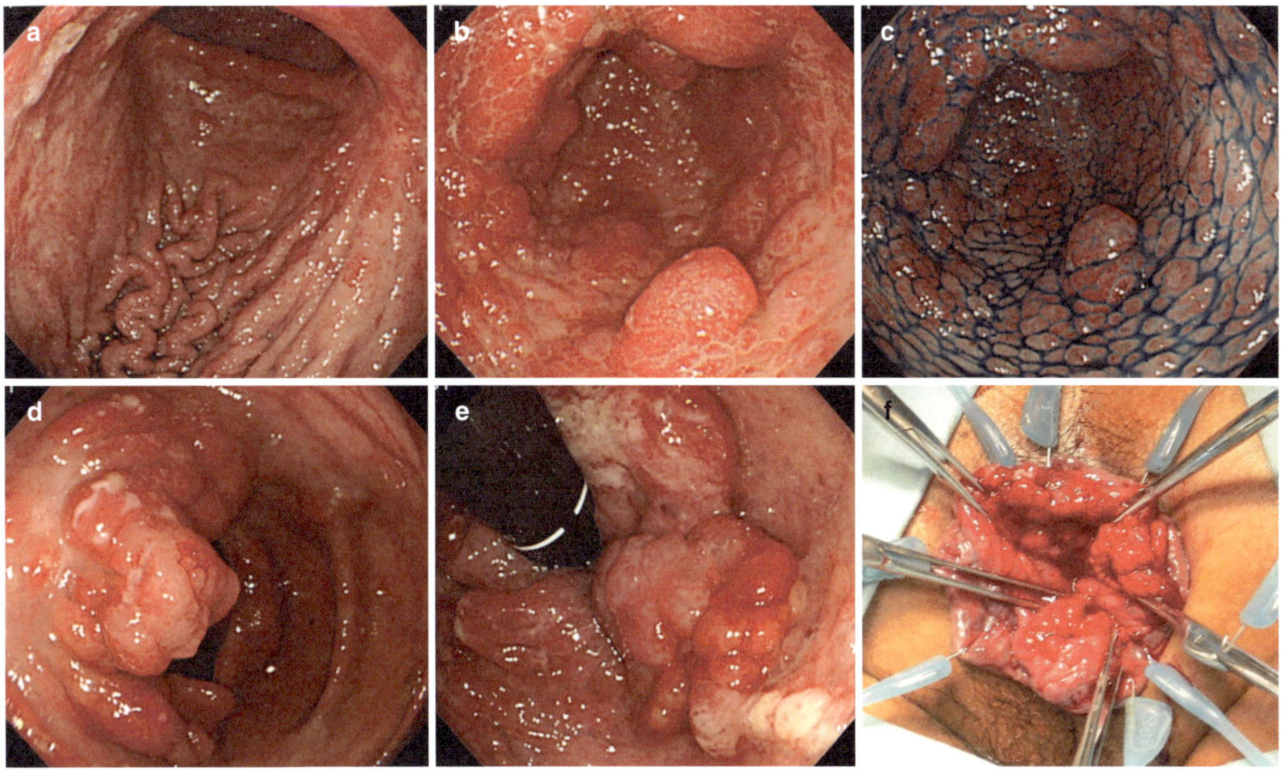

Fig. 24 (**a**), (**b**), (**c**) Stomach: Confluent type. Medium, edematous, and erythematous polyps. Edematous intervening mucosa. Open type atrophy. Multiple erythematous polyps through the whole stomach except the fornix. Scar with convergence of mucosal folds in the posterior and anterior walls of the angle. Indigocarmine dyeing in (**c**). (**d**) Colon: Sparse type. Large, erythematous, and erosive polyps. (**e**) Rectum: Circumferentially extending erythematous and erosive irregular polyps, which were soft and adhered with whitish mucus. (**f**) Transanal excision of rectal polyps. Pathological diagnosis: Non-neoplastic polyps

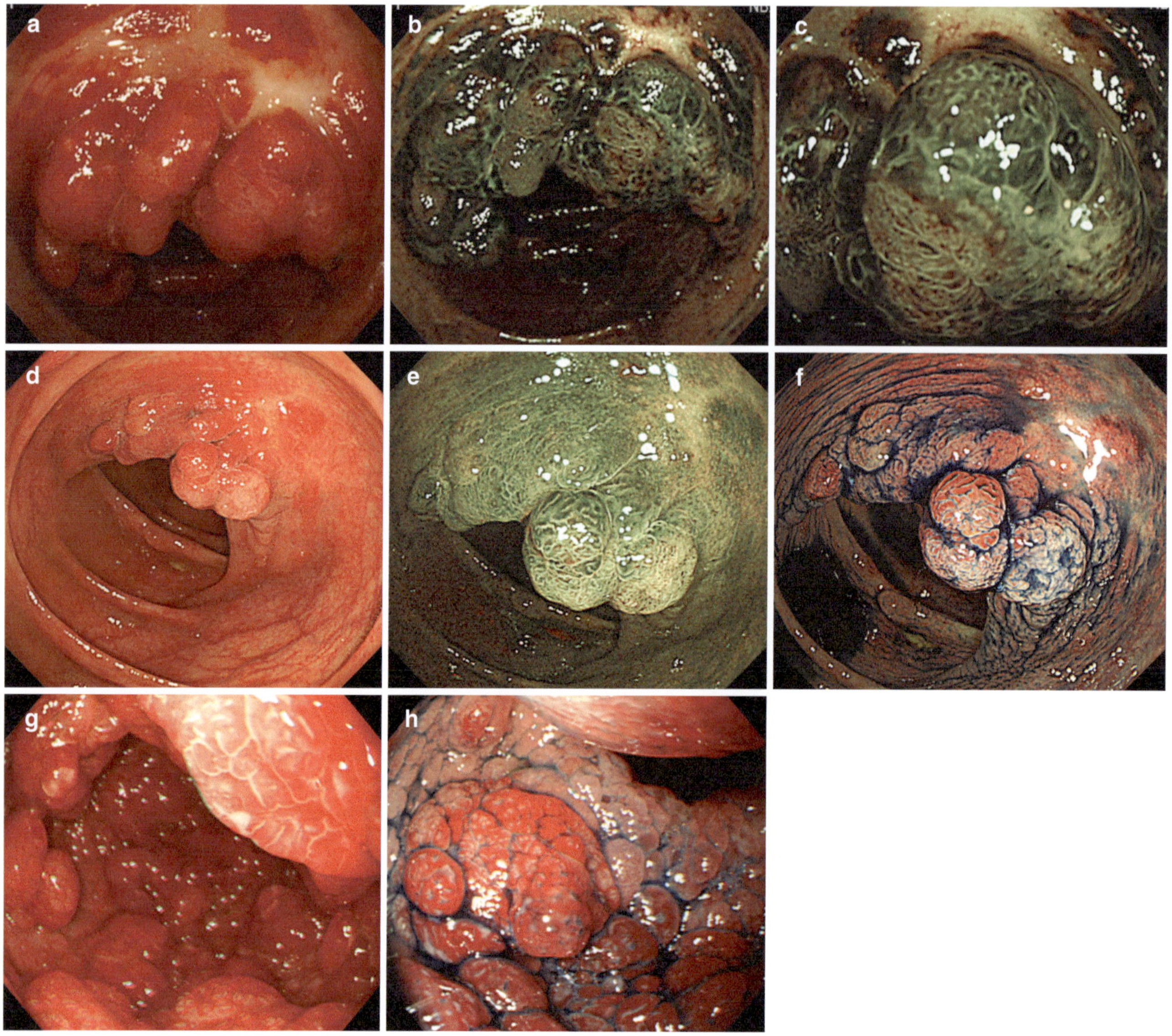

Fig. 25 (**a**) Colon (1 year after the treatment): Multiple erythematous, elevated, or flattened polyps through the entire colon. Semi-circumferential nodular polyps with some neoplastic type pit pattern within type I or type II pit pattern in ascending colon were revealed to be low-grade tubular adenoma by biopsy. (**b**) NBI observation of (**a**). (**c**) Close view of (**b**). (**d**) Colon (1.5 years after the treatment): The nodular polyps in the ascending colon shrunk, which still showed neoplastic type pit pattern partially. The polyps including the neoplastic lesion were endoscopically resected. Pathological diagnosis: Tubular adenoma in Cronkhite–Canada syndrome polyp. (**e**) NBI observation of (**d**). (**f**) Indigocarmine dyeing of (**d**). (**g**), (**h**) Stomach (2 years after the treatment): Both the size and number of polyps increased compared to the last examination. Some polyps were interconnected. Indigocarmine dyeing in (**h**)

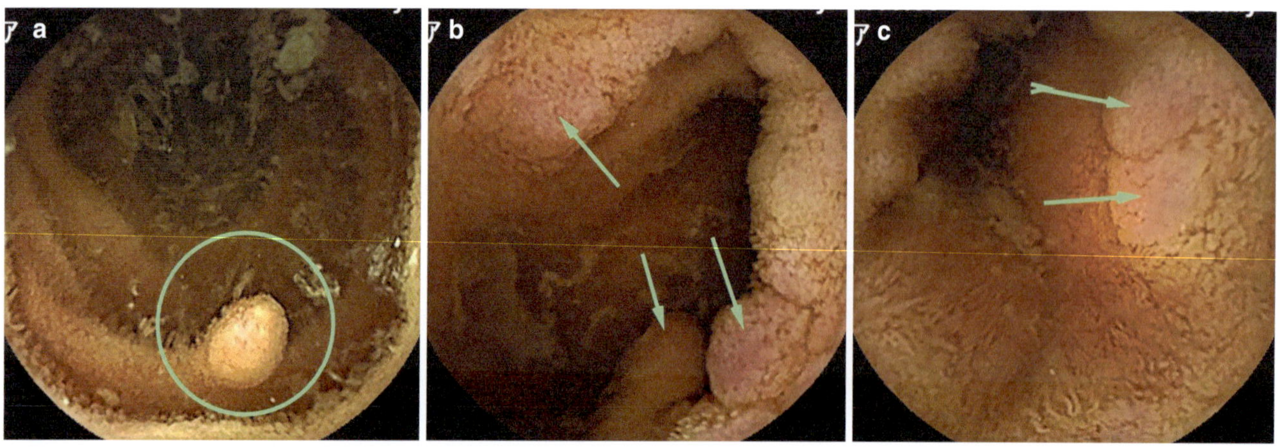

Fig. 26 (**a**), (**b**), (**c**) Small Intestine (SBCE): Sparse type. Medium polyps

Case 86: A case whose colorectal adenoma was detected after the initial treatment and was resected endoscopically

Provided by Kingo Hirasawa and Reiko Kunisaki

[Patient]

A 59-year-old male. CC: Dysgeusia, anorexia, diarrhea, epigastralgia.

[Clinical findings]

Alopecia (+), onychodystrophy (−), hyperpigmentation (+), dysgeusia (+), defecation: 2 times/day, mild edema.

[Laboratory findings]

Alb 3.6 mg/dL, CRP 0.77 mg/dL, Hb 18.5 g/dL.

[Endoscopic images 1] (Fig. 27a–g)

Glands became swollen and erythematous with slightly dilated interstitium.

[Clinical course]

Chronic continuous type.

Initial treatment: PSL 30 mg for 4 weeks.

Clinical response: 4 weeks.

Clinical remission: 6 weeks.

Therapeutic dose at relapse: PSL 30 mg.

Maintenance dose: PSL 0 mg.

[Endoscopic images 2] (Fig. 28a–e)

EGD and CS after the treatment.

All lesions improved.

[Endoscopic images 3] (Fig. 29a–c)

Polypectomy for two colorectal adenomas

Pathological diagnosis: Tubular adenoma, low to high grade.

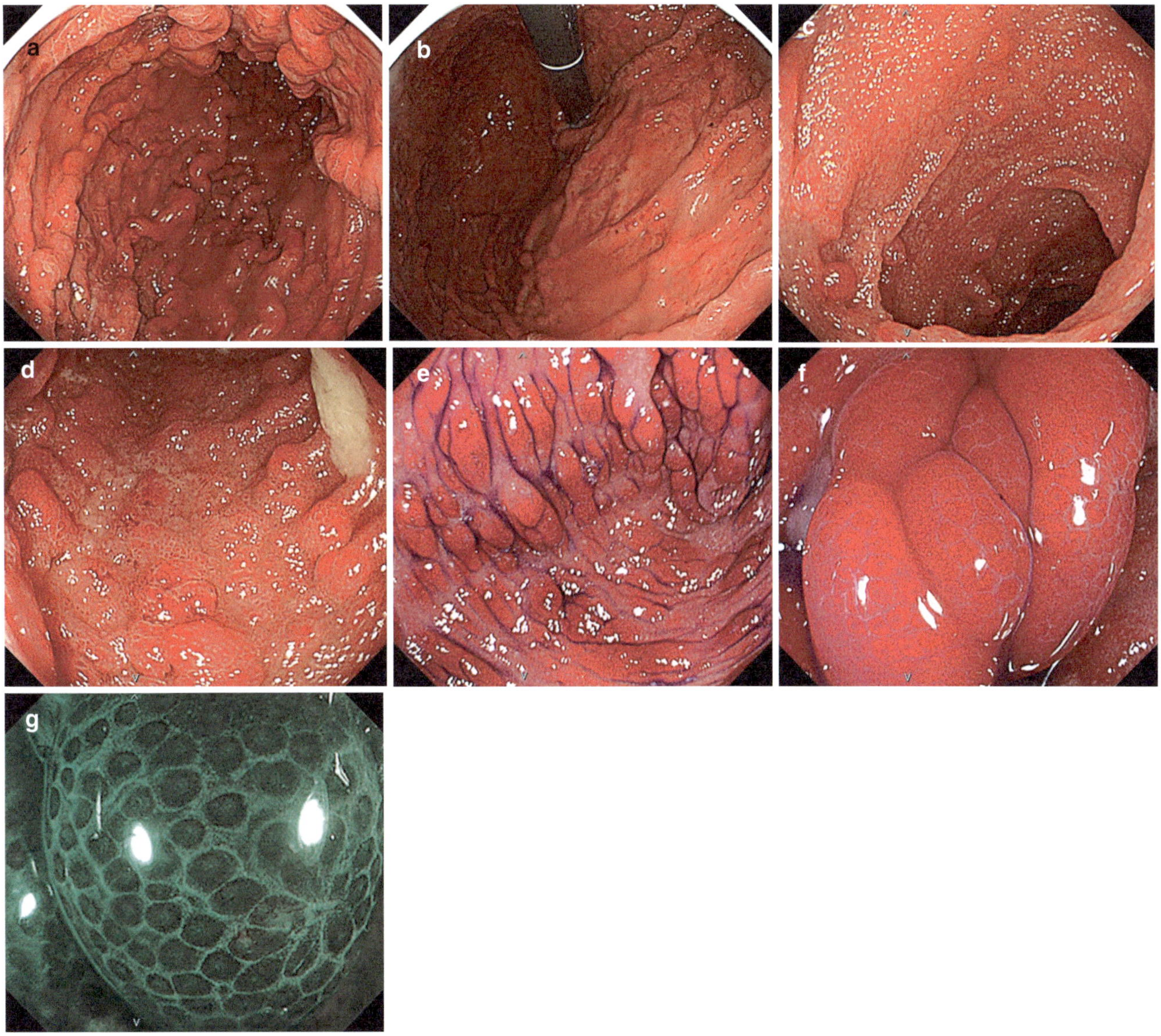

Fig. 27 (**a**), (**b**) Stomach: Semi-confluent type. Medium, edematous, and erythematous polyps. (**c**) Duodenum: Fold thickening type. (**d**) Ileum: Fold thickening type. (**e**) Colon (Indigocarmine dyeing): Confluent type. Medium, erythematous polyps. (**f**) Magnified observation of (**e**). (**g**) Magnified NBI observation of (**e**)

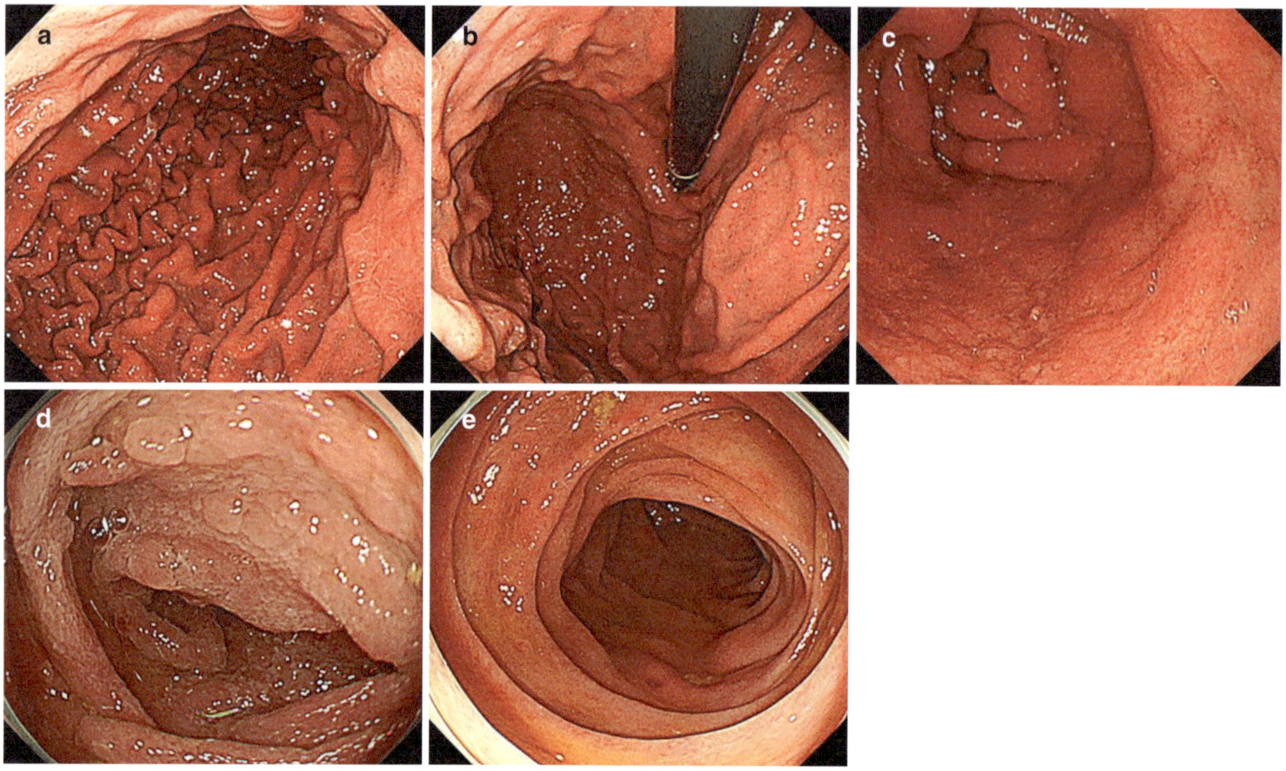

Fig. 28 (**a**), (**b**) Stomach. (**c**) Duodenum. (**d**) Ileum. (**e**) Colon

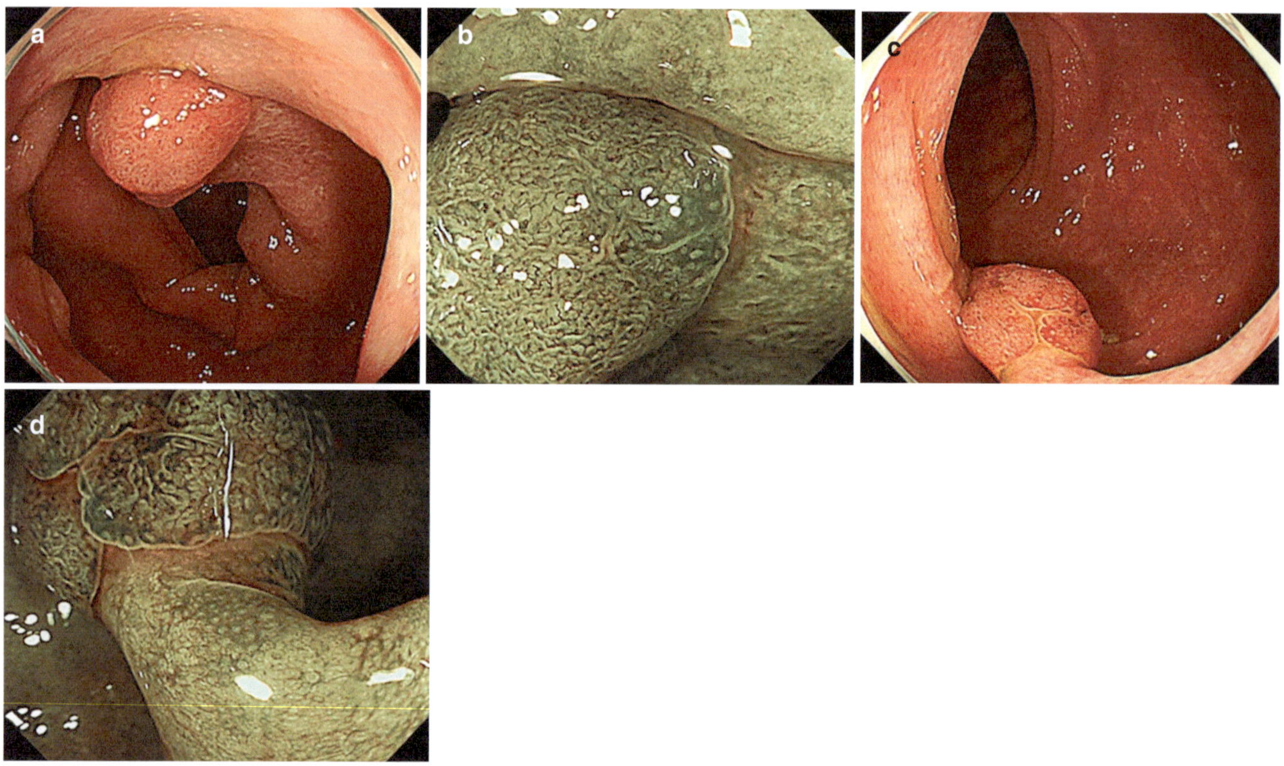

Fig. 29 (**a**) Ascending colon: Is polyp. (**b**) NBI observation of (**a**). JNET2A with predominantly neoplastic vascular structures, while there was an area with non-neoplastic vascular structures and open pits in the direction of 3 o'clock. Pathological diagnosis: Tubular adenoma, high grade. (**c**) Sigmoid colon: Ip polyp. (**d**) NBI observation of (**c**)

Case 87: A case whose colorectal adenoma was detected after the initial treatment

Provided by Rintaro Moroi and Atsushi Masamune

[Patient]

A 50-year-old male. CC: Dysgeusia, diarrhea.

[Clinical findings]

Alopecia (+), onychodystrophy (+), hyperpigmentation (+), defecation: 5 times/day

[Laboratory findings]

Alb 3.3 mg/dL, CRP 0.27 mg/dL, Hb 14.2 g/dL.

[Cutaneous manifestations and endoscopic images 1] (Fig. 30a–k)

[Clinical course]

First attack type.

Initial treatment: PSL 40 mg for 2 weeks.

Clinical response: 2 weeks.

Clinical remission: 12 weeks.

Maintenance dose: PSL 0 mg.

[Cutaneous manifestations and endoscopic images 2] (Fig. 31a–i)

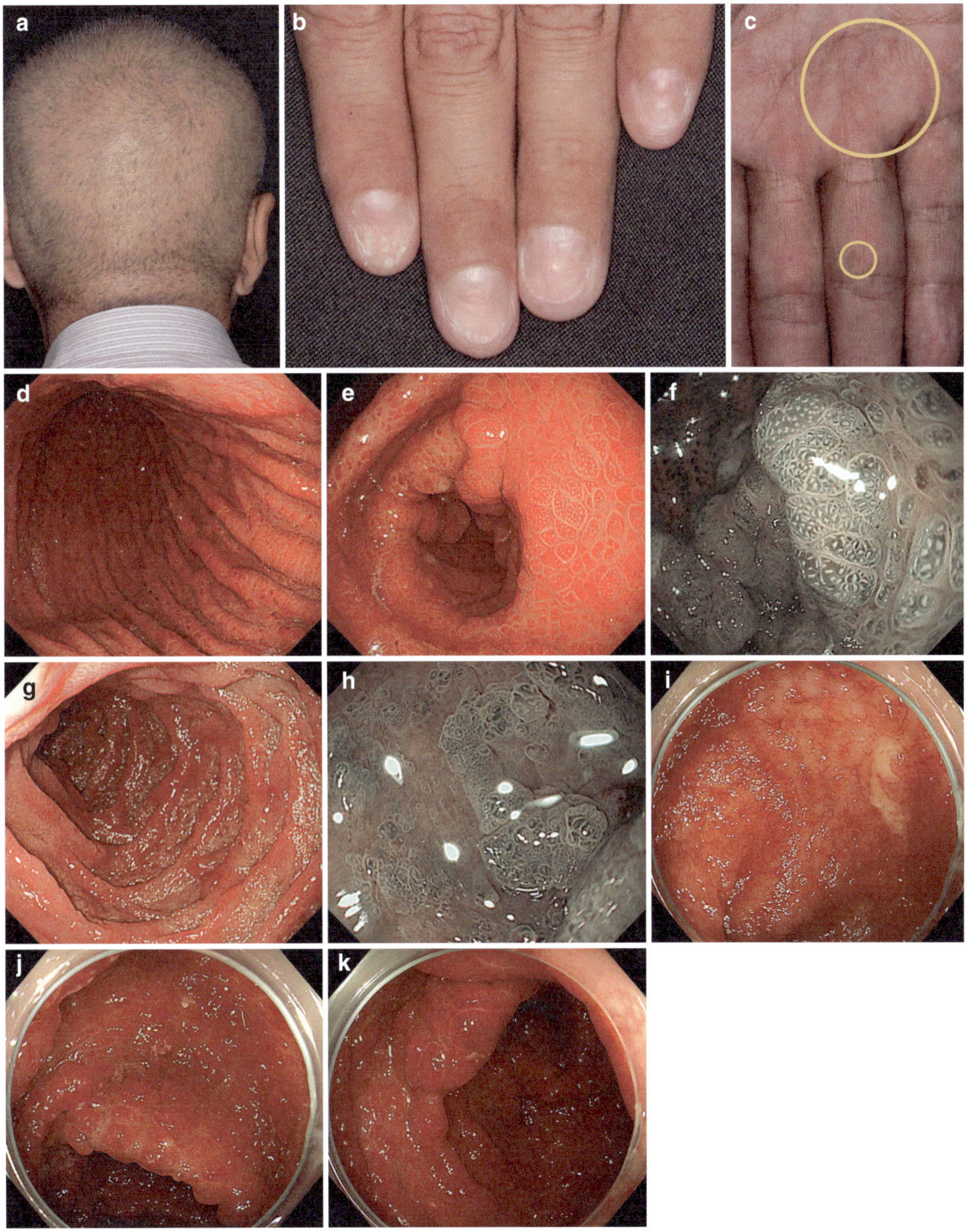

Fig. 30 (**a**) Head: Alopecia. (**b**) Fingers: Onychodystrophy. (**c**) Hand: Hyperpigmentation (yellow circles). (**d**), (**e**) Stomach: Confluent type. Small, edematous, and erythematous polyps. (**f**) Magnified NBI view of (**e**). (**g**) Duodenum: Fold thickening type with small polyps. (**h**) Magnified NBI view of (**g**). (**i**) Ileum: Folod thickening type with erythematous mucosa. (**j**), (**k**) Colon: Confluent type. Small, edematous, and erythematous polyps

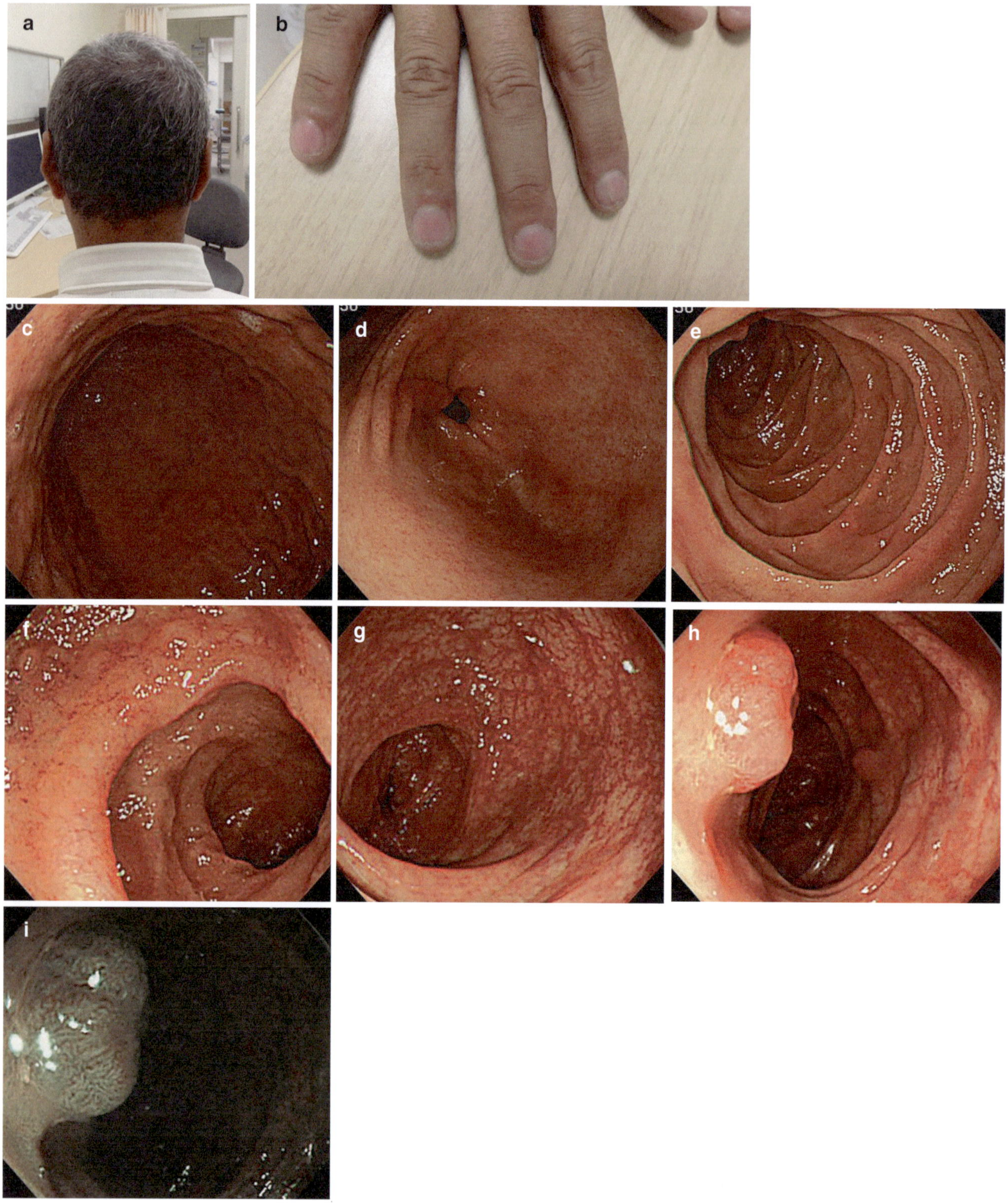

Fig. 31 (**a**) Head. (**b**) Fingers. (**c**), (**d**) Stomach. (**e**) Duodenum. (**f**) Terminal ileum. (**g**) Colon. All the cutaneous manifestations and endoscopic findings improved. (**h**), (**i**) Colon: The presence of adenomas was identified after the regression of surrounding polyps

Case 88: A case whose colorectal adenoma was detected after the initial treatment and resected endoscopically

Provided by Shigeki Bamba and Akira Andoh

[Patient]

A 73-year-old woman. CC: Anorexia, diarrhea.

[Clinical findings]

Alopecia (+), onychodystrophy (+), hyperpigmentation (+), defecation: 6 times/day, severe edema, weight loss: −5.7 kg/1 year.

[Laboratory findings]

Alb 2.5 mg/dL, CRP 0.44 mg/dL, Hb 11.6 g/dL.

Fecal alpha1-antitrypsin clearance: 134 mL/day

99Tc-human serum albumin scintigraphy: Abnormal leakage from the ileum and ascending colon.

[Endoscopic images 1] (Fig. 32a–k)

[Clinical course]

First attack type.

Initial treatment: PSL 30 mg for 1 week.

Clinical response: 1 week.

Clinical remission: 1 week.

Maintenance dose: PSL 0 mg.

[Endoscopic images 2] (Fig. 33a–d)

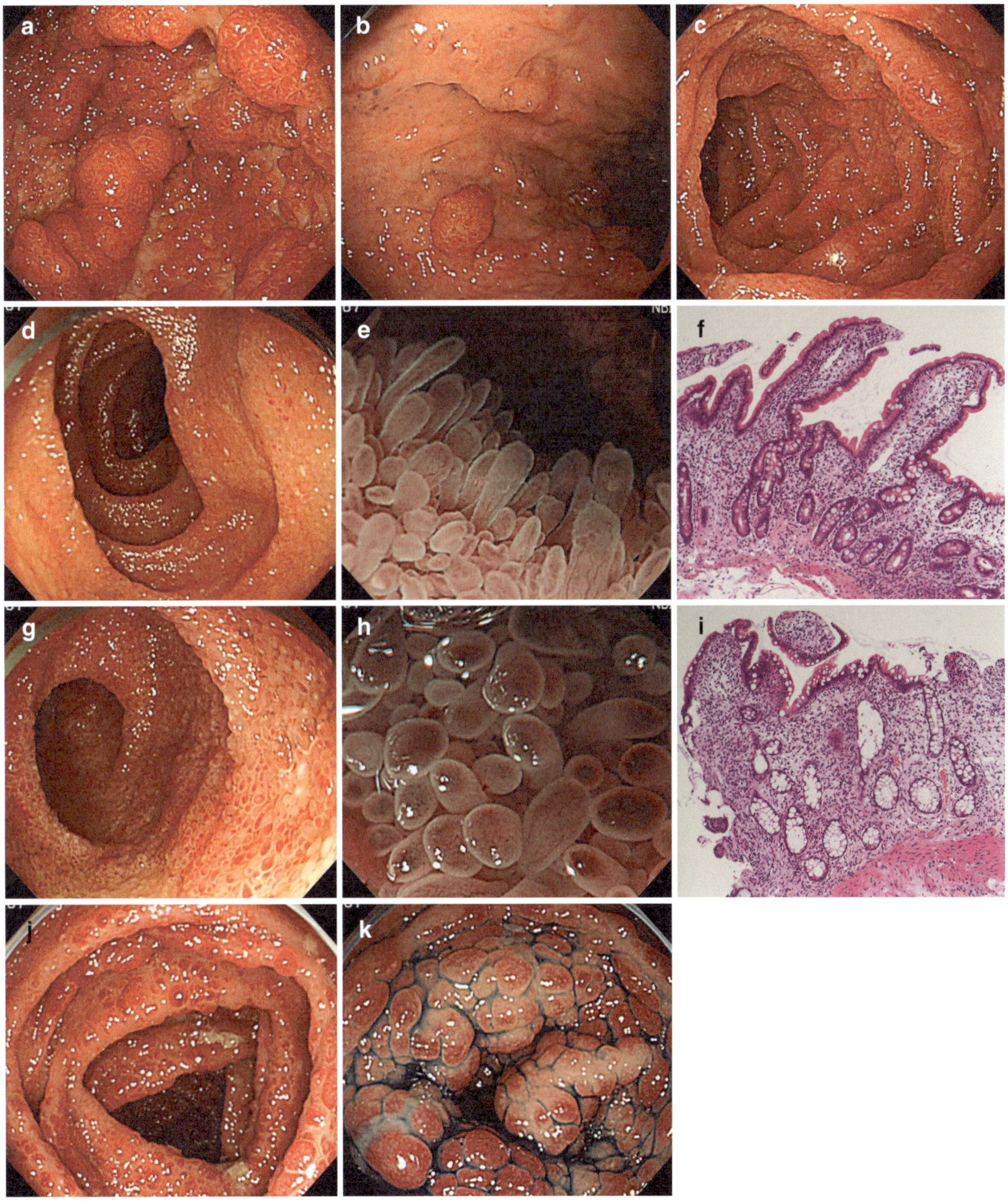

Fig. 32 (**a**), (**b**) Stomach: Confluent type. Medium, edematous, and erythematous polyps. (**c**) Duodenum: Fold thickening type. (**d**), (**e**), (**f**) Jejunum: Polyposis was not detected. Scattered white spots were detected, which was confirmed by magnified NBI as fine granules in the tips of the villi. Biopsy showed edematous changes and mild dilatation of lymphatic vessels. (**e**) Magnified NBI observation of (**d**). (**f**) Pathological image of (**e**). (**g**), (**h**), (**i**) Ileum: Fold thickening type with spherical swelling of villi, which showed severe edema pathologically. (**h**) Magnified NBI observation of (**g**). (**i**) Pathological image of (**h**). (**j**), (**k**) Colon: Confluent type. Medium, edematous, and erythematous polyps. Indigocarmine dyeing in (**k**)

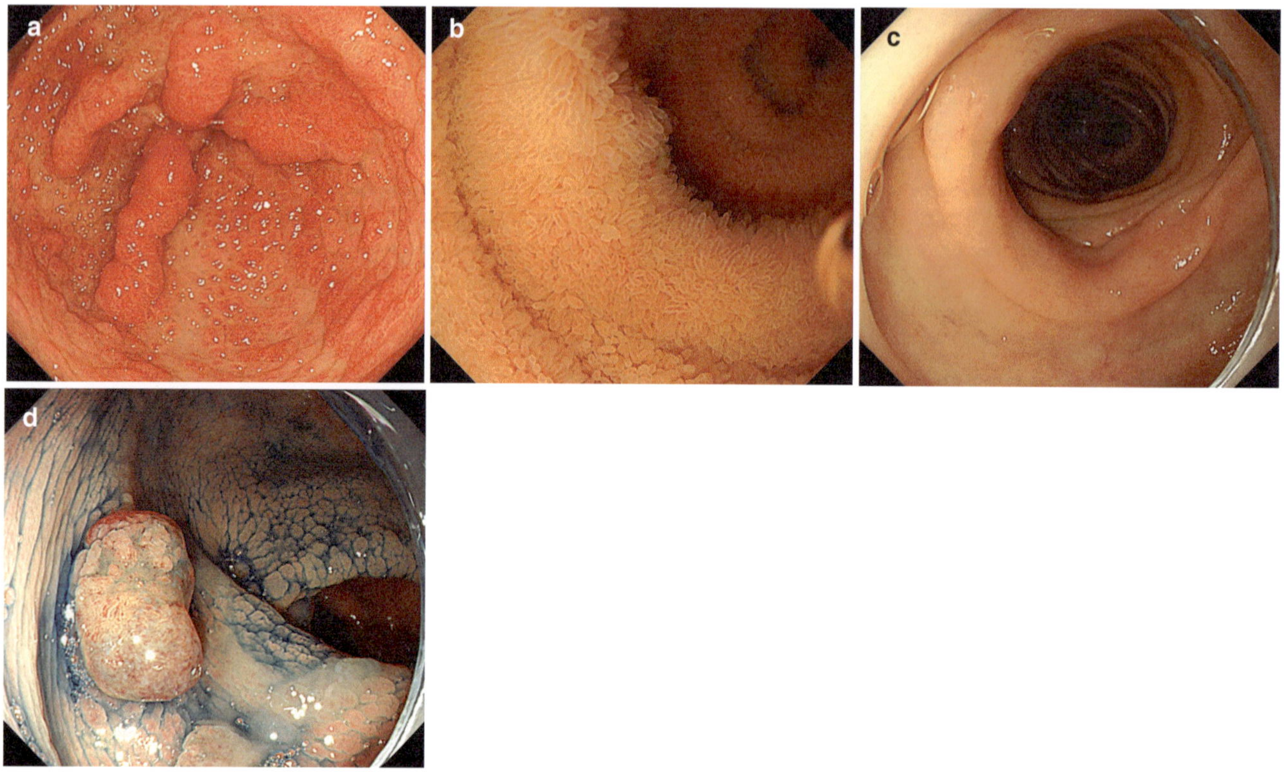

Fig. 33 (**a**) Stomach. (**b**) Jejunum. (**c**) Colon. (**d**) A colonic adenoma was detected and resected endoscopically

MIX
Papier aus verantwortungsvollen Quellen
Paper from responsible sources
FSC® C105338

If you have any concerns about our products,
you can contact us on
ProductSafety@springernature.com

In case Publisher is established outside the EU,
the EU authorized representative is:
Springer Nature Customer Service Center GmbH
Europaplatz 3, 69115 Heidelberg, Germany

Printed by Libri Plureos GmbH
in Hamburg, Germany